THE NEW DIMENSIONS
OF WARFARIN
PROPHYLAXIS

ADVANCES IN EXPERIMENTAL MEDICINE AND BIOLOGY

Recent Volumes in this Series

THE NEW DIMENSIONS OF WARFARIN PROPHYLAXIS

Edited by

Stanford Wessler

New York University School of Medicine
New York, New York

Carl G. Becker

Cornell University Medical College
New York, New York

and

Yale Nemerson

Mt. Sinai School of Medicine of the City University of New York
New York, New York

Springer Science+Business Media, LLC

Library of Congress Cataloging in Publication Data

International Symposium on the New Dimensions of Warfarin Prophylaxis (1986:
  New York University Medical Center)
  The new dimensions of warfarin prophylaxis.

  "Proceedings of the International Symposium on the New Dimensions of Warfarin
Prophylaxis, held October 16–18, 1986, at the New York University Medical Center in
New York"—T.p. verso.
  Includes bibliographies and index.
  1. Warfarin—Therapeutic use—Congresses. 2. Thrombosis—Chemotherapy—Con-
gresses. 3. Thrombosis—Prevention—Congresses. I. Wessler, Stanford, 1917–
II. Becker, Carl G. III. Nemerson, Yale. IV. Title. [DNLM: 1. Thromboembolism—
prevention & control—congresses. 2. Warfarin—pharmacodynamics—congresses. 3.
Warfarin—therapeutic use—congresses. QV 193 I613n 1986]
RC694.3.I575   1986   616.1′35061   87-20260

ISBN 978-1-4757-5987-7   ISBN 978-1-4757-5985-3 (eBook)
DOI 10.1007/978-1-4757-5985-3

Proceedings of the International Symposium on the New Dimensions of
Warfarin Prophylaxis, held October 16–18, 1986, at the New York University
Medical Center in New York

© 1987 Springer Science+Business Media New York
Originally published by Plenum Press, New York in 1987.
Softcover reprint of the hardcover 1st edition 1987

PREFACE

The International Symposium on The New Dimensions of Warfarin
Prophylaxis held on October 16-18, 1986 in New York City was conceived as
a forum to bring together physicians and other scientists knowledgeable
about the pharmacological effects of warfarin on the hemostatic mechanism
and the clinical usefulness of this compound in the prevention of
thromboembolic phenomena.

The coumarin compounds have commanded a striking breadth of interest
among members of the biomedical research community for almost one-half
century. Aspects of its effects on the vitamin K-dependent proteins, on
the laboratory recognition of the drug's pharmacologic action and its use
as a therapeutic agent in a variety of disease states have been actively
studied with increasing intensity in the past several decades. Thus, the
present state of these studies seemed to be a timely subject for
discussion, not only to gather together in one place representative
samples of the myriad of data on warfarin, but also to underscore the
ever increasing necessity for communication between basic research and
clinical practice.

The content and organization of this monograph reflect the scope and
importance of warfarin prophylaxis. One of the unique aspects of this
publication is that it spells out in one place the warfarin story from
molecular biology through clinical trials to future directions of
research and patient care.

The editors wish to thank DuPont Pharmaceuticals for a generous
educational grant in support of the symposium. Without their financial
backing this symposium would not have become a reality. We wish also to
thank both the American Heart Association, New York City Affiliate and
the National Heart, Lung and Blood Institute, National Institutes of
Health for their co-sponsorship.

Carl G. Becker
Yale Nemerson
Stanford Wessler

New York, NY
October 1986

CONTENTS

THE SCOPE OF THROMBOEMBOLISM

Stanford Wessler

Department of Medicine
New York University School of Medicine
550 First Avenue, New York, NY

Why, the question may be appropriately asked, should there be, in 1986, a 3-day symposium on warfarin prophylaxis--a drug, after all, that was introduced into clinical medicine 45 years ago?

It is because new knowledge concerning the pathophysiology of hemostasis, the effect of warfarin on an increasing number of vitamin K-dependent proteins and the results of recent clinical trials, have dramatically enhanced the usefulness of oral anticoagulants in both the primary and secondary prevention of thromboembolic episodes in an ever broader range of clinical conditions prone to intravascular coagulation.

The impact of thromboembolism unchecked, on mortality and morbidity in the U.S. is impressive. Thrombosis is a pathologic process that complicates the course and contributes to the lethal nature of several major killers in American society. Arterial thrombosis plays a role in the initiation, growth, and terminal occlusion of the atherosclerotic lesion and is a major contributor to mortality in acute myocardial infarction and stroke, the number 1 and 3 causes of death in the United States. In addition, thromboembolic events are frequently associated with cardiac arrhythmias, congestive failure, shock, valvular heart disease and intimal damage to arteries in the cerebral, cervical, aortoiliac, visceral, and peripheral areas of the circulation. Some inborn errors of metabolism, infections, blood dyscrasias, trauma, drugs, and certain diseases of unknown etiology are also associated with arterial as well as venous thrombosis.

Venous thromboembolism itself causes approximately 300,000 patients annually to be hospitalized in the United States, of whom more than 50,000 die, primarily in hospitals, rehabilitation centers, and nursing homes where prophylaxis would be feasible. Pulmonary embolism is a major threat to life in the postoperative state. It is the most frequent nonsurgical cause of death among patients hospitalized for hip fractures and major orthopedic reconstructive surgery; a common cause of mortality following neurosurgical procedures; the most frequent nonobstetrical cause of postpartum death; a major factor in mortality among the extensive population of patients with chronic cardiac and pulmonary disease, and among an equally large group who are subjected to prolonged immobilization because of a variety of medical and surgical conditions. Indeed, in hospitalized adult patients who die, careful autopsy examinations disclose evidence of antemortem pulmonary embolism in more than 60% of cases.

Thromboembolism induced by contact of blood with foreign surfaces is a major unresolved problem in the development of artificial organs either for extracorporeal circulation or for implantation within the heart and blood vessels. This phenomenon is a significant obstacle to advances in clinical care associated with prosthetic heart valves, extracorporeal cardiopulmonary bypass, cardiac assistance, respiratory assistance through extracorporeal circulation, intravascular catheters, electrodes, artificial hearts, artificial blood vessels, arteriovenous shunts, vascular sutures, and all other applications in which the blood comes into contact with a nonbiological surface.

Finally, thrombosis related to microcirculatory disturbances, unlike that of arteries and veins, cannot be expressed in precise terms, but is best appreciated by a partial listing of disciplines and diseases in which such disturbances are important. The microcirculation deranged by thrombosis is often a contributory and even a primary mechanism for the induction of pathology in hypertension, stroke, diabetes, cancer, infection, inflammation, autoimmune disease, host-graft rejection, hemolytic anemia, drug toxicity, mismatched blood transfusions, liver disease, pancreatitis, and glomerulonephritis.

Thus, clinically, thromboembolic obstruction to three major components of the circulation--arterial, venous, and microcirculatory--contributes materially to early death in our society. In many, but not all, of these conditions, warfarin is the drug of choice. It is one of the goals of this symposium to define these conditions.

It is hoped that the presentations made at this conference will suggest, in addition to guidelines for warfarin administration, future areas of research relative to thromboembolism--both basic and applied.

THE BIOCHEMICAL BASIS OF WARFARIN THERAPY

J. W. Suttie

Department of Biochemistry
University of Wisconsin-Madison
Madison, WI

INTRODUCTION

The necessity of a dietary nutrient to maintain normal blood coagulation function was discovered by Dam in the late 1920's during his efforts
to demonstrate the essentiality of cholesterol in the diet of the chick.
He noted a hemorrhagic condition in chicks fed lipid-free diets and demonstrated that the addition of alfalfa meal or a lipid extract of alfalfa
would prevent this condition. Continued study of this response in the
early 1930's by the research groups of Dam, Almquist, and Doisy led to the
isolation, characterization, and synthesis of the active compound, 2-Me-3-
phytyl-1,4-naphthoquinone (phylloquinone). These early studies also demonstrated that in addition to phylloquinone or vitamin K_1 in green plants,
vitamin K activity was present in many bacteria as a series of menaqui-
nones, 2-Me-1,4-naphthoquinones substituted at the 3-position with an un-
saturated polyisoprenoid chain. These historical aspects of the discovery
of vitamin K have been adequately reviewed.[1]

Dicoumarol

Warfarin

The reactions involving coagulation of plasma were not well understood
at that time, and fibrinogen and prothrombin were the only proteins involved in this response that were reasonably well characterized. Dam was
able to prepare a crude fraction of prothrombin from chick plasma and was
able to demonstrate that a similar fraction prepared from the plasma of
vitamin K-deficient chicks had less activity. The remaining three of the

3

four classical vitamin K-dependent clotting factors (factors VII, IX, and X) were discovered by clinicians as congenitally deficient proteins in the 1950's. Plasma proteins C, S, and Z were not discovered until the biochemical role of the vitamin was understood, and vitamin K is now known to be required for the synthesis of a limited number of non-plasma proteins.[1] The discovery of a naturally occurring antagonist of the vitamin by Link occurred at about the same time as the vitamin itself was discovered. A hemorrhagic disease of cattle which was prevalent in the American midwest and western Canada in the 1920's was traced to the consumption of improperly cured sweet clover hay. If serious hemorrhages did not develop, animals with "sweet clover disease" could be aided by transfusion with whole blood from healthy animals. By the early 1930's it was established that the cause of the prolonged clotting times was a decrease in the concentration of prothrombin in the blood. The compound which was present in spoiled sweet clover and was responsible for this disease was studied by a number of investigators, but was finally isolated and characterized as 3-3'-methyl-bis-4-(hydroxycoumarin) by Link's group and called dicoumarol.[2] Synthesis of a large number of 4-hydroxycoumarins in Link's laboratory led to a concentration of effort directed toward the use of warfarin (3-α-phenyl-β-acetylethyl-4-hydroxycouarin) as both an anticoagulant and a rodenticide.

Phylloquinone   Menaquinone-7

Although the ability of warfarin and other 4-hydroxycoumarins to antagonize the action of vitamin K was recognized by the early 1940's, the biochemical basis for this antagonism was not apparent until the nature of the vitamin K-dependent reaction was elucidated. This was established in the mid 1970's when Stenflo[3] and Nelsestuen[4] demonstrated that prothrombin contained a number of residues of a previously unidentified amino acid, γ-carboxyglutamic acid (Gla). Antagonism of the formation of this residue by the coumarin anticoagulants was the basis for this anticoagulant action.

THE VITAMIN K-DEPENDENT CARBOXYLASE

General Properties

Soon after the presence of Gla residues in prothrombin was reported, a rat liver microsomal activity that would fix $^{14}CO_2$ into glutamyl residues of endogenous precursor proteins to form ^{14}C-γ-carboxyglutamyl residues in

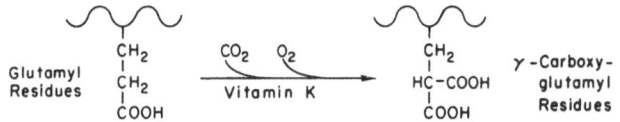

Figure 1. The reaction catalyzed by the vitamin K-dependent carboxylase.

the presence of vitamin K was described.[5] This activity (Fig. 1) required O_2, vitamin K, and HCO_3^-. The enzyme was stimulated by an energy source and factor(s) present in the postmicrosomal supernatant. Studies in this system demonstrated a requirement for NAD(P)H and/or a reduced pyridine nucleotide-generating system, and it was subsequently shown that vitamin KH_2 could substitute for these cytoplasmic factors. The general properties of the enzyme are now reasonably well understood and have recently been reviewed.[6] Crude liver microsomal preparations contain several vitamin K reductase activities, and the carboxylase activity has been studied with [NADH + vitamin K] or with vitamin KH_2 as a vitamin source. The enzymatic activity was soon solubilized, and solubilized preparations were shown to retain the basic requirement for reduced vitamin K and O_2 of the membrane-associated system. The enzyme does not require ATP, and it appears that the only energy needed to drive the carboxylation comes from the reoxidation of reduced vitamin K. The active species in the carboxylation reaction is CO_2 rather than HCO_3^-. The enzyme is usually studied at a pH of 7.2-7.4, and as most investigators have not controlled O_2 concentration, carboxylase assays have usually been carried out with a total CO_2 concentration of around 1 mM. there are relatively few measurements of the oxygen requirement of the enzyme available, but the K_m for O_2 appears to be in the range of 60 to 80 µM. Most investigators have studied the enzyme at a vitamin KH_2 concentration of 50 to 100 µM, and it is likely the vitamin concentration has not been initially limiting as other variables have been studied. The specificity of the enzyme for different forms of vitamin K has been studied in a number of systems, but an extensive investigation of the activity of various ring substituted forms of vitamin K as substrates for the carboxylase has not been carried out. The limited amount of available data suggest, however, that little deviation from the native

structure is allowed. Effective vitamin K activity at the active site appears to be limited to a 2-methyl-1,4-naphthoquinone with some degree of non-polar substitution on the 3-position.

Early studies of the detergent-solubilized carboxylase preparations demonstrated that a peptide comprising residues 5-9 (Phe-Leu-Glu-Glu-Val) of the bovine prothrombin precursor would serve as a substrate for the enzyme. This observation has led to the synthesis of a large number of low-molecular-weight peptide substrates designed to provide some assessment of binding site specificity.[7] In general, peptides with Glu-Glu sequences are better substrates than those with single Glu residues. Although the enzyme will carboxylate a derivatized Glu residue such as Boc-Glu-OBzl, compounds of this type are relatively poor substrates. Peptides containing Asp, D-Glu, Gln, or Homo-Glu residues were originally reported not to be carboxylated to any significant extent, but subsequent studies suggested that the enzyme can form β-carboxyaspartic acid at a very low rate. Most low-molecular-weight peptide substrates for the carboxylase have been reported to have K_m values in the range of a few mM, and this low apparent affinity of most peptide substrates suggests that some secondary or tertiary structure might be important in providing tight binding to the enzyme. The decarboxylated form of the vitamin K-dependent bone protein, osteocalcin, is a 6800 molecular weight protein which contains 3 Gla residues. This small protein has a reported K_m of 25 μM as a substrate for the hepatic carboxylase[8] and might be very useful in subsequent studies.

Inspection of the amino acid sequences of the vitamin K-dependent plasma proteins does not reveal any unique sequences that might serve as a signal for the carboxylation of Glu residues in these few hepatic secretory proteins. Sequencing of the cDNA for these proteins has now revealed that the primary gene product of these proteins contains a basic amino acid rich "propeptide" region between the amino terminal end of the secreted form of the protein and the signal or leader peptide sequence.[9] A similar homologous "propeptide" region has been shown to be present in the intracellular form of the vitamin K-dependent bone protein, osteocalcin.[10] This structural similarity in what are otherwise unrelated proteins has raised the possibility that this region may serve as a carboxylase enzyme recognition site. Preliminary studies utilizing altered constructs of protein C expressed in E. coli support this role,[11] but additional data will be needed to conclusively establish this interaction.

Reaction Mechanism

Speculations on the molecular action of vitamin K originally centered around two possibilities: that the vitamin was a cofactor utilized to labilize the hydrogen on the γ-position of the glutamyl residue to allow CO_2 attack at this position, or that it was involved as a CO_2 carrier. Evidence obtained in the last few years strongly supports the former hypothesis. Current ideas of the mechanism of the carboxylation reaction stress its relationship to a microsomal vitamin K epoxidase activity which converts vitamin KH_2 to the 2,3-epoxide of the vitamin and are consistent with the reaction mechanism shown in Figure 2. Over a period of time following the discovery of this microsomal internal mono-oxygenase, it became clear that this epoxidase activity was closely associated with the vitamin K-dependent carboxylase activity and had many properties in common. It has been shown[12] that at saturating concentrations of CO_2 there is an apparent equivalent stoichiometry between epoxide formation and Gla formation, but as the CO_2 concentration is lowered a large excess of vitamin K epoxide is produced. How epoxide formation is coupled to γ-hydrogen abstraction is not clear at this time, but one possibility would be through an oxygenated

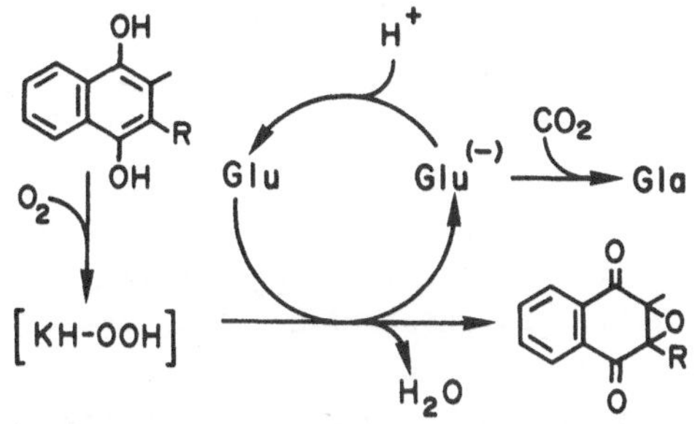

Figure 2. Proposed mechanism for the vitamin K-dependent carboxylase/
epoxidase system. The available data strongly support the vitamin K-
dependent formation of a carbanion on the γ-position of the Glu residue
followed by carboxylation in a step not involving the vitamin. Neither the
chemical nature of the proposed oxygenated intermediate nor the mechanism
by which hydrogen abstraction is linked to epoxide formation can be
determined from the available data.

intermediate such as a vitamin K hydroperoxide that would be on the pathway
of epoxide formation. Such an intermediate has not been directly demonstrated and the evidence for its presence is indirect.

Any detailed mechanism of how an oxygenated form of vitamin K could be
used to drive the carboxlation reaction is at the present time speculative.
Most investigators have suggested that hydrogen removal is an abstraction
of a proton to leave a formal carbanion on the glutamyl residue, and the
enzyme has been demonstrated to catalyze a vitamin KH_2 and oxygen-dependent
exchange of ^3H from ^3H_2O into the γ-position of a Glu residue in the substrate Boc-Glu-Glu-Leu-OMe.[13] Exchange of ^3H with the γ-carbon hydrogen is
decreased as the concentration of HCO_3^- in the media is increased. It has
also been demonstrated[14] that the fate of the activated Glu residue in
incubations carried out in the absence of CO_2 is to protonate rather than
form an adduct with some other component of the incubation that would
result in an altered Glu residue. These data place severe constraints on
any radical mechanism that might be postulated and are consistent with the
model shown in Figure 2, which indicates that the role of vitamin K is to
abstract the γ-hydrogen as a carbanion. Proof of this hypothesis will,
however, require a much clearer understanding of the mechanism by which
hydrogen abstraction is coupled to epoxide formation.

MECHANISM OF WARFARIN ACTION

Development of a Theory of Warfarin Action

As the 4-hydroxycoumarins were identified as anticoagulants and had
been shown to be antagonists of vitamin K action more than 30 years before
the molecular role of vitamin K was established, it is not surprising that

a number of theories of action of these important drugs have been put forth. Although seldom clearly expressed in the literature, it is apparent that many early investigators assumed that warfarin and similar compounds were direct antagonists of vitamin K at whatever site it mediated its effect. This view was consistent with the general agonist/antagonist relationship between the two compounds. Other investigators did recognize the noncompetitive nature of the antagonism[15] but were unable to produce a viable hypothesis of 4-hydroxycoumarin action based on the then limited understanding of the reactions involved. Early studies of the microsomal vitamin K-dependent carboxylase demonstrated that warfarin was not a potent antagonist of this system, and its action was clarified only after a more complete understanding of the metabolism and action of vitamin K within the liver was obtained.

Liver Vitamin K Metabolism

If, as shown in Figure 2, the co-product of Gla formation is vitamin K epoxide, microsomes must contain efficient mechanisms for recycling this metabolite to the active substrate form, vitamin KH_2. The microsomal-associated acivities that have been identified as being involved in these metabolic interconversions of the liver vitamin K pool are shown in Figure 3 and include a vitamin K epoxide reductase and at least two and possibly

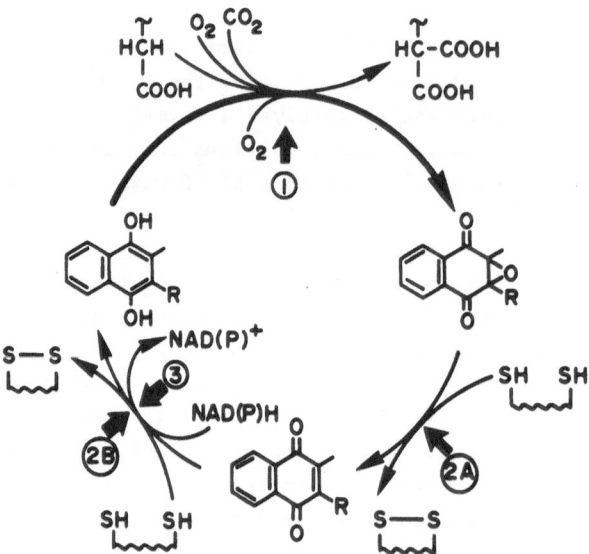

Figure 3. Vitamin K metabolism in hepatic microsomes. In addition to the carboxylase/epoxidase system (1), liver microsomes contain a dithiol-linked vitamin K epoxide reductase (2A) and a dithiol-linked vitamin K quinone reductase (2B). It is likely that these two dithiol-linked reductase activities which are strongly inhibited by the 4-hydroxycoumarin anticoagulants are catalyzed by the same enzyme or share a common subunit. The NAD(P)H linked quinone reductase activity (3) is catalyzed by at least two different enzymes.

other quinone reductases. The microsomal epoxide reductase requires a di-
thiol rather than a reduced pyridine nucleotide for activity and is commonly studied with DTT as a reductant. A cytosolic protein that enhances
the microsomal epoxide reductase activity has been purified,[16] but the
mechanism by which it stimulates the enzymatic activity has not been
clarified. The epoxide reductase activity has been solubilized,[17,18] and
preliminary kinetic studies carried out with both the solubilized[18] and
intact microsomal preparations[19] suggest that the reaction catalyzed by
vitamin K epoxide reductase is between the epoxide and a reduced disulfide
at the active site. These data and chemical model studies[20,21] are consistent with an enzymatic mechanism involving attack of a free sulfhydryl on
the enzyme to open the epoxide ring and form a thioether adduct. It is
suggested that this adduct is converted to an enzyme-bound enolate of 3-
hydroxy-vitamin K with the reformation of the disulfide form of the enzyme
and elimination of H_2O from this intermediate to form the reduction product, the quinone.

The reactions in Figure 3 indicate that there are a number of mechanisms by which the vitamin KH_2 needed for the carboxylase/epoxidase reaction can be generated. The relationship of the vitamin K reductase activity required for the microsomal vitamin K-dependent carboxylase system to
the extensively studied DT-diaphorase of liver has been investigated by
isolation of an oxidoreductase from both cytosol and microsomes that
appeared to be the same as DT-diaphorase.[22] Detergent-solubilized-micro-
somal preparations lacking this activity did not demonstrate a vitamin K-
dependent carboxylase activity unless purified reductase and NADH were
added, suggesting that this enzyme is one of the physiologically important
vitamin K activities in rat liver. It has also been demonstrated[23] that
DT-diaphorase can reduce vitamin K to vitamin KH_2. The importance of this
enzyme in human liver is much more questionable because of its low activity
in this organ.[24] Microsomes also contain two other NAD(P)H-linked reductase activities, cytochrome P-450 reductase and cytochrome b_5 reductase,
which do not appear[25,26] to be involved in vitamin K metabolism. Subsequent investigations of the in vitro carboxylase system demonstrated that
antibodies directed against DT-diaphorase would neutralize only part of the
[vitamin K + NADH]-dependent carboxylase activity in detergent-solubilized
microsomes suggesting that there is a second non-warfarin sensitive NADH-
linked dehydrogenase that can reduce vitamin K. This enzyme is membrane
bound and is probably of more physiological importance.[26] In intact microsomes, DTT will also serve as a reductant to drive a vitamin K quinone-
dependent carboxylase reaction,[27,28] and it has been clearly demonstrated[29,30] that intact microsomal preparations will catalyze a DTT-dependent
formation of vitamin KH_2 from either vitamin K epoxide or vitamin K quinone. The kinetics of formation from vitamin K epoxide[31] have suggested
that the quinone is an intermediate in this reaction.

Site of Warfarin Action

A real understanding of the mechanism of action of warfarin began when
Matschiner et al.[32] demonstrated that the 2,3-epoxide of vitamin K (vitamin

9

K oxide) was a normal metabolite in rat liver and that the ratio of vitamin
K oxide to vitamin K was increased by warfarin administration.[33]   Although
it was originally thought that the high levels of vitamin K oxide inhibited
the carboxylase, this was shown to be unlikely, and the general theory that
inhibition of vitamin K oxide reduction by warfarin would prevent efficient
recycling of the vitamin and limit the action of the carboxylase developed.
Acceptance of this theory was aided by the availability of a strain of wild
rats which were resistant to the action of the common 4-hydroxycoumarin
anticoagulants. It was demonstrated that the vitamin K epoxide reductase
preparation obtained from livers of the warfarin-resistant rats were relatively insensitive to inhibition by warfarin.[27,34]   These preparations
were, however, strongly inhibited by a second 4-hydroxycoumarin, Difenacoum, which had been developed as an effective rodenticide for control of
the warfarin-resistant rat population. These data appeared to provide the
final proof that the inhibiton of epoxide reductase by warfarin was related
to its anticoagulant action. The sensitivity of the other vitamin K-
dependent enzymes that might be involved in the anticoagulant response was
subsequently investigated,[35] and these data (Table 1) indicated that the
epoxide reductase was the most sensitive site and the most likely site of
action of the drug. One activity that was not assayed in the study shown
in Table 1 was the DTT-dependent vitamin K quinone reductase. This enzyme
has been reported[31] to be warfarin sensitive, and it has been shown[36] that
this activity, like that of the epoxide reductase, is less sensitive to
warfarin when assayed in tissues of the warfarin-resistant rat. It is,
therefore, likely that the effects of 4-hydroxycoumarins involve not only

Table 1.   4-Hydroxycoumarin Concentrations Giving 50% Inhibition

| | Warfarin | | Difenacoum | |
| | Normal Rat Liver | Resistant Rat Liver | Normal Rat Liver | Difenacoum Rat Liver |
Activity				
Vit. K Epoxide Reductase	4 μM	50 μM	2.5 μM	4.0 μM
Vit. K-dependent Carboxylase				
Vit. KH_2-dependent	3 mM	3 mM	1.4 mM	1.4 mM
[Vit. K + NADH]-dependent	2 mM	2 mM	1.0 mM	1.0 mM
Vit. K Epoxidase	4 mM	4 mM	2.0 mM	2.0 mM
DT-diaphorase				
Soluble Assay	33 μM	30 μM	49.0 μM	67.0 μM
Liposomal Assay	840 μM	540 μM	17.0 μM	17.0 μM

Difenacoum is a 4-hydroxycoumarin which is an effective rodenticide for
control of the warfarin-resistant strain of rats. The epoxide reductase is
not only the enzyme which is most sensitive to warfarin, but it is the only
one whose sensitivity is substantially altered in preparations from
warfarin-resistant rats. Data summarized from ref. 35.

the reduction of vitamin K epoxide to the quinone, but also the reduction
of the quinone to the hydroquinone. The NADH-dependent quinone reductases
are less sensitive to warfarin inhibition and constitute a pathway for
vitamin K quinone reduction in the anticoagulant-treated animal.[37] The
presence of this pathway explains the ability of administered vitamin K to
counteract the hemorrhagic condition resulting from a massive dose of
warfarin.

The alteration of two enzyme activities by what has been assumed to be
a single mutation responsible for the development of warfarin resistance in
the wild rat population raises some interesting questions in terms of the
structural relationship of the proteins involved. Whether or not the two
microsomal DTT-dependent activities, epoxide reductase and quinone reductase, are catalyzed by the same active site, two active sites on the same
protein, or on two different proteins is not clear at the present time, and
conflicting data have been presented[38,39]

The details of the interaction between warfarin and the epoxide reductase are still unsolved, although kinetic analysis[19] has provided some information. The structural similarity between an enzyme-bound hydroxyvita-
min K intermediate postulated to be an intermediate in the reductase of the
epoxide and the 4-hydroxycoumarins suggest that these anticoagulants are
acting as an analog of this transition state (Fig. 4). Other hypotheses
have, however, been suggested,[40] and if the site of coumarin action is not
at the catalytic site but rather at a subunit involved in transferring
electrons to the catalytic site, it is likely that this structural similarity is fortuitous.

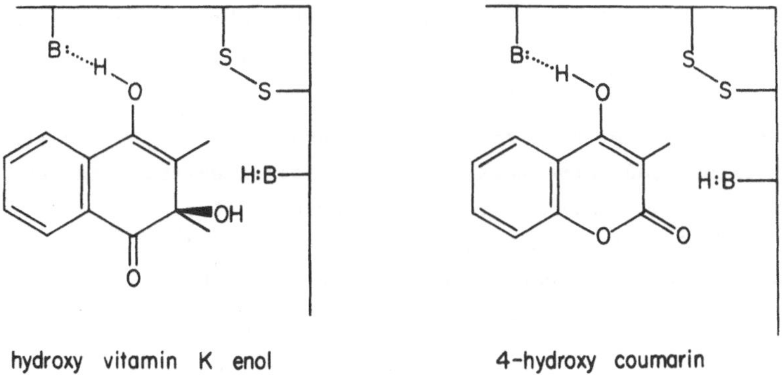

hydroxy vitamin K enol   4-hydroxy coumarin

Figure 4. Proposed interaction of 4-hydroxycoumarins with the vitamin K
epoxide reductase. A hydroxy half enol derivative of vitamin K has been
proposed as an intermediate in the reduction of vitamin K epoxide to vitamin K quinone. The structural similarity of 4-hydroxycoumarins to this
intermediate suggests that their inhibition might be due to competition for
this site on the enzyme.

The primary effect of warfarin administration is a decreased ability of the liver to effectively carry out the posttranslational conversion of glutamyl to γ-carboxyglutamyl residues during the intracellular processing of vitamin K-dependent proteins. Studies that led to the eventual discovery of Gla residues in prothrombin demonstrated that this resulted in the appearance of a des-γ-carboxy (abnormal) species of prothrombin in the plasma of the human and bovine. The appearance of abnormal prothrombin in the plasma occurred simultaneously with a decrease in the plasma concentration of native prothrombin. Significant concentrations of abnormal prothrombin do not appear in the plasma of other species when they are anticoagulated with warfarin, and the basis for this species difference has not been determined.

Although it was originally thought that plasma prothrombin in a warfarin-treated patient was either carboxylated or not, it was soon demonstrated that there is a complex mixture of partially carboxylated forms [41,42] and that any number of the ten potential Glu sites might be lacking in carboxylation. It is possible to separate the plasma abnormal prothrombin pool into fractions that contain on the average 1, 2, 5, or 7 moles of Glu per mole by heavy metal salt fractionation.[43] Studies of the metal-binding properties and biological activity of these partially carboxylated forms[44] have demonstrated that the rate of activation of these partially carboxylated forms to thrombin is dependent on the number of Gla residues in the molecule. The rate of thrombin generation from these species is greatly decreased by the loss of as few as 3 Gla residues per mole. This response has been shown to be related to an increase in the apparent K_m for the binding of prothrombin to the rest of the "prothrombinase" complex and is a function of the Ca^{++} and phospholipid binding properties of these proteins. The slower rate of thrombin generation from these species suggests that they are of little consequence in the rapid generation of thrombin catalyzed by the prothrombinase complex and that the loss of a few Gla residues effectively removes this fraction of prothrombin from participating in hemostatic control.

Warfarin therapy has traditionally been monitored by one-stage prothrombin times, and these measurements reflect a decrease in concentration or activity of the combined vitamin K-dependent clotting factors. It is usually assumed that because of the rapid biological turnover of factor VII, these measurements may often be as dependent on changes of factor VII concentration as they are on changes of prothrombin concentration. A ratio of the one-stage prothrombin time of a warfarin-treated patient plasma to that of a control plasma pool, "the therapeutic range," is commonly calculated in an effort to regulate warfarin dosage. Specific radioimmunoassays for circulating abnormal (des-γ-carboxy) prothrombin and for native prothrombin have been developed.[45] These assays have been used to monitor warfarin therapy,[46] and the available data would suggest that the important factor in predicting the possible risk of hemorrhagic or thrombotic complications is the level of native (normal, fully carboxylated) prothrombin

antigen present. Maintaining patients within a narrow range of native
plasma prothrombin concentration might have some advantage over current
practice in preventing the potential complications of warfarin therapy.
However, a great deal of additional investigation will be needed before
changes in standard practice can be recommended.

SUMMARY

Vitamin K is required for a liver microsomal enzyme that catalyzes the
posttranslational conversion of specific glutamyl residues in precursors of
the vitamin K-dependent clotting factors to γ-carboxyglutamyl residues in
the plasma form of these proteins. A second product of this carboxylation
reaction is the 2,3-epoxide of the vitamin. The anticoagulant warfarin
blocks the enzyme which reduces this epoxide to vitamin K quinone, and also
blocks one of the microsomal pathways which converts the quinone to the
active coenzyme form of the vitamin, the hydroquinone. Warfarin anticoagulation therefore reduces the activity of the vitamin K-dependent carboxylase and results in the secretion of vitamin K-dependent clotting
factors that are undercarboxylated. The presence of γ-carboxyglutamyl
residues is essential for the normal Ca^{++}/phospholipid-mediated activation
of prothrombin, and the des-γ-carboxy forms of prothrombin secreted by
patients receiving warfarin therapy lack biological activity and have a
reduced thrombotic potential.

REFERENCES

1. J. W. Suttie, Vitamin K, in: "The Fat-soluble Vitamins," A. T.
    Diplock, ed., p. 225, William Heinemann Ltd., London (1985).
2. K. P. Link, The discovery of dicumarol and its sequels, Circulation
    19:97 (1959).
3. J. Stenflo, P. Fernlund, W. Egan, and P. Roepstorff, Vitamin K de-
    pendent modifications of glutamic acid residues in prothrombin,
    Proc. Natl. Acad. Sci. USA 71:2730 (1974).
4. G. L. Nelsestuen, T. H. Zytkovicz, and J. B. Howard, The mode of
    action of vitamin K. Identification of γ-carboxyglutamic
    acid as a component of prothrombin, J. Biol. Chem. 249:6347 (1974).
5. C. T. Esmon, J. A. Sadowski, and J. W. Suttie, A new carboxylation
    reaction. The vitamin K-dependent incorporation of $H^{14}CO_3^-$ into
    prothrombin, J. Biol. Chem. 250:4744 (1975).
6. J. W. Suttie, Vitamin K-dependent carboxylase, Ann. Rev. Biochem.
    54:459 (1985).
7. D. H. Rich, S. R. Lehrman, M. Kawai, H. L. Goodman, and J. W. Suttie,
    Synthesis of peptide analogues of prothrombin precursor sequence
    5-9. Substrate specificity of vitamin K dependent carboxylase, J.
    Med. Chem. 24:706 (1981).
8. C. Vermeer, B. A. M. Soute, H. Hendrix, and M. A. G. de Boer-van den
    Berg, Decarboxylated bone Gla-protein as a substrate for hepatic
    vitamin K-dependent carboxylase, FEBS Lett. 165:16 (1984).

9. G. L. Long, R. M. Belagaje, and R. T. A. MacGillivray, Cloning and sequencing of liver cDNA coding for bovine protein C, Proc. Natl. Acad. Sci. USA 81:5653 (1984).

10. L. C. Pan and P. A. Price, The propeptide of rat bone γ-carboxy-glutamic acid protein shares homology with other vitamin K-dependent protein precursors, Proc. Natl. Acad. Sci. USA 82:6109 (1985).

11. J. W. Suttie, J. A. Hoskins, J. Engelke, A. Hopfgartner, H. Ehrlich, N. U. Bang, R. M. Belagaje, B. Schoner, and G. L. Long, Vitamin K dependent carboxylase: possible role of the "propeptide" as an intracellular recognition site (γ-carboxyglutamic acid/pro-tein C), Proc. Natl. Acad. Sci. USA (1987) in press.

12. A. E. Larson, P. A. Friedman, and J. W. Suttie, Vitamin K-dependent carboxylase: stoichiometry of carboxylation and vitamin K 2,3-epoxide formation, J. Biol. Chem. 256:11032 (1981).

13. J. J. McTigue and J. W. Suttie, Vitamin K-dependent carboxylase: demonstration of a vitamin K- and O_2-dependent exchange of ^{3}H from ^3H_2O into glutamic acid residues, J. Biol. Chem. 258:12129 (1983).

14. D. L. Anton and P. A. Friedman, Fate of the activated γ-carbon-hydrogen bond in the uncoupled vitamin K-dependent γ-glutamyl carboxylation reaction, J. Biol. Chem. 258:14084 (1983).

15. J. Lowenthal and J. A. MacFarlane, The nature of the antagonism between vitamin K and indirect anticoagulants, J. Pharmacol. Exp. Therap. 143:273 (1964).

16. C. M. Siegfried, Purification and properties of a factor from rat liver cytosol which stimulates vitamin K epoxide reductase, Arch. Biochem. Biophys. 223:129 (1983).

17. C. M. Siegfried, Solubilization of vitamin K epoxide reductase and vitamin K-dependent carboxylase from rat liver microsomes, Biochem. Biophys. Res. Commun. 83:1488 (1978).

18. E. F. Hildebrandt, P. C. Preusch, J. L. Patterson, and J. W. Suttie, Solubilization and characterization of vitamin K epoxide reductase from normal and warfarin-resistant rat liver microsomes, Arch. Biochem. Biophys. 228:480 (1984).

19. M. J. Fasco, L. M. Principe, W. A. Walsh, and P. A. Friedman, Warfarin inhibition of vitamin K 2,3-epoxide reductase in rat liver microsomes, Biochemistry 22:5655 (1983).

20. R. B. Silverman, Chemical model studies for the mechanism of vitamin K epoxide reductase, J. Am. Chem. Soc. 103:5939 (1981).

21. P. C. Preusch and J. W. Suttie, A chemical model for the mechanism of vitamin K epoxide reductase, J. Org. Chem. 48:3301 (1983).

22. R. Wallin, O. Gebhardt, and H. Prydz, NAD(P)H dehydrogenase and its role in the vitamin K (2-methyl-3-phytyl-1,4-naphthoquinone)-dependent carboxylation reaction, Biochem. J. 169:95 (1978).

23. M. J. Fasco and L. M. Principe, Vitamin K_1 hydroquinone formation catalyzed by DT-diaphorase, Biochem. Biophys. Res. Commun. 104:187 (1982).

24. R. Wallin and L. F. Martin, Vitamin K-dependent carboxylation and vitamin K metabolism in liver. Effects of warfarin, *J*. *Clin*. *Invest*. 76:1879 (1985).

25. R. Wallin and J. W. Suttie, Vitamin K-dependent carboxylation and vitamin K epoxidation. Evidence that the warfarin-sensitive microsomal NAD(P)H dehydrogenase reduces vitamin K_1 in these reactions, *Biochem*. *J*. 194:983 (1981).

26. R. Wallin, Vitamin K antagonism of coumarin anticoagulation. A dehydrogenase pathway in rat liver is responsible for the antagonistic effect, *Biochem*. *J*. 236:685 (1986).

27. D. S. Whitlon, J. A. Sadowski, and J. W. Suttie, Mechanism of coumarin action: significance of vitamin K epoxide reductase inhibition, *Biochemistry* 17:1371 (1978).

28. R. Wallin and S. Hutson, Vitamin K-dependent carboxylation. Evidence that at least two microsomal dehydrogenases reduce vitamin K_1 to support carboxylation, *J*. *Biol*. *Chem*. 257:1583 (1982).

29. M. J. Fasco and L. M. Principe, Vitamin K_1 hydroquinone formation catalyzed by a microsomal reductase system, *Biochem*. *Biophys*. *Res*. *Commun*. 97:1487 (1980).

30. P. A. Sherman and E. G. Sander, Vitamin K epoxide reductase: evidence that vitamin K dihydroquinone is a product of vitamin K epoxide reduction. *Biochem*. *Biophys*. *Res*. *Commun*. 103:997 (1981).

31. M. J. Fasco and L. M. Principe, R- and S-warfarin inhibition of vitamin K and vitamin K 2,3-epoxide reductase activities in the rat, *J*. *Biol*. *Chem*. 257:4894 (1982).

32. J. T. Matschiner, R. G. Bell, J. M. Amelotti, and T. E. Knauer, Isolation and characterization of a new metabolite of phylloquinone in the rat, *Biochim*. *Biophys*. *Acta* 201:309 (1970).

33. R. G. Bell and J. T. Matschiner, Warfarin and the inhibition of vitamin K activity by an oxide metabolite, Nature 237:32 (1972).

34. A. Zimmerman and J. T. Matschiner, Biochemical basis of hereditary resistance to warfarin in the rat, *Biochem*. *Pharmacol*. 23:1033 (1974).

35. E. F. Hildebrandt and J. W. Suttie, Mechanism of coumarin action: sensitivity of vitamin K metabolizing enzymes of normal and warfarin-resistant rat liver, *Biochemistry* 21:2406 (1982).

36. M. J. Fasco, E. F. Hildebrandt, and J. W. Suttie, Evidence that warfarin anticoagulant action involves two distinct reductase activities, *J*. *Biol*. *Chem*. 257:11210 (1982).

37. R. Wallin, S. D. Patrick, and J. O. Ballard, Vitamin K antagonism of coumarin intoxication in the rat, *Thromb*. *Haemostas*. (Stuttg.) 55:235 (1986).

38. P. C. Preusch and J. W. Suttie, Relationship of dithiothreitol-dependent microsomal vitamin K quinone and vitamin K epoxide reductases: inhibition of epoxide reduction by vitamin K quinone, *Biochim*. *Biophys*. *Acta* 798:141 (1984).

39. J. J. Lee and M. J. Fasco, Metabolism of vitamin K and vitamin K 2,3-epoxide via interaction with a common disulfide, Biochemistry 23:2246 (1984).

40. R. B. Silverman, A model for a molecular mechanism of anticoagulant activity of 3-substituted 4-hydroxycoumarins, J. Am. Chem. Soc. 102:5421 (1980).

41. P. A. Friedman, R. D. Rosenberg, P. V. Hauschka, and A. Fitz-James, A spectrum of partially carboxylated prothrombins in the plasmas of coumarin-treated patients. Biochim. Biophys. Acta 494:271 (1977).

42. M. P. Esnouf and C. V. Prowse, The gamma-carboxy glutamic acid content of human and bovine prothrombin following warfarin treatment, Biochim. Biophys. Acta 490:471 (1977).

43. O. P. Malhotra, Dicoumarol-induced prothrombins, Ann. N. Y. Acad. Sci. 370:426 (1981).

44. O. P. Malhotra, M. E. Nesheim, and K. G. Mann, The kinetics of activation of normal and γ-carboxyglutamic acid-deficient prothrombins, J. Biol. Chem. 260:279 (1985).

45. R. A. Blanchard, B. C. Furie, S. F. Kruger, G. Waneck, M. J. Jorgensen, and B. Furie, Immunoassays of human prothrombin species which correlate with functional coagulant activities, J. Lab. Clin. Med. 101:242 (1983).

46. B. Furie, H. A. Liebman, R. A. Blanchard, M. S. Coleman, S. F. Kruger, and B. C. Furie, Comparison of the native prothrombin antigen and the prothrombin time for monitoring oral anticoagulant therapy, Blood 64:445 (1984).

WARFARIN AND THE BIOCHEMISTRY OF THE

VITAMIN K DEPENDENT PROTEINS

Edwin G. Bovill and Kenneth G. Mann

University of Vermont
Departments of Biochemistry and Pathology
Given Building
Burlington, Vt. 05405

The vitamin K-dependent proteins are a diverse group of molecules, all sharing the unique amino acid gamma carboxy glutamic acid (Gla). Gla is produced by the vitamin K-dependent post translational gamma carboxylation of selected glutamic acid residues, a step blocked by warfarin (Fig. 1). Gla-containing proteins have been most thoroughly studied in the blood coagulation system and bone but are found in other tissues such as the kidney. This review will focus on the blood coagulation system but will also touch on other Gla-containing proteins which shed light on common structural and functional features.

Most of the vitamin K-dependent coagulation proteins are serine proteases. A number of recent reviews, combining information from traditional protein biochemistry and molecular genetics, have traced the structural evolution of the serine proteases (1,2). These proteases vary from the low molecular weight, rather indiscriminate digestive protease trypsin to the high molecular weight, highly specific regulatory proteases of the coagulation, fibrinolytic and complement systems. Trypsinogen consists of a polypeptide domain containing the elemental serine protease structure. Analysis of protease evolution suggests that over time a number of modular functional domains have been inserted between the signal peptide and the zymogen domain which have conferred upon these proteins their high degree of specificity. These functional domains, defined by sequence homology, can be found in the noncatalytic regions of many of the serine protease zymogens and interestingly in nonproteases; for example, fibronectin (2). The occurrence of these homologous regions amongst diverse proteins has been suggested by some investigators (3,4) to have resulted from exon shuffling. The concept of shuffling of similar functional domains among diverse proteins led them to propose an evolutionary scenario for the serine proteases of coagulation and forms a basis for comparison amongst these proteins.

The noncatalytic region of the vitamin K-dependent serine proteases of the coagulation system contain varied combinations of three different domains:
  1. The Gla domain contains the sites of carboxylation of selected glutamic acid residues in the gamma position. The Gla residues found at the amino terminal end of the molecule bind metal ions,

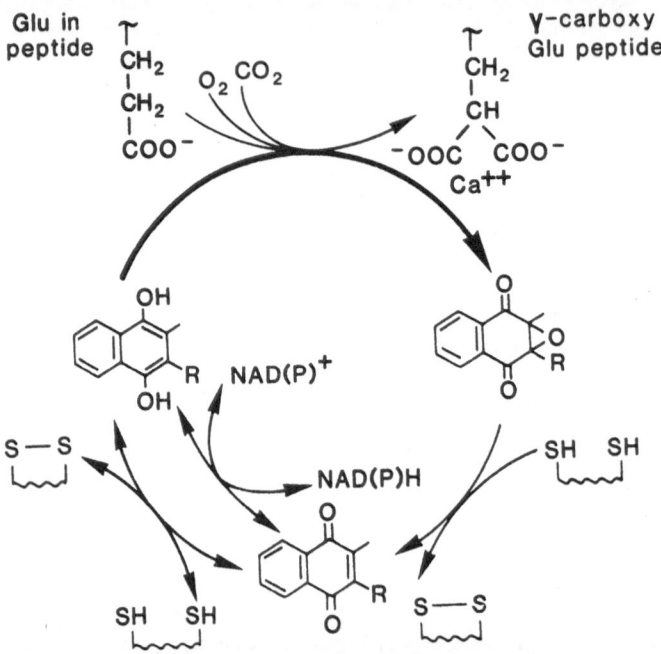

Fig. 1 Vitamin K metabolism in rat liver microsomes. In addition
to the carboxylase/epoxidase system, liver microsomes contain a
dithiol-linked epoxide reductase and quinone reductase and at least
two NAD(P)H-linked quinone reductases. It is likely that the two
dithiol-linked reductase activities represent the same enzyme or
that they share a common subunit. These two activities are strongly
inhibited by the 4-hydroxycoumarin anticoagulants. (Reproduced with
permission from the Annual Review of Biochemistry, Vol. 54, p. 472
1985.)

especially Ca^{+2}, and, as a result of this binding, mediate binding of the
protein to negatively charged phospholipid surfaces such as phospholipid
vesicles and platelets (5,6).

2. An epidermal growth factor (EGF) domain shows varying
degrees of homology with EGF.(7)

3. A Kringle domain consisting of a complex, folded disulfide
linked region is thought to provide a binding function in some proteins
(8). As yet, there are no studies explicitly describing such a function
in the vitamin K-dependent proteases.

Of these various areas of homology, with their postulated functions,
only the Gla regions have established functional roles at this time.

Another recently described area of homology amongst the vitamin
K-dependent proteins is in the leader peptide. Nine amino acid residues
proximal to the amino terminus of bone gla protein (BGP) show strong
similarity to similar peptides in the other vitamin K-dependent proteins
(9). It is speculated that this leader sequence may play a role in the
post translational carboxylation of these proteins. Recent observations
by Suttie's and Long's laboratories support this notion. They

demonstrated that protein products of plasmids of protein C complete with
a propeptide region were substrates for a cell free carboxylase system
whereas protein products of plasmids lacking the propeptide region were
not carboxylated (10). They concluded that their data support the role
of the leader sequence in initiating carboxylation.

Figure 2 diagrammatically illustrates those vitamin K-dependent
proteins whose structures are sufficiently known to demonstrate the areas
of similarities and differences in the previously mentioned domains
including the catalytic active site and the leader sequence.

The genes have been isolated for most of the proteins shown in
figure 2. Analysis of the genes has revealed that the position of
intervening sequences (introns) within the genes generally correspond to
structure function domain boundaries in these proteins. It is apparent
from this diagram that factors VII, IX, X, Z and protein C are quite
similar with respect to the domain insertions in their noncatalytic
regions. Protein S shows significant similarities but is not a serine
protease and has four rather than two growth factor domains. The large
region of protein S carboxy terminal to the growth factor domains showed
no extensive regions of homology to other proteins following a search of
the Protein Identification Resource protein sequence database (11). The
noncatalytic domains of prothrombin share only the Gla domain with the
other factors (12). Instead of the growth factor domains, prothrombin
has two kringle regions. In spite of this latter finding, thrombin is
the only coagulation protein with established growth factor activity

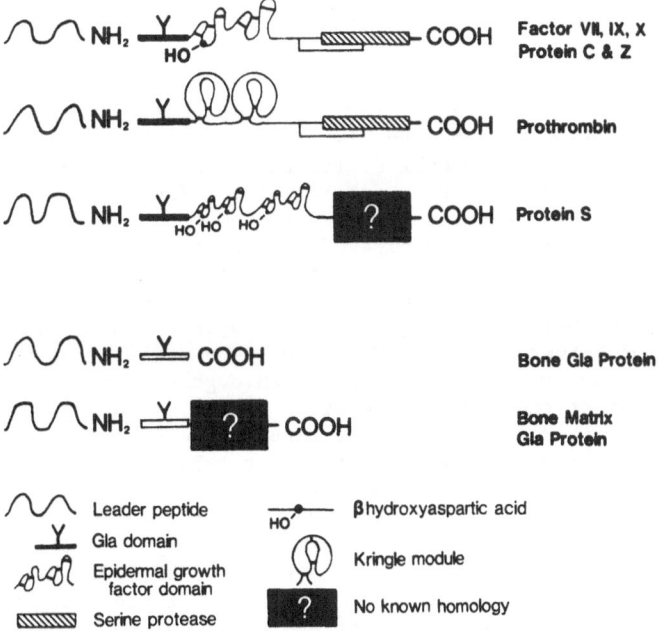

Fig. 2 Demonstrates the relative positions of the homologous
domains present in the non catalytic regions of the vitamin
K-dependent proteins.

which has been recently described in the B-loop region of the molecule (13).   These dissimilarities between the structures of prothrombin and the other vitamin K-dependent serine proteases suggest that one must be cautious in extrapolating the properties of prothrombin to these other molecules. This caution is especially important since we know significantly more about prothrombin due to its more ready availability in plasma. The precise functions of proteins Z and M are not known at this time although protein Z does not appear to be an active serine protease zymogen (14).

The bone proteins share homology in their leader sequence with the rest of the vitamin K-dependent proteins. The Gla region of these two proteins are homologous one to the other but not to the rest of the vitamin K-dependent proteins (15).

The differences between prothrombin and the other vitamin K-dependent serine proteases and the lack of established roles for the domains described above point out the need for more fundamental investigation of this family of proteins.

BIOCHEMISTRY OF THE VITAMIN K-DEPENDENT PROTEINS AND THEIR COFACTORS

Line drawings of the known vitamin K-dependent factors are illustrated in figure 3. The location of the Gla residues are identified by the symbol Y. Each of these protein molecules contains 10-13 gamma-carboxyglutamic acids. In addition, the location of carbohydrate in the protein is illustrated by the symbol CHO. Other structural features of significance, such as disulfide bonds and the location of the active site serines expressed after activation of the zymogens, are also identified.

Factor VII

Factor VII has been identified as the initiating enzymatic component of blood coagulation mediated by tissue factor (16). Factor VII has been studied extensively by a number of laboratories, and it has been isolated from both bovine (17) and human species (18). The amino acid sequence of human factor VII has recently been elucidated from a cDNA coding for human factor VII (19). The uncleaved form of factor VII has been reported to be biologically active. The uncleaved single chain factor VII can incorporate DFP into the active site serine under mild conditions. The molecular weight of the single chain molecule is reported to be between 45,000 and 54,000. The activity of the single chain protein can be further stimulated through cleavage by other proteases of the blood coagulation system. Cleavage at site A (figure 3) by either factor Xa or by thrombin results in an approximately 100 fold stimulation of factor VII activity. The resulting two chain molecule is disulfide bridged, and no activation peptide is lost. Active site serine has been placed in the COOH-terminal peptide by DFP incorporation studies. The heavy chain containing the active site serine has been reported to have a molecular weight of 29,500, while the light chain, derived from the amino terminal portion of the zymogen contains the vitamin K-dependent modification and has a molecular weight of 23,500.

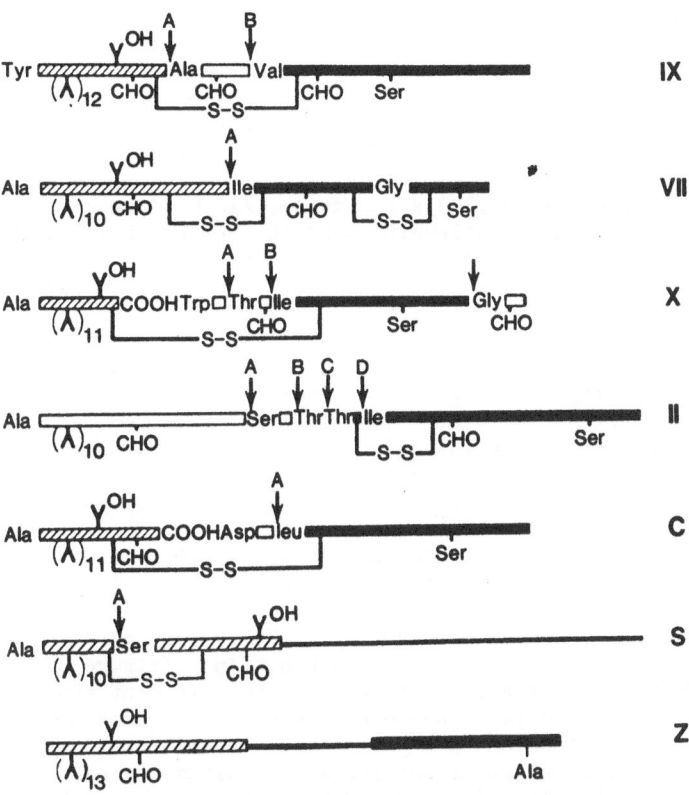

Fig. 3. The vitamin K-dependent blood clotting factors. For each
factor, the locations of proteolytic cleavages in the proenzymes are
identified, as are also the resulting products. The peptide chain
that contains the proteolytic machinery is identified in boldface,
while activation peptides that are not covalently attached to
resulting enzyme products are represented by open boxes. Hatched
areas represent covalently attached peptide chains associated with
the protease products. gamma-carboxylglutamic acid is represented
by γ, and the subscripts represent the quantitative level of Gla in
each of the vitamin K-dependent proteins. CHO represents carbohydrate
side chains, while γ^{OH} represents beta-hydroxyaspartate. The desig-
nation Ser, as a subscript to the chains, represents the location of
the active site serine in the trypsin-like enzymes. The carboxy
terminal half of the protein S molecule is represented without detail.

Factor IX

Factor IX is a single chain zymogen with a molecular weight of
55,000 (20). The amino acid sequence has been deduced from a cDNA coding
for human factor IX (21). The zymogen can be activated by factor XIa or
factor VIIa (22,23). Both activation processes require calcium and two
bond cleavages. Bond A (figure 3) is cleaved to yield a two-chain
disulfide-linked protein. Cleavage of bond B releases a 9,000-dalton
peptide containing carbohydrate and produces a two chain active form of
factor IXa. The active site serine placed by DFP incorporation is in the
carboxyl terminal 27,000-dalton peptide. The amino terminal of the
zymogen remains covalently linked to the remainder of the enzyme by
disulfide bonds. Since factor IXa lacks the 9,000-dalton activation
peptide, the resulting molecular weight of factor IXa is about 46,500.

Factor X

Factor X is a substrate in both the intrinsic and extrinsic pathways of coagulation (24,25). Factor X is a two chain molecule, composed of a heavy chain of 37,000-daltons and a light chain of 17,000-daltons. The two chains are bridged by disulfide bonds. The light chain corresponds to the amino terminal of the other vitamin K-dependent coagulation factors, and it contains 12 Gla residues. Factor X is activated by the cleavage of an arginine-isoleucine bond at site B (figure 3) by either factor VII or factor IXa, yielding factor Xa-alpha. Once factor Xa activity is expressed, there is an autocatalytic cleavage of the enzyme at site C, producing factor Xa-beta. Factor Xa can also cleave the factor X molecule at site A. This hydrolysis occurs slowly and may not be of physiologic significance. After cleavage to produce factor Xa-alpha, the molecular weight of the heavy chain becomes 30,000 and a 7,000-dalton peptide is lost. Cleavage at sites B and C to produce factor Xa-beta leads to a molecular weight of 27,000 for the heavy chain.

Prothrombin

Prothrombin is a substrate for factor Xa (26,27). This vitamin K-dependent protein is the most extensively studied of the group, primarily because of its relatively high concentration in plasma. Prothrombin has a molecular weight of 72,000. During activation by factor Xa, the molecule is cleaved at position D (figure 3) and at position B, yielding the amino terminal "pro" fragment and active alpha-thrombin, which is composed of two disulfide linked chains, an A chain of 5,700-daltons and a B chain of 31,000-daltons. Inspection of figure 3 demonstrates that alpha thrombin, unlike the other vitamin K-dependent procoagulant factors, is no longer connected by a covalent bridge to its Gla containing "pro" portion of the molecule.

In addition to the factor Xa-mediated cleavages of the prothrombin molecule, the zymogen is also a substrate for thrombin. Thrombin can cleave prothrombin at position A, yielding prothrombin fragment 1 (23,000-daltons) from the amino terminal of the molecule. The other product of this reaction is termed prethrombin 1, and it has a molecular weight of 55,000. When this reaction occurs, the entire vitamin K-dependent portion of the molecule is deleted, and the efficacy of prothombin as a substrate for phospholipid bound Factor Xa is decreased. In addition to the cleavage site, which is present in both bovine and human prothrombin, and resides between fragment 1 and prethrombin 1, there is another thrombin sensitive site in the human prothrombin molecule. This cleavage site is located 13 residues carboxyl terminal to the cleavage site that results in the formation of the A chain, and since this cleavage is autocatalytic, isolated human thrombin always has these 13 residues deleted. The significance of this thrombin cleavage has not been established. A recent observation made in our laboratory with respect to alternative mechanisms of prothrombin activation via meizothrombin may have important implications for the activation of warfarinized prothrombin and is reviewed in the warfarin section below.

Park et al. (12) have recently crystallized prothrombin fragment 1 which contains the Gla residues and submitted this to x-ray crystallography. They were able to elucidate the three dimensional structure of the kringle region and noted that the amino terminal region containing the 10 Gla residues exhibited disorder in the crystal structure. They postulated that this disorder might be due to a requirement for more flexibility in the Gla region due to its membrane binding function.

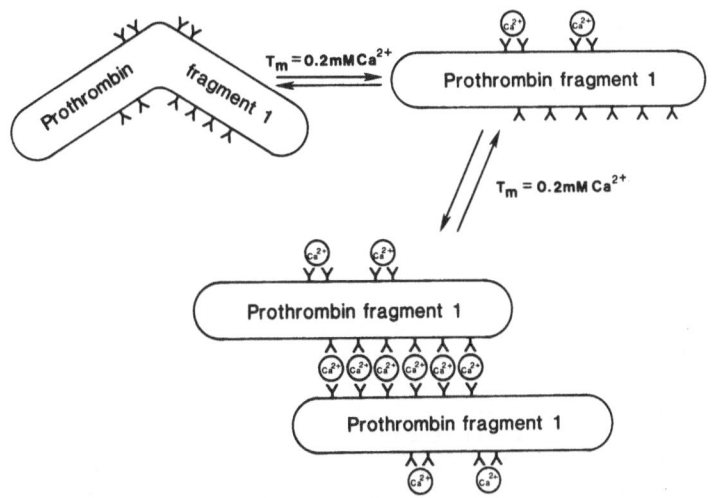

Fig 4. Model for prothrombin fragment 1 metal ion binding.
Prothrombin fragment 1 is represented as a prolate ellipsoid with an
axial ratio of 6/1. The symbols Y represent gamma-carboxyglutamic
acid residues. (Reprinted with permission, Mann KG, Bloom J,
Biochemistry 1978, No. 17, p 4437.)

With respect to possible Gla related shape changes - fully
carboxylated prothrombin has been demonstrated to undergo two transitions
in the presence of Ca^{2+} ions, one of which involves a conformational
change and the other of which involves self association and lipid binding
(5,6) Figure 4 represents a model for the effect of metal binding on
prothrombin fragment 1 (the gla containing portion of prothrombin), based
on circular dichroism and intrinsic fluorescence experiments. These
studies were done initially with prothrombin fragment 1 (6) and
subsequently were expanded to intact prothrombin (5).

Protein C

Protein C has a peptide molecular weight of 45,000 and is composed
of two disulfide linked chains of molecular weights 17,000 and 28,000.
The entire sequence is known for both the human (28) and bovine protein
(29). Unlike the other vitamin K-dependent proteins identified in the
classic coagulation scheme, protein C zymogen activation leads to the
generation of an anticoagulant enzyme. The protein can be cleaved by
thrombin in the amino terminal region of the heavy chain at position A
(figure 3). The release of the 14 amino acid activation peptide results
in the formation of activated protein C (APC) which inactivates both
factors Va and VIIIa (30,31).

Protein S

Protein S has a molecular weight of 69,000 (32). The entire sequence
of human protein S has recently been deduced from a human liver cDNA (8).
The protein contains 10 Gla residues and 3 beta hydroxyaspartate residues
and is not a serine protease. Isolated protein S migrates at 69,000
daltons on an unreduced polyacrylamide gel but forms a doublet with bands
at 69,000 and 64,000 daltons on a reduced gel with the presence of a
6-8000 dalton peptide containing the amino terminal Gla domain of the
intact molecule. Protein S has been shown to accentuate the inactivation

of factor Va and VIIIa by APC in human and bovine systems (33,34), apparently by acting as a cofactor for APC. Thrombin cleaves protein S at site A and leads to loss of its anticoagulant activity (35). In plasma about 60% of protein S is bound to complement component C4 binding protein. The bound protein S does not appear to be an active cofactor for APC (36). Recently another binding protein has been described in plasma which appears to accentuate the anticoagulant activity of protein S (37).

Protein Z

Protein Z has a molecular weight of 43,700 and contains 13 Gla residues and one beta hydroxyaspartic acid (14). The protein is homologous to the other factor X-like vitamin K-dependent proteases. However, in the active site, residues corresponding to histidine-57 and serine-195 in trypsin are replaced by threonine and alanine respectively. These changes in the active site render the molecule inactive as a serine protease. The role of protein Z is unknown at the present time.

Other Vitamin K-dependent plasma proteins

An additional protein has been identified which may correspond to a vitamin K-dependent molecule. Protein M has been identified by Seeger's laboratory through DEAE chromatography of the bovine vitamin K-dependent proteins (38). Protein M has an apparent molecular weight of 50,000 and appears to be procoagulant in nature, influencing the conversion of prothrombin to thrombin.

Protein cofactors for vitamin K-dependent enzymes

Each of the vitamin K-dependent serine proteases described above requires a cofactor protein whose participation is vital for the expression of maximal activity. The following paragraphs are a brief review of these cofactors. The cofactor group includes tissue factor, factor V, factor VIII, thrombomodulin and protein S. Protein S has already been described above. Factor V was the first cofactor isolated to homogeneity and is present in greatest abundance (39). Factor V circulates in plasma as a single chain, high molecular weight pro-cofactor that must be cleaved by thrombin or factor Xa to give rise to factor Va (40). It is factor Va that participates in the prothrombinase reaction. A line drawing representation of the activation of factor V is illustrated in figure 5. During activation by thrombin, factor V is cleaved to produce intermediates and ultimately final product peptide chains of 74,000 and 94,000, which make up factor Va activity and appear to be self associated in the presence of calcium ions (41).

Recent studies on factor VIII activation suggest that factor VIII also exists in plasma as a high molecular weight precursor of factor VIIIa activity (42,43). The cleavage of factor VIII by thrombin results in a more active species (factor VIIIa) and present data suggest the model shown in figure 6. Like factor Va, the peptide chains that make up factor VIIIa appear to be self associated in the presence of calcium ions (44,45).

Tissue factor and thrombomodulin have been isolated (46,47). In contrast to factor Va and factor VIIIa, both tissue factor and thrombomodulin appear to be single chain proteins. Both of these proteins bind to phospholipids in a manner similar to those of factors Va and VIIIa, and appear to form the receptors for their respective enzymes, factor VIIa and thrombin.

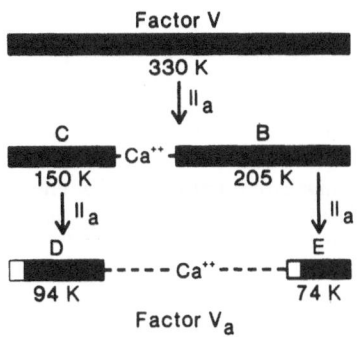

Factor V

330 K

$\downarrow$ II_a

C   -Ca⁺⁺-   B
150 K   205 K $\downarrow$ II_a

$\downarrow$ II_a

D   E
94 K - - - - Ca⁺⁺ - - - -   74 K

Factor V_a

Fig. 5. The activation of Factor V represented schematically.
Procofactor Factor V is cleaved by thrombin first to give rise to
two intermediate peptide chains that are noncovalently associated in
the presence of calcium ions. These chains are subsequently cleaved
to give rise to two polypeptide chains, D and E, that are obtained
from the NH_2- and COOH-terminal of the parent molecule,
respectively. These two chains are noncovalently associated with
the process involving calcium ion. The open areas indicated at the
NH_2-termini of the D and C chain represent areas that have been
shown to be homologous to similar areas of the Factor VIIIa peptide
chains (see Fig 6) [modified from Higgins DL, Mann KG: The
interaction of bovine factor V and factor V-derived peptides with
phospholipid vesicles. J. Biol. Chem. 258:6503, 1983 with
permission.]

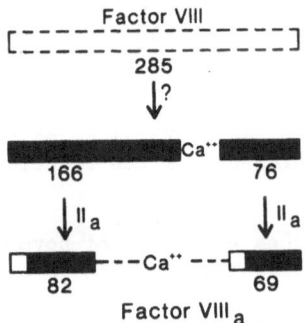

Factor VIII

285

$\downarrow$?

166   Ca⁺⁺   76

$\downarrow$ II_a $\downarrow$ II_a

82   - - Ca⁺⁺ - -   69

Factor VIII_a

Fig. 6 A schematic representation of the process of Factor VIII
activation. The present physical data obtained on porcine Factor
VIII indicate that the isolated molecule is composed of two chains
of apparent molecular weights 166,000 and 76,000 with Ca^{2+} involved
in the noncovalent association of these chains. A hypothetical
precursor is shown by a dotted line with an apparent molecular
weight of 285,000. The products obtained from the two chains of the
isolated Factor VIII molecule upon thrombin treatment are
illustrated at M_r values of 82,000; 69,000; and associated in the
presence of calcium ions. The open segments at the NH_2-termini of
each of these chains represent regions of the peptides that are
homologous to Factor Va. (Reprinted with permission from Mann KG,
Membrane-bound complex in blood coagulation, In: Progress in
Hemostasis and Thrombosis, Vol. 7 (c) 1984 by Grune & Stratton,
Orlando, Fla.)

The coagulation proteins described above play a central role in hemostasis. The hemostatic response is an integrated network of reactions involving the blood vessel wall, the blood platelet, and the plasma blood clotting proteases which lead to localized expression of procoagulant activity at the site of vascular damage. Central to the development of local procoagulant activity is the activation of blood coagulation zymogens to their respective enzymes and the membrane-associated expression of blood clotting activity.

Of importance in the development of the fibrin clot and the regulation of procoagulant activity are the vitamin K dependent blood clotting enzyme complexes (48,49,50). These enzyme complexes (see figure 7) provide for the rapid expression of the enzymatic activities which activate the proenzymes, prothrombin, factors VII, IX, X and protein C to their respective enzymes. These are subsequently expressed in the procoagulant and anticoagulant enzyme cascades. Two vitamin K-dependent enzyme complexes are known to activate factor X. The extrinsic X activator is composed of the serine protease factor VII (which can be proteolytically activated to a more active species factor VIIa), the membrane associated tissue factor cofactor, a phospholipid surface and calcium ion. The intrinsic factor X activator is composed of the serine protease factor IXa, the cofactor factor VIII (factor VIIIa), a phospholipid membrane surface and calcium ion.

The division between intrinsic and extrinsic factor X activators is not explicit as evidenced by the capacity of the extrinsic Factor X activator to activate factor IX to factor IXa (73) as well as the ability of factor IXa to activate factor VII to VIIa (51). Factor Xa, resulting from either pathway, activates prothrombin as part of a complex enzyme system prothrombinase which is composed of the serine protease factor Xa, the cofactor factor Va, a membrane surface and calcium ion. This enzyme complex cleaves two peptide bonds in prothrombin to produce alpha thrombin at a rate approximately 5 orders of magnitude greater than that which could be obtained with factor Xa alone at physiologic concentrations of the constituents of the reaction system (52,53).

Thrombin (factor IIa) has a variety of potential physiologic substrates. The action of thrombin results in several clotting and cellular events including fibrin generation, platelet activation, factor XIII activation and cofactor factors V and VIII activation. In addition, as represented in figure 7, thrombin complexed with the cofactor thrombomodulin, a membrane surface and calcium ion, activates the anticoagulant vitamin K-dependent zymogen protein C to activated protein C (55). Activated protein C, the vitamin K-dependent cofactor protein S, a membrane surface and calcium ion then form an anticoagulant enzyme complex which inactivates the procoagulant cofactors Va and VIIIa (56).

The most extensively studied of these enzyme complexes is prothrombinase. Consequently, the following discussion will focus on this complex. Work in Seeger's (38) laboratory led to the identification of the five components required for this reaction: prothrombin; the enzyme factor Xa; a cofactor protein, factor Va; calcium ions and phospholipid. The availability of purified factor V and factor Va, as well as the other constituents of the prothrombinase complex, have made it possible in recent years to provide a reasonably compelling description of how the complex is assembled and why assembly of the complex appears to be a significant event in the regulation of the blood

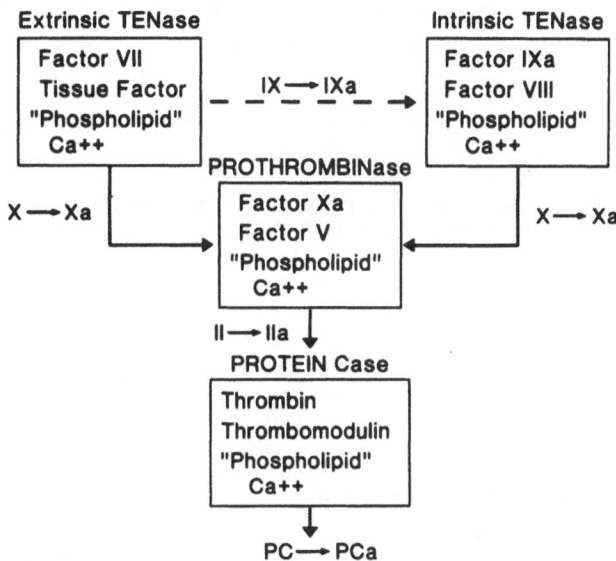

Fig 7. Vitamin K-dependent complex enzymes of blood coagulation.
Each complex enzyme is represented by a box containing the
appropriate constituents which make up the complex enzyme. The top
component of each list is a serine protease which catalyzes the
respective bond cleavages. The second component identified is the
cofactor protein required. All of the reactions require a membrane
surface which may be replaced by purified phospholipid preparations.
The assembly of all catalysts require calcium ions. The arrows
between the complex enzymes represent the proteolytic
transformations catalyzed by the respective catalysts.
(Reprinted by permission of John Wiley and Sons, Inc., Mann KG, Fass
DN, The molecular biology of blood coagulation, In: Current
Hematology, Vol. 2, 1983, Fairbanks, V.S., ed) Copyright^{c} John Wiley
& Sons, Inc.)

Table 1. Rates of Prothrombin Activation in the Presence of Various
Combinations of the "Prothrombinase" Complex

Components Present*	Rate[+]
Xa	0.0044
Xa, Ca^{2+}	0.010
Xa, Ca^{2+}, Phospholipid	0.092
Xa, Ca^{2+}, Va	1.55
Xa, Ca^{2+}, Phospholipid, Va	1210

*Proteins are present at potential physiological concen-
tration; prothrombin ~ 10^{-6}M, Factor Va, ~10^{-8} M, Factor Xa,
~10^{-9} M. Phospholipid is present at a concentration adequate
to saturate the reaction. [+]Rates expressed as moles of thrombin per
minute per mole of Factor Xa.
(Reprinted with permission from Mann KG, Membrane-bound complexes in
blood coagulation, In: Progress in Hemostasis and Thrombosis, Volume
7 Edited by Theodore H. Spaet, M.D. 1984 by Grune & Stratton, Inc.)

coagulation process. The influence of complex formation is illustrated in table 1. This table shows the relative rate of prothrombin conversion by factor Xa in conjunction with saturating levels of other cofactors in the prothrombinase complex and factor Xa by itself or with any incomplete mixture of prothrombinase components (56). This table illustrates that the dramatic acceleration occuring upon complex formation is evident only when all the complex constituents are present. The deletion of any constituent leads to at least a 1,000-fold decrease in the reaction rate. The formation of the prothrombinase complex has been examined in our laboratory in a variety of physical and chemical studies. The bimolecular interactions of enzyme with cofactor, and enzyme and substrates with phospholipid vesicles in the presence of calcium ions have been evaluated. The molecular interactions of factor Xa and Va with platelets and with phospholipid vesicles in the presence of calcium ions have also been evaluated. In the case of platelets, the binding of radiolabeled enzyme and cofactor protein to the cell was measured (57). The binding of fluorescent active site labelled Xa to phospholipid vesicles in the presence of Va was also studied (58). In addition, we conducted extensive kinetic analyses of the influence of complex formation on the hydrolysis rate of prothrombin in producing thrombin and on the hydrolysis rate toward synthetic substrates (59). All of the studies completed thus far are consistent with the notion that factor Va is the platelet or phospholipid bound receptor for factor Xa, and factor Va is the principle vehicle leading to the partitioning of factor Xa to the cell or phospholipid vesicle surface.

In the case of phospholipid studies, partitioning of prothrombin and its utilization as a substrate appears principally related to the binding of prothrombin to acidic phospholipids by a calcium ion mediated interaction. As a consequence of the lipid and cofactor interactions, substrate and enzyme are condensed in a limited microenvironment, leading to accelerated catalysis through the concentration of enzyme and substrate. In addition, by virtue of unknown interactions between enzyme, phospholipid bound factor Va and substrate, the catalytic efficiency of factor Xa toward prothrombin is increased by three orders of magnitude.

There appear to be two components to this dramatic increase in reaction rate. One of these leads to a reduction in the apparent K_m for the reaction, while the other leads to an increase in the k_{cat}. We and others have hypothesized that the so called "K_m effect" is related to the co-condensation of enzyme and substrate on the membrane surface, and have attempted to rationalize the influence of this phenomenon on reaction rate (60,61). Table 2 provides a description of the distribution of reaction components as might be expected to occur under physiological conditions. Using the collection of dissociation constants which have been determined in our laboratory from equilibrium binding measurements and enzyme kinetics, one may conclude that when the reaction mixture is saturated with respect to the cofactors, approximately 95% of the enzyme is bound to the membrane surface. We conclude that the reaction observed is occurring by virtue of the membrane bound enzyme. Under sets of conditions in which the membrane component is saturating (with respect to rate), only a fraction of the substrate(prothrombin) is bound; however, this fraction is the principle occupant on the surface of the lipid vesicle.

Membrane binding by prothrombinase components brings about a dramatic increase in local concentration of reactants and is illustrated in figure 8. From dynamic light scattering measurements, one may

Table 2. Distribution of Components Between Bulk Solution and Phospholipid Vesicles at Onset of Activation

Component*	Solution	Vesicle	Fractional Saturation of Vesicle
II	0.97	0.03	~0.50
Xa Va	0.05	0.95	~0.10
(II)/(Va Xa)	10^4	~3/1	----

*Physiologic concentrations of proteins, [II] = 1.4×10^{-6}M, [Xa] = 5×10^{-9}M, [Va] = 1.5×10^{-8}M. (Reprinted with permission of Mann KG, Membrane-bound complexes in blood coagulation, In: Progress in Hemostasis and Thrombosis, Vol. 7, Ed. Theodore H. Spaet, M.D., 1984, Grune and Stratton, Inc.)

conclude that the lipid vesicles increase by approximately 100 A in radius when the proteins are bound to their surface (62). It is possible to describe apparent local concentrations of enzyme and substrate at the membrane surface if one assumes that an interfacial volume exists at the vesicle surface. These apparent concentrations can be deduced from bulk concentrations of reactants and the dissociation constants of the

CONCENTRATION DISTRIBUTION OF PROTEINS FOLLOWING COMPLEX FORMATION

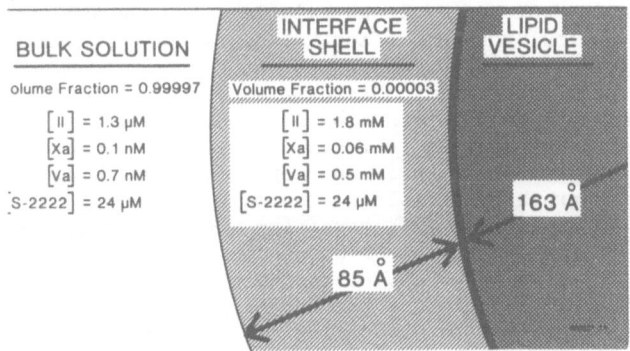

Fig. 8 A representation of the micro environment around a phospholipid vesicle involved in the assembly and function of the prothrombinase complex. The region designated "interface shell" is presumed in which enzyme, Factor Va, and substrate concentrate, and in which catalysis occurs. The dimensions of the lipid vesicle of the interface shell are taken from light scattering data. The concentrations indicated are those that would apply at equilibrium from a calculation based upon nominal concentration of prothrombin at approximately 1.4×10^{-6}M (the plasma concentration) and Factor Xa at approximately 2×10^{-9} M. Factor Va and lipid are present at optimum levels to saturate the reaction. The term S2222 represents a synthetic Factor Xa substrate that is not concentrated by virtue of lipid or Factor Va binding, hence, its concentrations in the interface shell and in bulk solution are equal (from Nesheim ME, Eid S, Mann KG: Assembly of the prothrombinase complex in the absence of prothrombin. J.Biol.Chem. 256:9874, 1981 with permission).

prothrombinase constituents. This representation is crude, as in reality one would have a continuous concentration gradient extending from the interface to some point in bulk solution. For simplicity we represent the interface shell as represented in figure 8, containing high local concentrations of enzyme and substrate. Hence, at least part of the reaction rate increase illustrated in table 1 can be conceived as being related to local concentrations of enzyme and substrate.

The concentration of reactants on the membrane surface provides some notion of the peculiar dependence of the apparent Km of prothrombin activation on membrane binding phenomenon. Recent evidence for an alternative pathway to thrombin generation by complexed prothrombin would have a similar effect and is reviewed below in the warfarin section. However, the sort of model represented in figure 8 provides no insight as to why the k_{cat} of this reaction is increased by three orders of magnitude upon complex formation. Potentially, the change in k_{cat} can be divided into two components. One is purely statistical and may be a consequence of physical orientation of substrate with respect to enzyme. The second component is mechanistic in nature. The possibility exists that the susceptibility of the peptide bonds in the substrate or the active site of the enzyme are altered by complex formation. Evidence for this latter mechanism exists for factor Xa following complex formation (63).

A model illustrating the hypothetical structure of the microenvironment in which catalysis takes place is illustrated in figure 9 a-c. The large curved space illustrates the surface of a phospholipid vesicle. From hydrodynamic (64) and electron microscopic (65,66) considerations we may represent factor V as an asymmetric molecule with multiple domains. As the binding of the molecule to phospholipids is primarily the responsibility of the carboxy terminal domain, this region of factor Va is represented in association with the membrane surface in figure 9a. Following thrombin activation (figure 9b), the central region of the molecule is deleted and the D and E chains remain bound to the membrane. The D chain remains associated with the membrane only through its metal ion-dependent interaction with component E. The prothrombinase complex (figure 9c) appears to function by factor Xa interacting with the membrane, the factor Va E chain and potentially also the D chain. Factor Xa cleaves the prothrombin molecule bound to the factor Va heavy chain. Prothrombin is implicated as interacting with the factor Va heavy chain through the fragment 2 region, a point deduced from earlier kinetic studies (67,68). As noted above, following the cleavage of prothrombin by the prothrombinase complex, the thrombin produced is no longer bound to the surface through its Gla region and is free to leave the membrane surface.

While similar detailed information is not available for the extrinsic and intrinsic factor X activating complexes on the thrombomodulin/thrombin protein C activating complex, they appear to be similar to prothrombinase (50). A summary of the events in complex formation associated with factor Va and factor VIIIa, tissue factor and thrombomodulin is illustrated in table 3, in which the principle features of complex formation in blood clotting are restated, such as: localization of the reaction, amplification of procoagulant reactivity and modulation of the overall reaction. Presumably the localization process that makes the reaction system relevant to the hemostatic defect is accomplished by binding interactions of the plasma proteins with subendothelial components and/or activated cells bound at the site of injury. Amplification occurs to provide rapid delivery of activity. This occurs by virtue of processes in which reagents are concentrated at the site of injury through binding interactions and by increased

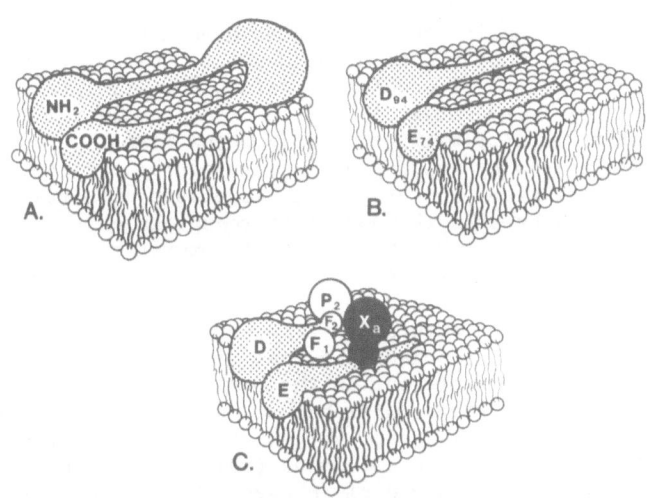

Fig. 9a-c Assembly of the prothrombinase complex. a) Factor V is
shown as a multi-domainal molecule embedded in the membrane lipid
bilayer predominantly through the COOH-terminal region of the
molecule. b) Following thrombin activation, the Factor Va
molecule, composed of the COOH-terminal derived peptide (component
E) and the NH_2-terminal derived peptide (component D), remains bound
to the membrane surface through component E.   c) Factor Va forms at
least part of the Factor Xa receptor through interactions in which
Factor Xa binds to membrane-bound component E in a 1:1 molar
stoichiometry. Prothrombin, composed of fragment 1(F1), fragment 2
(F2) and prethrombin 2 (P2) domains, interacts with component D of
the Factor Va molecule through its F2 region. Factor Xa cleaves the
prothrombin molecule bound to Factor Va.
(Reproduced with permission from Mann, et al. Expression of blood
clotting enzymes on natural and synthetic membranes, In: Proceedings
of UCLA Symposium on Proteases and Biological Control 1986, J.
Cellular Biochemistry (1986 in press).

efficiency of the enzyme-substrate complexes themselves, leading to
increases in k_{cat} and decreases in "apparent Km" of the enzymatic
reactions.

Table 3.   Complex Formation in Blood Coagulation

Feature	Significance	Accomplished by
Localization	Relevant to hemostatic defect; nonsystemic	Binding interactions of subendothelium, cells, and humoral factor
Amplification	Rapid delivery of activity	Concentration of reagents; increased efficiency (k_{cat}/K_m) of enzymes
Modulation	Multiple triggering; Extent of response related to defect	Feedback activation of enzymes, cofactors, and inhibitors; inhibition; resistance to inhibition

(Reprinted with permission from Mann KG, Membrane-bound enzyme
complexes in blood coagulation, In: Progress in Hemostasis and
Thrombosis, Volume 7 Edited by Theodore H. Spaet, M.D. 1984 by
Grune & Stratton, Inc.)

The events of complex formation also have a significant impact with respect to modulation of the reaction system. Complex formation corresponds to an event of modulation, since for all intents and purposes, the complexed enzyme is switched "on" while the uncomplexed enzyme is "off". Multiple triggers of complex formation occur through a variety of mechanisms by which procofactors can be activated to cofactors. In addition, the process is modulated with respect to the extent of response because the number of receptors organized at the site of injury ultimately dictate the extent of enzymatic reaction. The response is thus directly related to the extent of damage.

Negative modulation occurs by virtue of dissociation of complex constituents leading to a coincident loss of reactivity. In addition, the various constituents present in the complex that may be protected within the confines of the complex become exposed to potential inhibitors in plasma. In the case of factor Va and VIIIa, inactivation occurs by virtue of APC cleavage of the molecules (30). In the case of factor Va, it is the 94,000 dalton heavy chain cleavage by APC that gives rise to the most significant loss of activity. This cleavage reaction is inhibited by factor Xa binding to factor Va; thus, in complex, factor Va is relatively immune from APC cleavage. Dissociated factor Va, however, becomes "fair game" for APC. Similarly, antithrombin III inhibition of factor Xa is markedly inhibited when factor Xa is present in the factor Va membrane complex (66). However, free factor Xa is directly subject to inhibition. Constituents escaping by virtue of dissociation from the site of injury are thus rapidly eliminated. Thrombin escaping from the site of injury becomes a negative regulator by binding to thrombomodulin and by activating plasma protein C to provide negative feedback.

THE BIOCHEMICAL EFFECT OF WARFARIN

Biochemistry

Sodium Warfarin anticoagulation interferes with the post ribosomal gamma carboxylation of the vitamin K-dependent proteins described in figure 1. In man it leads to the production of uncarboxylated proteins and a spectrum of partially carboxylated proteins (71,72,73,74). The functional role of prothrombin which has been carboxylated to varying degrees has been elucidated recently by our laboratory in collaboration with Malhotra (75). It appears that the loss of as few as three Gla residues inactivates prothrombin by increasing its K_m in the prothrombinase complex and by severely decreasing its calcium and phospholipid binding capacity. Figure 10 shows the Lineweaver-Burke plots of the prothrombinase catalyzed activation of normal and Gla deficient prothrombin. Table 4 summarizes the kinetic parameters obtained both by initial rate and by the integrated Michaelis-Menten-Henri equation. From these data it is evident that the defect in the Gla deficient prothrombin appears primarily in K_m rather than k_{cat}. In addition, the defect reflected in the increased K_m values coincide with the deletion of as few as three Gla residues.

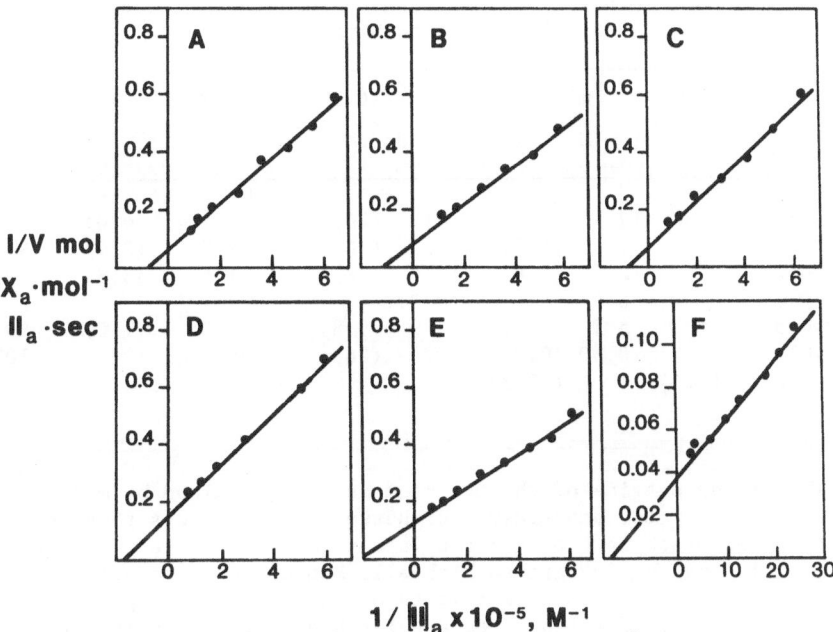

I/V mol

$X_a \cdot mol^{-1}$

$II_a \cdot sec$

$1/\, II_a \times 10^{-5},\ M^{-1}$

Fig. 10 Lineweaver-Burk plots of the prothrombinase-catalyzed activation of normal and Gla-deficient prothrombins. Initial rates of prothrombin activations were measured by the fluorescence intensity of the DAPA-thrombin complex. Reciprocals of initial rates (vertical axes) are plotted against the reciprocals of the initial concentrations of prothrombin (horizontal axes). The substrates were prothrombins 0-Gla (A), 1-Gla (B), 2-Gla (C), 5-Gla (D), 7-Gla (E) and 10-Gla (F). Kinetic parameters are summarized in Table 4. (Reprinted with permission from Malhotra, Nesheim, and Mann, The Kinetics of Activation of Normal and -Carboxyglutamic Acid-deficient Prothrombins Journal of Biological Chemistry Vol. 260 No. 1, 1985 pp 279-287.)

Table 4 K_m and k_{cat} values for the conversion of normal and gla-deficient prothrombins to thrombin*

Sample	K_m μM		k_{cat} s^{-1}		$k_{cat}/K_m \times 10^{-6}$		Thrombin Yield**
0-Gla	12	(4.9)	17	(20)	1.4	(4.0)	%
1-Gla	7	(5.5)	12	(16)	1.7	(2.9)	91
2-Gla	10	(4.8)	14	(18)	1.4	(3.8)	90
5-Gla	6.9		7.7		1.1		75
7-Gla	5.1	(7.1)	9.4	(9.8)	1.8	(1.4)	99
10-Gla	0.60	(0.94)	27	(26)	45	(28)	100
10-Gla(no PCPS)		(22.3)					

*The values outside of the parentheses were obtained by measurements of initial rates and Lineweaver-Burke plots, whereas those enclosed by parentheses were obtained by analysis of complete reaction profiles by the integrated Michaelis-Menten-Henri equation. The values obtained from measurements of initial rates represent best (least-square) fits to a rectangular hyperbola ($y = ax/(b - x)$). The standard deviation of these values for data from any single set of experiments was <10% of the tabulated values. Each value represents the average of at least two experiments performed on separate isolates of the corresponding sample of prothrombin.

**Based on the fluorescence of the DAPA-thrombin complex at completion of the reaction compared to the yield from an equivalent concentration of activated 10-Gla prothrombin. Prothrombin concentrations were determined by absorbance at 280 nm. Yields of less than 100% most likely reflect residual prothrombin 2 at the time chosen as the end of the reaction.

(Reprinted with permission from The Kinetics of Activation of Normal and gamma-Carboxyglutamic Acid-deficient Prothrombins. Malhotra, Nesheim, Mann, JBC, Vol 260 No. 1 pp. 282. 1985.)

Figures 11 and 12 demonstrate similar changes for calcium and lipid binding with the loss of as few as three Gla residues.

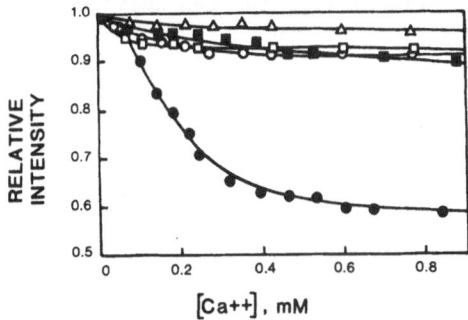

Fig. 11 Ca^{2+}-induced changes in the intrinsic fluorescence of the fragment 1 domains isolated from normal and Gla-deficient prothrombins. Solutions of fragment 1 derived from prothrombins with 0- and 1-Gla (□), 2-Gla (○), 5-Gla (△), 7-Gla (■) and 10-Gla(●) were titrated with Ca^{2+} and intrinsic fluorescence was measured. Fragment 1 from normal prothrombin exhibited an approximate 40% reduction in intrinsic fluorescence whereas small and most likely insignificant changes were observed with each of the fragment 1 regions isolated from the Gla-deficient prothrombins. (reprinted with permission from Malhotra, Nesheim, and Mann, The Kinetics of Activation of Normal and -Carboxyglutamic Acid-deficient Prothrombins Journal of Biological Chemistry Vol. 260 No. 1, 1985 pp 279-287)

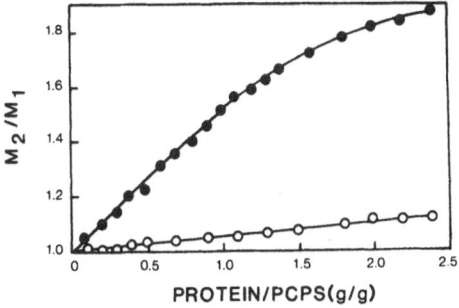

Fig 12 Phospholipid binding of 10-Gla and 7-Gla prothrombins. The interaction of 10-Gla (●) and 7-Gla (○) prothrombin with uniformly sized vesicles of phosphatidylcholine-phosphatidylserine (3:1) was inferred by right-angle light scattering. The results are plotted as relative molecular weight of the phospholipid-protein complex (verticle axis) versus the mass of prothrombin added to the vesicles (horizontal axis). (reprinted with permission from Malhotra, Nesheim, and Mann, The Kinetics of Activation of Normal and -Carboxyglutamic Acid-deficient Prothrombins Journal of Biological Chemistry Vol. 260 No. 1, 1985 pp 279-287)

Furthermore, preliminary data from our laboratory (76) indicate that
Gla residues at selected positions may be retained preferentially in
warfarinized bovine prothrombin. The identification of the specific Gla
residues involved their chemical modification by activation of the
carboxyl groups with water-soluble carbodiimide, followed by quantitative
addition of glycine ethyl esther. After chemical modification of the
Glu/Gla residues in the protein, prothrombin was subjected to sequence
analysis using conventional spinning cup Edman degradation. At each
position where Gla was known to occur, the resulting thiazolanone was
hydrolyzed with hydrogen iodide and the relative composition of glutamic
acid to glycine was evaluated. The results of such analyses are
presented in figure 13 for normal prothrombin and for prothrombin
decarboxylated by the method of Tuhy et al. (77).

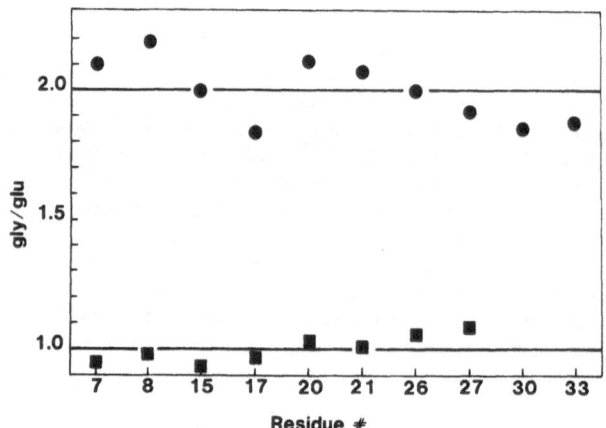

Fig. 13 The presence or absence of Gla at the appropriate amino
acid residues in fully carboxylated and fully decarboxylated
prothrombin fragment 1. The x-axis represents the specific amino
acid residue by number and the y-axis represents the Gly/Glu ratio
as an index of carboxylation. A ratio of 2.0 represents a
gamma-carboxylated residue. (Reprinted with permission of Bovill,
et al., Future directions in monitoring oral anticoagulant therapy.
In: Advances in Coagulation Testing (Triplett D, ed.) pp 79-89,
College of American Pathologists Press, Skokie, Ill.)

Figure 14 contrasts the results of a similar analysis of 7-Gla and
5-Gla prothrombin fragment 1. The x-axis represents the specific
residues by number, and the y axis represents the presence or absence of
Gla. Although these data are preliminary, they indicate that selective
positions (residues 7,8,20,30 and 33) may be obtained preferentially in
warfarinized prothrombin. Recent data from Furie's laboratory on
abnormal, partially decarboxylated human prothrombin demonstrated a
selective absence of Gla residues and was accompanied by dramatic loss of
function associated specifically with the lack of Gla at residue sixteen
(78).

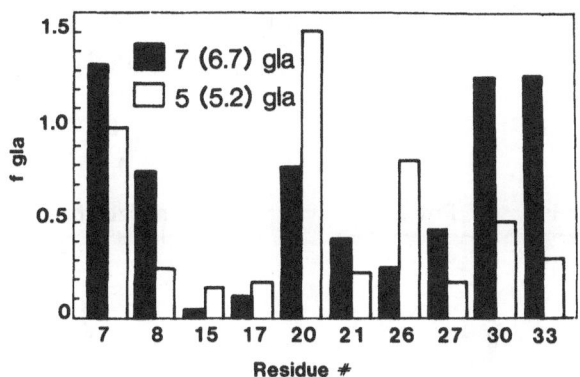

Fig. 14 The presence or absence of Gla at the appropriate amino acid residues in 7-Gla versus 5-Gla prothrombin fragment 1. The x-axis represents the amino acid residue by number; the y-axis represents the presence (f Gla = 1) versus the absence (f Gla = 0) of gamma-carboxylation (f Gla = fraction of carboxylated glutamates). (Reprinted with permission of Bovill, et al., Future directions in monitoring oral anticoagulant therapy. In: Advances in Coagulation Testing (Triplett D, ed.) pp 79-89, College of American Pathologists Press, Skokie, Ill.)

Few studies have been done on decarboxy vitamin K-dependent coagulation proteases other than prothrombin. However, Stenflo's laboratory recently evaluated protein C in bovine plasma after warfarin therapy (79). They demonstrated decreased calcium binding and an absence of anticoagulant activity.

There is a recent major observation relevant to discussion of the rate increase associated with vitamin K-dependent enzyme complex formation; namely, an alteration in the gross reaction pathway of prothrombin activation which is directly related to the carboxylation state of prothrombin. Figure 15 illustrates potential pathways which may account for the two cleavages that occur during prothrombin activation to alpha thrombin. Pathway 1 provides prothrombin fragment 1·2 and prethrombin-2 in the first step, followed by alpha thrombin in a second step. As an alternative, pathway 2 is possible in which meizothrombin would be produced in the first step and subsequent cleavage of meizothrombin would result in alpha thrombin and prothrombin fragment 1·2.

In earlier studies conducted in this laboratory (80) and by Jackson's laboratory (81) using isolated prothrombin and factor Xa, it was concluded that prothrombin activation proceeds by pathway 1, giving rise to prothrombin fragment 1•2 and prethrombin 2 in a first step, followed by the production of alpha-thrombin. When these studies were conducted, our insights into the formation of prothrombinase were limited by the unavailability of purified factor Va. Our laboratory began to reevaluate the pathway of prothrombin activation in a study which made use of the observation that prethrombin-2 and meizothrombin were all capable of binding dansylarginine-N-(3-ethyl-1,5 pentanediyl) and each dansylarginine-N-(3-ethyl-1,5 pentanediyl) protein complex exhibited unique spectral properties (82). In an initial study (83) of the kinetics of the individual bond cleavages in prothrombin (steps a-b and b-a), we deduced that neither pathway would be favored (1 or 2 of figure 15). Subsequently, using energy transfer fluorescence measurements of

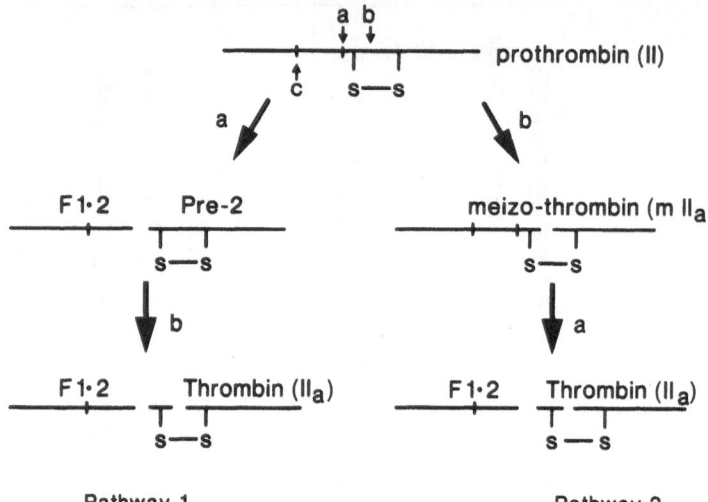

Fig. 15   Potential pathways and intermediates of bovine prothrombin.
activation catalyzed by the prothrombinase complex.   Two factor
Xa-catalyzed cleavages convert prothrombin to thrombin.   These occur at
Arg_{274}-Thr_{275} (a) and at Arg_{323}-Ile_{324} (b).   A third cleavage, at
Arg_{156}-Ser_{157} (c), can be catalyzed by either thrombin or meizothrombin.
(Modified from Nesheim ME, Mann KG: J. Biol. Chem. 258:5286,1983.)

the DAPA-protein complexes produced during prothrombin activation, we
have obtained conclusive evidence that membrane bound catalyst
(prothrombinase) activates membrane bound substrate (fully carboxylated,
normal prothrombin) exclusively by a mechanism in which meizothrombin is
the only intermediate (84,85).   In contrast, Factor Xa in solution
produces alpha-thrombin by pathway 1 as previously concluded.   Studies
conducted with partially carboxylated prothrombins which are not capable
of binding to membranes also give evidence of the formation of
alpha-thrombin by pathway 1 (85).   Thus, pathway 2 represents a unique
mechanism available for only <u>membrane-bound</u> prothrombin being <u>bound</u>
by membrane bound catalyst.

The production of alpha thrombin by an ordered sequential recation
in which meizothrombin is the first product is an exciting discovery
since the active site of meizothrombin remains covalently attached to the
membrane and factor Va binding sites present in the prothrombin fragment
1·2 region of the protein.   Since meizothrombin is a competent enzyme,
its formation may have great significance in the ultimate localization of
the expression of thrombin activity from normal prothrombin and
conversely lack of activity with decarboxy prothrombin.

Clinical Monitoring

With the exception of a few studies focusing on the procoagulant vitamin K-dependent proteins following Warfarin reversal (88) it has been over 15 years since the last systematic analysis of sodium warfarin pharmacology with respect to the concentrations of the vitamin K-dependent proteins (86,87). The foregoing discussion demonstrates the recent advances made in our understanding of these proteins and points out that at the very least a thorough accounting of the anticoagulant proteins C and S is needed.

Our laboratory and Furie's laboratory have begun to evaluate warfarinized individuals using monoclonal and polyclonal antibodies which can distinguish between the abnormal des-carboxy forms of the vitamin K-dependent proteins and the fully carboxylated forms. Our laboratory has an extensive collection of monoclonal antibodies directed against the vitamin k dependent proteins (89) with varying degrees of calcium dependence which can be used as probes for the Gla/Ca2+ dependent and independent epitopes on the vitamin K dependent proteins. A related approach has been developed by Furie's lab. (90). They have done extensive work with monoclonal and polyclonal antibodies to abnormal des-carboxy prothrombin. In a recent clinical study, they demonstrated that there was good correlation between their immunoassay of native prothrombin and traditional hemostatic tests (91). One of the obvious advantages of an immunoassay in this setting is that serum can be used making the special specimen handling inherent in coagulation assays unnecessary. Stenflo's laboratory in Sweden (97) and Aoki's laboratory in Japan (93) have also characterized antibodies specific to calcium induced conformational changes in vitamin K-dependent proteins.

SUMMARY

We have reviewed the biochemistry of the normal and warfarinized vitamin K-dependent coagulation proteins, both individually and as members of their respective macromolecular enzyme complexes. Much has been learned in the past 10-15 years about the molecular mechanisms of coagulation. However, we have only scratched the surface and are beset by a number of interesting challenges. Clearly, we must begin to dissect the other vitamin K-dependent macromolecular enzyme complexes as has been done for prothrombinase. Prothrombin differs in fundamental ways from the other vitamin K-dependent proteins and we can anticipate significant differences as well as similarities in the other complexes. The presence of potentially functional domains in the non-catalytic portions of the vitamin K-dependent proteins and their similarities within this family of proteins should prove a fruitful area of future research. Finally, the evaluation of warfarinized vitamin K-dependent proteins, both in fundamental studies with purified systems and using uniquely engineered immunoassays, should shed light on basic molecular mechanisms and modes of monitoring warfarin therapy.

REFERENCES

1. Neurath, H., Proteolytic Enzymes, past and present, Federation
    Proceedings, Vol. 44, No. 14, November 1985 p 2907-2913.

2. Patthy, L., Evolution of the proteases of blood coauglation and
    fibrinolysis by assembly from modules. Cell, Vol. 41, pp 657-663
    July 1985.

3. Banyai, L, Varodi, A., Patthy, L. Common evoluntionary origin of
    the fibrin-binding structures of fibronectin and tissue-type
    plasminogen activator. FEBS Letter 163 37-41 1983.

4. Patthy, L., Trexler, M., Vali, Z., Banyai, L., Varadi, A. Kringles:
    modules specialized for protein binding. Homology of the gelatin
    binding region of fibronectin with the kringle structures of
    proteases. FEBS Letter, 171 131-136 1984.

5. Bloom, J.W., Mann, K.G. Metal ion induced conformational transition
    of prothrombin and prothrombin fragment 1. Biochemistry 1978;
    17:4430-4438.

6. Prendergast, F.G., Mann, K.G. Differentiation of metal ion-induced
    transitions of prothrombin fragment 1. J. Biol. Chem. 1977,
    252:840-850.

7. Yoshitake, S. Schach, B.G., Foster, D.C., Davie, E.W. Hurachi, K.
    The complete nucleoside sequence of the gene for human Factor IX.
    Biochemistry 1985, 24, 3736-3750.

8. Zonneveld, A.J., Veerman, H., Pannekoek, H. Autonomous functions of
    structural domains of human tissue-type plasminogen activator.
    Proc. Nat'l. Acad. Sci. USA. Vol 82 pp 4670-4674 July 1986.

9. Pan, L.C. Price, P.A. The propeptide of rat bone -carboxyglutamic
    acid protein shares homology with other vitamin K-dependent protein
    precursors. Proc. Nat'l. Acad. Sci. USA. Vol. 82 pp 6109-6113 Sept.
    1983.

10. Suttie, J.W., Hoskins, J.A. et al., Vitamin k-dependent carboxylase;
    a possible role of the "propeptide" as an intracellular recognition
    site, Proc. Nat'l. Acad. Sci. USA (in press 1986)

11. Hoskins, J. Norman, D.K., Beckman, R.J., Long, G.L. Cloning and
    characterization of human liver cDNA encoding a Protein S precursor.
    Proc. Nat'l. Acad. Sci. USA (in press 1986).

12. Park, C.H., Tulinsky A., Three dimensional structure of the kringle
    sequence: structure of prothrombin fragment 1. Biochemistry Vol. 25
    No. 14 July 1986 pp 3977-3982.

13. Bar-Shavit, R., Kahn, A.J., Mann, K.G., Wilner, G.D., Identification
    of a thrombin sequence with growth factor activity on Macrophages.
    Proc. Nat'l. Acad. Sci USA, Vol. 83 pp 976-980. February 1986.

14. Hojrup, P., Jensen, M.S., Petersen, T.E., Amino acid sequence of
    bovine protein Z: a vitamin K-dependent serine protease homolog,
    FEBS Letters, Vol. 184 No. 2, May 1985 pp 333-338.

15. Price, P.A., Williamson, M.K., Primary Structure of Bone Matrix Gla Protein, a new vitamin K-dependent bone protein. J. Biol. Chem., Vol. 260, No. 28, 14971-14975 Sec 5, 1985.

16. Jesty, J., Spencer, A.K., Nemerson, Y. The mechanism of activation of factor X. Kinetic control of alternative pathways leading to the formation of activated factor X. J. Biol. Chem. 249: 5614-5622, 1974.

17. Redclifte, R., Nemerson, Y. The activation and control of factor VII by activated factor X and Thrombin. J. Biol. Chem. 250: 388-395, 1975.

18. Bajaj, S.P., Rapaport, S.I., Brown, S.F., Isolation and characterization of human factor VII. J. Biol.Chem. 256: 283-259 1981.

19. Hagen, F.S., Gray, C.L. et al, Characterization of a cDNA coding for human factor VII, Proc. Nat'l. Acad. Sci. USA Vol 83, pp 2412-2416, April 1986.

20. Fujikawa, K., Davie, E.W. Bovine Factor IX. Methods Enzymol. 45: 74-83,1974.

21. Kurachi, K. Davie, E.W. Isolation and characterization of a cDNA coding for human factor IX, Proc. Nat'l. Acad. Sci. USA Vol 79 pp 6461-6464 Nov. 1982.

22. Jesty, J., Silverberg, S.A. Kinetics of the tissue factor dependent activation of coagulation factors IX and X in a bovine plasma system. J. Biol. Chem. 254: 12337-12345, 1979.

23. Osterud, B., Rapaport, S.I.: Activation of [125]-I factor IX and ^{125}I-Factor X: effect of tissue factor and factor VII, factor Xa and thrombin. Scand. J. Haem. 24:213-276 1960.

24. Titani, K., Fujikawa, A.L., Enfield, D.L., et al, Bovine factor X, (Stuart factor): amino acid sequence of heavy chain. Proc. Nat'l. Acad. Sci. USA 72:3982-3086 1975.

25. Jackson, C.M., Factor X, in CRC Handbook series in clinical laboratory science, Section I: Hematology, edited by Seligson D. Boca Raton, CRC Press pp 101-107 1980.

26. Mann, K.G., Elion, J., Prothrombin, in CRC Handbook series in Clinical Laboratory Science, Section 1: Hematology, Edited by Seligson, D., Boca Raton, CRC Press 1980 pp. 15-21.

27. Magnusson, S. Peterson, T.E., Sottrup-Hensen, L. et al, Complete primary structure of prothrombin: Isolation, Structure and reactivity of ten carboxylated glutamic acid residues and regulation of prothrombin activity by thrombin, in Proteases and Biological Control, edited by Reich, E., Ritkin, D.B., Shaw, E. New York, Cold Spring Harbor Laboratories, 1975 pp 123-149.

28. Beckman, R.J., Schmidt, R.J., Santerre, R.F., Plutzky, J., Crabtree, G., Long, G.L. The structure and evolution of a 461 amino acid human protein C precursor and its messenger RNA, based upon the DNA sequence of cloned human liver DNAs. Nucleic Acids Research Vol. 13 No. 14 1985 pp 5233-5247

29. Long, G.L., Belagaje, R.M., MacGillivray, R.T. Cloning and sequencing of liver cDNA coding for bovine protein C. Proc. Nat'l. Acad. Sci. USA Vol. 81 pp 5653-5656 September 1984.

30. Kisiel, W., Canfield, W.M., Ericsson, L. H. et al. Anticoagulant properties of bovine plasma protein C following activation by thrombin. Biochemistry 16:5824-5881, 1977.

31. Vehar, G.A., Davie, E.W., Preparation and Properties of bovine factor VIII (anti-hemophitic factor) Biochemistry 19: 401-410 1980.

32. Di Scipio, R.G., Davie, E.W. A characterization of protein S, a -carboxyglutamic acid containing protein from bovine and human plasma. Biochemistry 18: 899-904 1979.

33. Suzuki, K. Nishioka, J. Matsuda, M. Murayama, H. Hashimoto S, Protein S is essential for the activated protein C-catalyzed inactivation of platelet associated Va J. Biochem. 96, 455-460 1984

34. Walker, F. Regulation of activated protein C by protein S. J. Biol. Chem. 256: No. 21 pp 11128-11131 1986.

35. Suzuki, K., Nishioka, J. Hushimoto, S., Regulation of activated protein C by thrombin modified protein S. J. Biochem. 94 699-705 1983

36. Dahlback, B. Inhibition of Protein C cofactor function of human and bovine protein S by C4b-binding protein. J. Biol.Chem. 261: 26 pp 12022-12027.

37. Walker, F. Identification of a new protein involved in the regulation of the anticoagulant activity of activated Protein C. J. Bio. Chem. 261 No. 23: pp 10941-10944.

38. Seegers, W.H., Ghosh, A. Way V-Y. Function of previously unrecognized plasma protein M in thrombin generation. In Vitamin K metabolism and vitamin K-dependent proteins. Edited by Suttie, J.W., Baltimore, Universityy Press, 1980 pp 96-101.

39. Katzmann, J.A., Nesheim, M. Hibbard, L.S. eta al. Isolation of functional human coagulation factor V using a hybridoma antibody. Proc. Nat'l. Acad. Sc. USA 78: 162-166, 1981.

40. Nesheim, M., Mann, K.G. Thrombin catalyzed activation of single chain bovine factor V. J. Biol. Chem. 254: 1226-1234, 1979.

41. Hibbard, L.S., Mann, K.G. The calcium binding properties of bovine factor V. J. Biol. Chem. 255: 638-645, 1980.

42. Hoyer, L.W., Trabold, N.C. The effect of thrombin on human factor VIII J. Lab. Clin. Med. 8-97: 50-64 1981.

43. Rotblat, F. Obrien, D.P., Middleton, S.M. Purification and characterization of human factor VIII C Thrombin, Haemost. 50:108 (abstract 19) 1983.

44. Fass, D.N., Knutson, G.J., Katzmann, J.A. Monoclonal antibodies to porcine factor VIII coagulant and their use in isolation of active coagulant protein. Blood 59, 594-600 1982.

45. Fulcher, C.A., Roberts, J.R., Zimmerman, T.S.   Thrombin proteolysis of purified factor VIII procoagulant protein: Correlation of activation with generation of a specific polypeptide.   Blood 61: 807-811 1983.

46. Bach, R., Nemerson, Y., Konigsberg, W.   Purification and characterization of bovine tissue factor.   J. Biol. Chem. 256: 8324-8331, 1981.

47. Esmon, N.L., Owen, W.R., Esmon, C.T.   Isplation of a membrane-bound cofactor for thrombin-catalyzed activation of protein C. J. Biol. Chem. 257:859-864, 1982.

48. Davie, E.W., Ratnoff, O.D. Waterfall sequence for intrinsic blood clotting Science 145: 1310 1965.

49. Macfarlane, R.B.   An enzyme cascade in the blood clotting mechanism, and its function as a biochemical multiplier.   Nature 202,498 1964.

50. Mann, K.G.   Membrane bound enzyme complexes in blood coagulation in Progress in Hemostasis and Thrombosis ed. Spaet, T., vol. 7 p 1-24, 1984.

51. Rao, M.V., Rapaport, S.I., Bajaj, P.S.   Activation of human factor VII in the initiation of tissue factor dependent coagulation.   Blood 1986, 68 No. 3, pp 685-691.

52. Nesheim, M., Taswell, J.B., Mann, K.G.   The contribution of bovine Factor V and Factor Va to the activity of prothrombinase.   J. Biol. Chem.   254:10952, 1979.

53. Miletich, J.P., Jackson, C.M., Majerus, P.W.   Interaction of coagulation factor Xa with platelets.   Proc. Nat'l. Acad. Sci. USA 74: 4033, 1983.

54. Mann, K.G., Downing, M.R., Thrombin generation.   In: Lundblad R.L., Fenton, J.W., Mann, K.G. (eds) Chemistry and Biology of Thrombin, Ann Arbor, Michigan, Ann Arbor Press, 1977, pp 11-22.

55. Esmon, C.T., Owen, W.G.: Identification of an endothelial cell cofactor for thrombin catalyzed activation of Protein C. Proc. Nat'l Acad. Sci. USA 78:2249 1981.

56. Nesheim, M.E. Taswell, J.B., Mann, K.G.   The contribution of bovine factor V and factor Va to the activity of prothrombinase J.Biol. Chem 254: 10952-10962, 1979.

57. Tracy, P.B., Nesheim, M.E., Mann, K.G.   Coordinate binding of factor Va and factor Xa to the unstimulated platelet.   J. Biol. Chem. 256: 743-751, 1981.

58. Nesheim, M.E., Kettner, C. Shaw, E. et al Cofactor dependence of factor Xa incorporation into the prothrombinase complex.   J. Biol. Chem. 256: 6537-6540 1981.

59. Nesheim, M.E., Eid, S., Mann, K.G.   Assembly of the prothrombinase complex in the absence of prothrombin.   J. Biol. Chem. 256, 9874 1981.

60. Rosing, J., Tan, G. Grovers-Riemslag, J.W.P., Zwaal, R.F.A., Hemker, H.C. The role of phospholipids and factor Va in the prothrombinase complex. J. Biol. Chem. 255:274, 1980.

61. va Rijn, J.L. M.C., Grovers-Riemslag, J.W.P., Zwaal, R.F.A. Kinetic studies of prothrombin activation: effect of factor Va and phospholipids on the formation of the enzyme substrate complex. Biochemistry 23: 4557, 1984.

62. Lim, T.K., Bloomfield, V.A., Nelsestuen, G.L. Structure of the prothrombin and blood clotting factor X-membrane complexes. Biochemistry 16: 4177, 1977.

63. Mann, K.G., Odegaard, B.H., Krishnaswamy, S., Tracy, P.B., Nesheim, M. Expression of blood clotting enzymes on natural and synthetic membranes in Proceedings of UCLA Symposium on Proteases and Biological Control 1986, J. Cellular Biochemistry (1986 in press).

64. Mann, K.G., Nesheim, M.E., Tracy, P.B.: The molecular weight of undegraded plasma Factor V. Biochemistry 20:28-33, 1981.

65. Mosesson, M.W., Nesheim. M.E., Di Orio, J., Hainfield J.F., Wall, J.S., Mann, K.G: Studies on the structure of bovine Factor V by scanning transmission electron microscopy.(STEM) Blood 65: 1158, 1985.

66. Lampe, P.D., Pusey, M.I., Wei, G.J., Nelsestuen, G.L. Electron microscopy and hydrodynamic properties of blood clotting factor V and activation fragments of factor V with phospholipid vesicles. J. Biol. Chem. 259: 9959, 1984.

67. Bajaj, S.P., Butkowski, R.J., Mann, K.G: Prothrombin fragments. Ca2+ binding and activation kinetics. J. Biol. Chem. 250:2150-2156, 1975.

68. Esmon, C.T., Jackson, C.M.: The conversion of prothrombin to thrombin: IV the function of the fragment 2 region during activation in the presence of factor V. J. Biol. Chem. 249: 7791 1974.

69. Nesheim, M.E., Canfield, W.M., Kisiel, W.M. et al. Studies of the capacity of factor Xa to protect factor Va from inactivation by activated protein C. J. Biol. Chem. 247: 1443, 1982.

70. Miletich, J.P., Kane, W.H., Hofmann, S.L. et al. Deficiency of factor Xa-factor Va binding sites on the platelets of a patient with a bleeding disorder. Blood 54: 1015 1979.

71. Malhotra, O.P. Dicoumarol-induced prothrombins. Ann.N.Y. Acad. Sci. 1981; 370: 426-437.

72. Malhotra, O.P. Partially carboxylated prothrombins I Comparison of activation properties and purification of 1 and 0 carboxyglutamyl variants. Biochem. Biophys. Acta. 1982: 702, 178-184.

73. Malhotra, O.P. Partially carboxylated prothrombins II. Effect of gamma carboxyglutamyl residues on the properties of prothrombin fragment 1. Biochem. Biophys. Acta. 1982, 702:185-192.

74. Friedman, P.A. Rosenberg, R.D., Hanschka, P.V., Fitz-James, A., A spectrum of partially carboxylated prothrombins in the plasma of coumarin treated patients. Biochem. Biophys Acta. 1977, 494, 271-276.

75. Malhotra, O.P., Nesheim, M.E., Mann, K.G. The kinetics of activation of normal and carboxyglutamic acid deficient prothrombins. J. Biol. Chem. 260:279-287, 1985.

76. Bovill, E., Malhotra, O.P., Nesheim, M.E., Mann, K.G. Future Directions in Monitoring Oral Anticoagulant Therapy. In: Advances in Coagulation Testing (Triplett, D. ed.) pp. 79-89, College of American Pathologist Press, Skokie, IL (in press 1986).

77. Tuhy, P., Bloom, J., Mann, K.G. Decarboxylation of bovine prothrombin fragment 1 and prothrombin. Biochemistry 1979; 18, 5842-5848.

78. Borowsi, M. Furie, B.C., Furie, B. Distribution of carboxyglutamic acid residues in partially carboxylated human prothrombins, J. Biol. Chem., Vol. 261 No. 4 Feb 5 pp 1624-1628.

79. Sugo, T. Ulla, P., Stenflo, J. Protein C in Bovine Plasma after Warfarin Treatment Journal of Biol. Chem. Vol. 260 No. 19 September 5 pp 20453-10457.

80. Mann, K.G.: Prothrombin. In: Methods in Enzymology, Proteolytic Enzymes, Part B, (Lorand, L. ed.) p. 123,Academic Pres, New York, 1976.

81. Jackson, C.M., Esmon, C.T., Owen, W.G. The activation of bovine prothrombin. in Reich, E., Rutkin, D.B., Shaw, E.(ed.): Proteases and Biological Control, Cold Spring Harbor 1975, p 95.

82. Hibbard, L.S., Nesheim, M.E.,Mann, K.G.: Progressive development of a thrombin inhibitor binding site. Biochemistry 21: 2285-2292, 1982.

83. Nesheim, M.E., Mann, K.G., The kinetics and cofactor dependence of two cleavages involved in prothrombin activation. J. Biol. Chem. 258: 5386-5391, 1983.

84. Krishnaswamy, S., Mann, K.G., Nesheim, M.E., The prothrombinase-catalyzed activation of prothrombin proceeds through the intermediate meizothrombin in an ordered, sequential reaction. J.Biol. Chem. 261: No. 19, pp 8977-8984 1986.

85. Malhotra, O.P., Nesheim, M.E., Mann, K.G. The kinetics of activation of normal and GLA-deficient prothrombins. J. Biol. Chem. 260:279-287, 1985.

86. Kazmier, F.J., Spittell, J.A., Thompson, J.J., Owen, C.A., Effect of oral anticoagulantson factors VII, IX, X and II. Arch. Int. Med. 1965 115, pp 667-673.

87. O'Reilly, R.A., Aggeler, P.M., Studies on Courmarin Anticoagulant drugs. Initiation of warfarin therapy without a loading dose. Circulation 1968; 38, 169-177.

88. Taberner, D.A., Thompson, J.M., Poller, L., Comparison of prothrombin complex concentrate and vitamin K in oral anticoagulant reversal. Br. Med. J. 1976, 2, 83-85.

89. Mann, K., Katzmann, J.A., Foster, W.B., Fass, D.N., Monoclonal Antibodies and Coagulation in Handbook of Monoclonal Antibodies ed. Ferrone, S. and Dierich, M., Noyes, Inc., 1985 Chap. 11 pp 166-194.

90. Lewis, R.M., Furie, B.C., Furie, B. Conformation-specific monoclonal antibodies directed against the calcium-stabilized structure of human prothrombin. Biochemistry 1983, 22, pp. 948-954.

91. Blanchard, R.A., Furie, B.C., Kruger, S.F. Waneck, G., Jorgensen, M.J., Furie, G. Immunoassays of human prothrombin species which correlated iron functional coagulation activities. J. Lab. Clin. Med. 1983, 101, 24.

92. Laurell, M., Ikeda, K., Lindgren, S., Stenflo, J. Characterization of monoclonal antibodies against human protein C specific for the calcium ion. FEBS Letters Vol. 191 No. 1 Oct5ober 1985 pp 75-81.

93. Wakabayashi, K., Sakata, Y., Aoki, N., Conformation specific monoclonal antibodies to the calcium induced structure of protein C. J. Biol. chem. 261:24 pp 11097-11105 1986.

ANTICOAGULATION PROTEINS C AND S

Charles T. Esmon, Silvana Vigano-D'Angelo, Armando D'Angelo
and Philip C. Comp

Thrombosis/Hematology, Oklahoma Medical Research Foundation
and Department of Medicine, University of Oklahoma Health
Sciences Center, Oklahoma City, OK

ABSTRACT

Proteins C and S are two vitamin K-dependent plasma proteins that work
in concert as a natural anticoagulant system. Activated protein C is the
proteolytic component of the complex and protein S serves as an activated
protein C binding protein that is essential for assembly of the anticoagulant complex on cell surfaces. The anticoagulant activity is expressed
through the selective inactivation of Factors Va and VIIIa. Many patients
deficient in proteins C and S have been described and have an associated
thrombotic tendency, but not all heterozygous protein C and S deficient individuals experience thrombotic complications. Multiple mechanisms and/or
drugs can lead to acquired deficiencies of these proteins: oral anticoagulation, liver disease, DIC and in the case of protein S, lupus erythematosus,
nephrotic syndrome, pregnancy and certain hormones. The anticoagulant activity of protein C decreases rapidly after administration of warfarin (i.e.,
with a time course similar to Factor VII). This rapid decrease may lead
to a transient imbalance and contribute to coumarin induced skin necrosis.
Protein S antigen levels do not decrease as rapidly, but protein S functional levels are often low in patients with an acute thrombus. The discrepancy
between antigen and function results from elevations in C4b-binding protein,
which complexes reversibly with protein S. Unlike free protein S, the complex does not function in the anticoagulant pathway. The available information all suggest that deficiency of protein C and protein S should be considered a risk factor contributing to recurrent thrombotic disease and that
the function of these proteins is altered by many common clinical conditions
which have associated an increased risk of thrombosis.

INTRODUCTION

For many years, it has been commonly believed that the hypercoaguable
state contributes to thrombosis in patients. Attempts to identify the coagulation factor(s) responsible have met with limited success. Alternatively,
deficiencies in anticoagulant factors or changes in cellular receptors might
constitute mechanisms to shift the hemostatic balance toward coagulation.
Potential cellular contributors would be tissue factor formation, or loss
of cell surface anticoagulant activities. These include potential loss of
vascular heparins[1] or components of the protein C anticoagulant pathway,
i.e., endothelial cell thrombomodulin[2] or cell surface protein S binding

sites[3]. In the plasma, potential molecular abnormalities which could lead to a hypercoaguable state are decreases in circulating antithrombin III, increases in plasminogen activator inhibitor[4], or decreases in functional protein C or protein S levels[5-7]. This chapter will focus on the protein C anticoagulant pathway and will not consider the potential interplay of these regulatory systems in any significant detail. For individuals interested in more detailed review of this system, these can be found in references 1,2,4,5,6,7,8,9.

Expression of Activated Protein C Anticoagulant Activity

To begin to understand the potential involvement of the protein C anticoagulant pathway in the genesis of thrombosis, DIC and/or skin necrosis, it is useful to review the current knowledge of the mechanisms by which this system functions. Protein C is a vitamin K-dependent zymogen of the natural anticoagulant protein, activated protein C. Activated protein C exerts its anticoagulant activity through the inactivation of Factors Va[10-13] and VIIIa[12,14,15]. At least two additional requirements must be met for the system to function effectively. Activated protein C must bind to membrane surfaces[10,11,16] and for this binding to be of sufficient affinity to be biologically relevant, a second vitamin K-dependent factor is required. This second factor, protein S, is a plasma protein that increases the affinity of activated protein C for either artificial[16] or natural membrane surfaces[3,17]. Very recently an additional factor, termed protein S binding protein, has been identified which appears to further augment the assembly of the anticoagulant complex on artificial membrane surfaces[18].

Regulation of Protein C Activation

For protein C to function as an anticoagulant, the zymogen must be activated. Although thrombin can activate protein C, the rate of activation under physiological conditions is too slow to provide a significant anticoagulant response. Rapid activation requires an endothelial cell specific regulatory protein, thrombomodulin (TM), which binds thrombin reversibly and accelerates protein C activation several thousand-fold[19-21]. While accelerating protein C activation, complex formation also decreases the procoagulant functions of thrombin[22-23] and in a very recent report Factor Xa[24]. Thus, thrombomodulin serves as a vascular focal point to switch procoagulant enzymes into an anticoagulant generating system. From this perspective, it is apparent that significant decreases in TM concentration might alter the hemostatic balance in favor of a hypercoaguable state. As will be discussed in later sections, mechanisms for down-regulating TM have now been described.

Regulation of Protein S Activity

A second class of regulatory mechanisms potentially involved in control of this anticoagulant pathway involves an extremely unusual interaction between C4b binding protein (C4BP) and protein S[25,26]. C4BP interacts reversibly with protein S (Kd $\sim 0.9 \times 10^{-7}$ M). With normal plasma concentrations of these two proteins, between 50 and 65% of the protein S is complexed with C4BP. Only the free form of protein S is functional in the anticoagulant pathway, raising the possibility that protein S activity might be controlled by both changes in protein S levels and by changes in the percent in complex. This second mechanism for regulating functional levels of protein S could involve alterations in the affinity of protein S for C4BP (or vice versa) or alterations in C4BP levels.

Clinical Studies of Protein S Deficiency

Familial protein S deficiencies have been identified[27,30,31] and in all cases affected family members appeared to be at greater risk of thrombosis than unaffected members. Although these studies suggest that protein S deficiency is a risk factor in the development of thrombotic disease, the extent of the risk is uncertain. Several family members with significant reductions in protein S levels have no history of thrombotic disease[32]. Similar observations have been made with protein C deficiency[33-35]. Most recently, an extensive study of ostensibly normal individuals revealed that several had reduced protein C levels without any personal or familial history of thrombosis. Thus, while deficiencies of these proteins is likely a significant risk factor, ultimate establishment of the relationship between protein levels and the risk of thrombosis must await extensive epidemiological studies.

What Determines Which Deficient Patients Develop Thrombosis?

Assuming that reduced protein C and protein S levels do contribute to an increased risk of thrombotic disease, then it is of interest to attempt to explain why some patients develop thrombotic complications and others do not. The most obvious answer is that we do not know at the present time, but some information is beginning to emerge which could provide possible answers.

One observation that provides a potential mechanism for clinical variability is that protein S levels appear to be affected significantly by several common clinical conditions and/or selected drugs. For instance, patients with lupus erythematosus[36], nephrotic syndrome[36], or either women on birth control pills[37] or during pregnancy[38] have reduced levels of free protein S. The basis for this decrease is either elevation of C4BP in some of the lupus patients or decreases in protein S levels in pregnancy. In addition, we have noticed that functional protein S levels are low in patients with thrombophlebitis primarily because their C4BP levels are elevated. Although not yet proven unambiguously, most of the observations with C4BP suggest that it is an acute phase reactant. With these considerations, multiple mechanisms associated with the inflammatory response could transiently depress protein S levels. In individuals with reduced protein C or protein S activity on a hereditary or acquired basis, this transient fluctuation could provide some or all of the additional impetus required to initiate thrombus formation.

Regulation of Thrombomodulin and Protein S Function on the Endothelium

These inflammatory processes can compromise the protein C pathway in other ways. Thrombomodulin and the endothelial-protein S binding sites required for Factor Va inactivation[3] both decrease when rabbits are exposed to interleukin 1 in vivo[39]. Cultured endothelial cells decrease their thrombomodulin and protein S binding site concentrations when exposed to tumor necrosis factor[40] or endotoxin[41] (only thrombomodulin was measured in this latter study). Thus, in response to an inflammatory stimulus it is possible to compromise the protein C pathway by three distinct mechanisms: 1) inhibition of protein C activation; 2) inhibition of activated protein C anticoagulant activity; and 3) transient decreases in free protein S. In concert with the generation of vascular[41] or macrophage[42] tissue factor this response might be sufficient to alter the hemostatic balance favoring either thrombus formation or DIC.

Oral Anticoagulants and the Function of Protein C and Protein S

One of the most unusual features of this pathway is that both protein C and protein S require vitamin K for their biosynthesis. Of particular interest, protein C levels decrease rapidly with the onset of oral anticoagulant therapy. Protein C and Factor VII levels decrease at similar rates and to similar extents[2,43]. While protein C antigen decreases to 40-50% of normal, the anticoagulant activity decreases further to 10% or less of normal. Protein S levels decrease more slowly than protein C and follow a time course similar to that of Factor X[44]. It is interesting, however, that the free protein S levels are often low in patients at the time oral anticoagulants are initiated. Presumably, this is due to an increase in C4BP which results from the thrombus formation and concomitant acute phase response. The elevated C4BP then complexes an additional fraction of the free protein S leading to reduced protein S activity. Thus, although protein S levels decrease rather slowly, the levels are already compromised at the onset of oral anticoagulant therapy.

Protein C Deficiency and Coumarin Induced Skin Necrosis

The rapid decline of protein C following initiation of oral anticoagulation suggested that there might be a transient imbalance in the regulation of coagulation favoring clot formation. Many clinicians believe that it takes 3-5 days to achieve the antithrombotic effect of warfarin, even though Factor VII levels and the prothrombin time increase much earlier. One of many potential explanations for this is that only when the levels of all coagulation and anticoagulation factors are depressed to about the same level do you achieve a stable antithrombotic influence of the oral anticoagulant. Assuming that this hypothesis is correct, then patients with hereditary protein C deficiency should experience a greater imbalance at the onset of oral anticoagulant therapy than normal individuals. In rare instances, patients experience coumarin induced skin necrosis shortly after

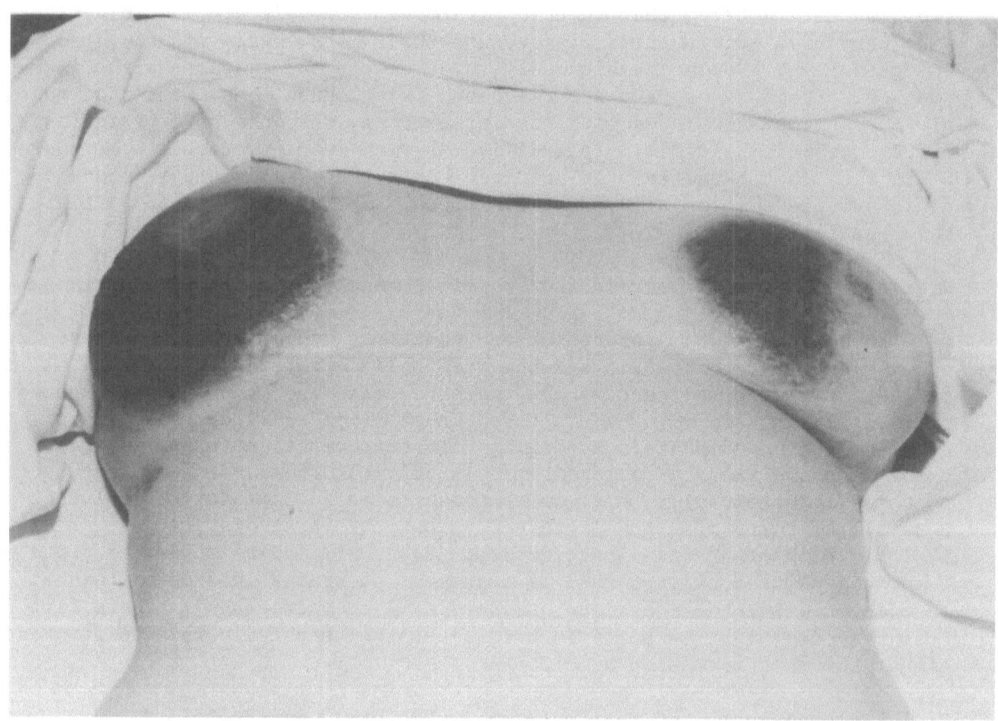

Fig. 1. Warfarin-induced skin necrosis in a 19-year-old woman. The patient had a baseline protein C level of 51%. Skin necrosis over the breasts started on the third day of warfarin therapy. (Photograph and history courtesy of Dr. Jack B. Alperin.)

administration of coumarin. This led several investigators[45-49] to test
the hypothesis that the skin necrosis might occur more frequently when patients with protein C deficiency were treated with coumarin than in normal
individuals. Four reports of protein C deficiency associated with coumarin
induced skin necrosis have now been published and we are aware of several
additional patients whose cases have not been published. These data suggest
that protein C deficiency is likely to be a significant risk factor in the
development of skin necrosis. An example of the lesions which form in the
deficient individuals is shown in Figure 1.

It is interesting that several of the patients either have been treated
previously with coumarin or have been treated subsequently without obvious
complications[45-48]. Indeed, most family members with protein C deficiency
are treated with coumarin without complication[6,7]. Potential mechanisms to
account for this clinical variability are summarized in Figure 2. In this
hypothetical model, deficiency of protein C alone usually causes relatively
little problem. When secondary changes occur, as in the case of a major inflammatory response, the protein C system is further compromised since both
activation and expression mechanisms are impaired. If coumarin is administered when tissue factor levels are high, it is possible that the rapid
decrease in protein C will result in impaired control and skin necrosis may
result. Although this scenario is purely hypothetical, the model can be
tested in both clinical studies and in animal models and may help to explain
the clinical variability.

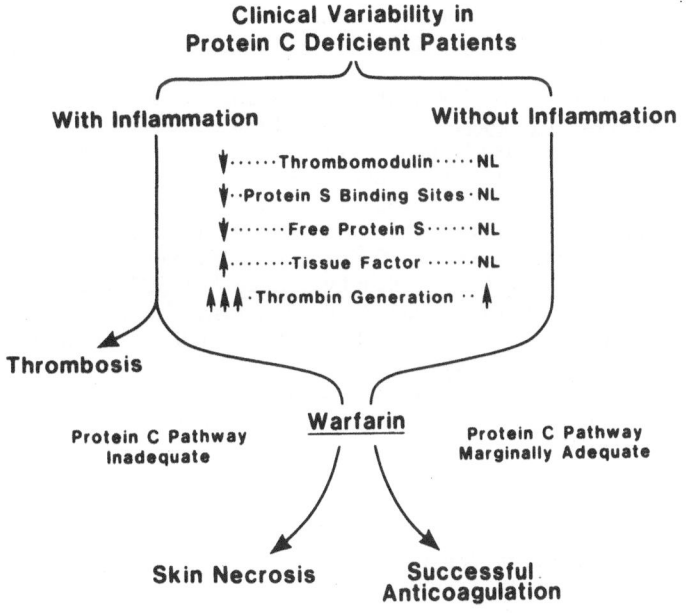

Fig. 2. Factors which may affect the clinical response of
protein C deficient patients to warfarin.

PERSPECTIVES

The protein C anticoagulant pathway serves as a natural control mechanism for blood coagulation. At the present time, many factors and/or clinical conditions are known which impair the function of the pathway. This information suggests that inhibition of the function of this pathway may place patients at increased risk of thrombosis. It is clear that additional clinical information will be required to test this hypothesis. With improved diagnostic tests it may be possible to understand in greater detail how or whether perturbations in the system predispose to a thrombotic state.

REFERENCES

1. R. D. Rosenberg, and J. S. Rosenberg, Natural anticoagulant mechanisms, J. Clin. Invest. 74:1 (1984).
2. C. T. Esmon, Protein C, in: "Progress in Hemostasis and Thrombosis," T. Spaet, ed., Vol. 7, pp. 25-54, Grune & Stratton, New York, NY (1984).
3. D. M. Stern, P. P. Nawroth, K. Harris, and C. T. Esmon, Cultured bovine aortic endothelial cells promote activated protein C- protein S- mediated inactivation of factor Va, J. Biol. Chem. 261:713 (1986).
4. I. M. Nilsson, H. Ljungner, and L. Tengborn, Two different mechanisms in patients with venous thrombosis and defective fibrinolysis: low concentrations of plasminogen activation or increased concentration of plasminogen activator inhibitor, Br. Med. J. 290:1453 (1985).
5. P. C. Comp, Hereditary disorders predisposing to thrombosis, in: "Progress in Hemostasis and Thrombosis," B. Coller, ed., Grune & Stratton, New York, NY (in press).
6. J. H. Griffin, Clinical studies of protein C, Sem. Thromb. Hemostas. 10:162 (1984).
7. A. W. Broekmans, and H. M. Bertina, Protein C, in: "Recent Advances in Blood Coagulation," L. Pollen, ed., pp. 127-137, Churchill Livingstone, New York, NY (1980).
8. B. Laemmli, and H. J. Griffin, Formation of the fibrin clot: the balance of procoagulant and inhibitory factors, Clinics in Hematol. 14:281 (1985).
9. L. H. Clouse, and P. C. Comp, The regulation of hemostasis: The protein C system, N. Engl. J. Med. 314:1298 (1986).
10. W. Kisiel, W. M. Canfield, E. H. Ericsson, and E. W. Davie, Anticoagulant properties of bovine plasma protein C following activation by thrombin, Biochemistry 16:5824 (1977).
11. F. J. Walker, P. W. Sexton, and C. T. Esmon, Inhibition of blood coagulation by activated protein C through selective inactivation of activated factor V, Biochem. Biophys. Acta 571:333 (1979).
12. R. A. Marlar, A. J. Kleiss, and J. H. Griffin, Mechanism of action of human activated protein C, a thrombin-dependent anticoagulant enzyme, Blood 59:1067 (1982).
13. K. Suzuki, J. Stenflo, B. Dahlback, and B. Teodorsson, Inactivation of human coagulation factor V by activated protein C, J. Biol. Chem. 258:1914 (1983).
14. G. A. Vehar, and E. W. Davie, Preparation and properties of bovine factor VIII, Biochemistry 19:410 (1980).
15. C. A. Fulcher, J. E. Gardiner, J. H. Griffin, and T. S. Zimmerman, Proteolytic inactivation of human factor VIII procoagulant protein by activated protein C and its analogy with factor V, Blood 63:486 (1984).
16. F. J. Walker, Regulation of activated protein C by protein S: The role of phospholipid in factor Va inactivation, J. Biol. Chem. 256:11128 (1981).

17. K. W. Harris, and C. T. Esmon, Protein S is required for bovine plate-
    lets to support activated protein C binding and activity, J. Biol.
    Chem. 260:2007 (1986).
18. F. J. Walker, Identification of a new protein involved in the regula-
    tion of the anticoagulant activity of activated protein C: Protein
    S binding protein, J. Biol. Chem. 261:10941 (1986).
19. C. T. Esmon, and W. G. Owen, Identification of an endothelial cell co-
    factor for thrombin-catalyzed activation of protein C, Proc. Natl.
    Acad. Sci. (USA) 78:2249 (1981).
20. N. L. Esmon, L. E. DeBault, and C. T. Esmon, Proteolytic formation and
    properties of γ-carboxyglutamic acid-domainless protein C, J. Biol.
    Chem. 258:5548 (1983).
21. H. H. Salem, I. Maruyama, H. Ishii, and P. W. Majerus, Isolation and
    characterization of thrombomodulin from human placenta, J. Biol.
    Chem. 259:12246 (1984).
22. C. T. Esmon, N. L. Esmon, and K. W. Harris, Complex formation between
    thrombin and thrombomodulin inhibits both thrombin-catalyzed fibrin
    formation and factor V activation, J. Biol. Chem. 257:7944 (1982).
23. I. Maruyama, H. H. Salem, H. Ishii, and P. W. Majerus, Human thrombo-
    modulin is not an efficient inhibitor of procoagulant activity of
    thrombin, J. Clin. Invest. 75:987 (1985).
24. E. A. Thompson, and H. H. Salem, Inhibition by human thrombomodulin of
    factor Xa-mediated cleavage of prothrombin, J. Clin. Invest. 78:13
    (1986).
25. B. Dahlback, and J. Stenflo, High molecular weight complex in human
    plasma between vitamin K-dependent protein S and complement compo-
    nent C4b-binding protein, Proc. Natl. Acad. Sci. (USA) 78:2512
    (1981).
26. B. Dahlback, Interaction between vitamin K-dependent protein S and the
    complement protein, C4b-binding protein: a link between coagulation
    and the complement system, Sem. Thromb. Haemost. 10:139 (1984).
27. P. C. Comp, R. R. Nixon, M. R. Cooper, and C. T. Esmon, Familial pro-
    tein S deficiency is associated with recurrent thrombosis, J. Clin.
    Invest. 74:2082 (1984).
28. R. M. Bertina, A. van Wijngaarden, J. Reinalda-Poot, and V. J. J. Bomm,
    Determination of plasma protein S -- the protein cofactor of acti-
    vated protein C, Thromb. Haemost. 53:268 (1985).
29. B. Dahlback, Inhibition of protein Ca cofactor function of human and
    bovine protein S by C4b-binding protein, J. Biol. Chem. 261:12022
    (1986).
30. A. W. Broekmans, R. M. Bertina, J. Reinalda-Poot, L. Engesser, H. P.
    Muller, J. A. Leeuw, J. J. Michiels, E. J. P. Brommer, and E. Briet,
    Hereditary protein S deficiency and venous thromboembolism: A study
    in three Dutch families, Thromb. Haemost. 53:273 (1985).
31. H. P. Schwartz, P. Fischer, M. A. Batard, and J. H. Griffin, Plasma
    protein S deficiency in familial thrombotic disease, Blood 64:1297
    (1984).
32. P. C. Comp, D. Doray, D. Patton, and C. T. Esmon, An abnormal plasma
    distribution of protein S occurs in functional protein S deficiency,
    Blood 67:504 (1986).
33. U. Seligsohn, A. Berger, M. Abend, L. Rubin, D. Attias, A. Zivelin,
    and S. I. Rapaport, Homozygous protein C deficiency manifested by
    massive venous thrombosis in the newborn, N. Engl. J. Med. 310:559
    (1984).
34. E. Marciniak, H. D. Wilson, and R. A. Marlar, Neonatal purpura fulmi-
    nans: a genetic disorder related to the absence of protein C in
    the blood, Blood 65:15 (1984).
35. J. P. Miletich, and G. J. Broze, Jr., Plasma protein C antigen in the
    normal population: What is deficiency? Circulation (abstr.),
    (in press).

36. P. C. Comp, S. Vigano, A. D'Angelo, G. Thurnau, C. Kaufman, and C. T. Esmon, Acquired protein S deficiency occurs in pregnancy, the nephrotic syndrome and acute systemic lupus erythematosus, Blood 66:348a (abstr. #1279) (1985).

37. L. M. Boerger, P. Morris, G. Thurnau, C. T. Esmon, and P. C. Comp, Oral contraceptives and gender influence protein S status, Blood (in press).

38. P. C. Comp, G. R. Thurnau, J. Welsh, and C. T. Esmon, Functional protein S levels are reduced during pregnancy, Blood 68:881 (1986).

39. P. P. Nawroth, D. A. Handley, C. T. Esmon, and D. M. Stern, Interleukin 1 induces endothelial cell procoagulant while suppressing cell surface anticoagulant activity, Proc. Natl. Acad. Sci. (USA) 83:3460 (1986).

40. P. P. Nawroth, and D. M. Stern, Modulation of endothelial cell hemostatic properties by tumor necrosis factor, J. Exp. Med. 163:740 (1986).

41. K. L. Moore, S. P. Andreoli, N. L. Esmon, C. T. Esmon, and N. U. Bang, Endotoxin enhances tissue factor and suppresses thrombomodulin expression on human vascular endothelium in vitro, J. Clin. Invest. (in press).

42. F. R. Rickles, J. Levin, J. A. Hardin, C. F. Barr, and M. E. Conrad, Tissue factor generation by human mononuclear cells: Effects of endotoxin and dissociation of tissue factor generation from mitogenic response, J. Lab. Clin. Med. 89:792 (1977).

43. S. V. D'Angelo, P. C. Comp, C. T. Esmon, and A. D'Angelo, Relationship between protein C antigen and anticoagulant activity during oral anticoagulation and in selected disease states, J. Clin. Invest. 77:416 (1986).

44. A. D'Angelo, C. T. Esmon, P. C. Comp, C. Boyer, P. M. Mannucci, and S. Vigano-D'Angelo, The half life of protein S is much longer than protein C, Blood 66:349a (abstr.) (1985).

45. A. W. Broekmans, R. M. Bertina, E. A. Loeliger, V. Hofmann, and H.-G. Klingemann, Protein C and the development of skin necrosis during anticoagulant therapy, Thromb. Haemost. 49:244 (1983).

46. W. G. McGehee, T. A. Klotz, D. J. Epstein, and S. I. Rapaport, Coumadin necrosis associated with hereditary protein C deficiency, Ann. Int. Med. 100:59 (1984).

47. M. Samama, M. H. Horellou, J. Soria, J. Conard, and G. Nicolas, Successful progressive anticoagulation in a severe protein C deficiency and previous skin necrosis at the initiation of oral anticoagulation treatment, Thromb. Haemost. 51:132 (1984).

48. N. P. Zauber, and M. W. Stark, Successful warfarin anticoagulation despite protein C deficiency and a history of warfarin necrosis, Ann. Intern. Med. 104:659 (1986).

49. F. J. Kazmier, Thromboembolism, coumarin necrosis and protein C, Mayo Clin. Proc. 60:673 (1985).

WARFARIN AND BONE: IMPLICATIONS FOR RATIONAL STRATEGIES TO SELECTIVELY

ANTAGONIZE THE ACTION OF VITAMIN K IN TARGET TISSUES

Paul A. Price

Department of Biology (B-022)
University of California at San Diego
La Jolla, CA 92093

INTRODUCTION

We have recently reported that vitamin K counteracts the action of
Warfarin on blood coagulation but not on the synthesis of bone Gla protein (BGP; osteocalcin) (1). The purpose of this paper is to describe
the observations which led to this discovery and the implications of
this discovery for Warfarin prophylaxis.

Bone synthesizes the only well characterized class of vitamin K-
dependent proteins other than the blood coagulation factors. We have
recently reviewed the structure and properties of BGP (2), a 49 residue
protein which contains 3 residues of γ-carboxyglutamic acid (Gla) (3).
The newly discovered matrix Gla protein (MGP) is a 79 residue protein
which contains 5 Gla residues (4). There is sufficient homology between
BGP and the C-terminal region of MGP to conclude that they arose from a
common ancestor by gene duplication and subsequent divergent evolution
(4). Thus MGP and BGP represent a class of evolutionarily-related vitamin K dependent bone proteins much as the blood coagulation factors
represent a class of evolutionarily related vitamin K-dependent liver
proteins.   It is noteworthy that there is no sequence homology between
these two classes of vitamin K dependent proteins at the level of the
secretion product.

Because vitamin K-dependent bone proteins are unrelated structurally to the blood coagulation factors, we have been able to use the bone
system to investigate the common themes in vitamin K metabolism.   The
complete cDNA structure for rat BGP revealed the existence of remarkable
homology between residues −16 to −1 in the BGP propeptide and the
corresponding propeptide region of the vitamin K-dependent blood coagulation factors (5). We have postulated that this homologous propeptide
structure targets BGP and the vitamin K-dependent coagulation factors
for γ-carboxylation, as shown schematically in Figure 1. As required by
this model, the homologous region of the BGP propeptide is indeed part
of the intracellular BGP precursor (6) which is the substrate for the
γ-carboxylase (7).

We have more recently taken advantage of the fact that BGP is made
by osteoblasts (2) while vitamin K-dependent coagulation factors are
made by hepatocytes to compare the metabolism of vitamin K and of

vitamin K antagonists in these two tissues. The methods we have developed to assess the vitamin K status of osteoblasts is based on the fact that BGP binds strongly to hydroxyapatite only if it is γ-carboxylated (8). Thus, it is possible to separately measure the fraction of normally γ-carboxylated BGP, which binds to and can be subsequently desorbed from hydroxyapatite, and the faction of under-γ-carboxylated BGP, which does not bind.

Before reviewing the BGP response to vitamin K antagonists, it is necessary to first discuss serum BGP and its relationship to BGP in bone. BGP is the most abundant non-collagenous protein in the extracellular matrix of bone and dentine, and is anchored in these tissues by virtue of its ability to bind to hydroxyapatite (2). Serum BGP is a quantitatively minor component which was first discovered after the development of specific radioimmunoassays for the protein (9). Serum BGP arises from new synthesis by osteoblasts, and appears to represent that faction of BGP secreted from the osteoblast which fails to bind to bone mineral and so diffuses into serum (8). These relationships are also illustrated schematically in Figure 1.

THE BGP RESPONSE TO WARFARIN

Shortly after the administration of Warfarin to a vitamin K-replete rat, serum BGP loses its ability to bind hydroxyapatite strongly (Figure 2). This reflects the undercarboxylation of the protein (8), although it is not presently known whether one, two, or all three of the Gla residues are in fact required for hydroxyapatite binding. If Warfarin is administered daily, bone levels of BGP decrease to 2 percent of normal over several weeks (Figure 3), essentially at the rate at which bone matrix turns over. Bone levels of BGP remain at this decreased level as long as Warfarin treatment is continued (10).

These observations indicate that Warfarin affects the γ-carboxylation status of new BGP synthesis soon after its administration. Since normal γ-carboxylation is required for BGP to anchor to hydroxyapatite in bone, nearly all new BGP synthesized by osteoblasts escapes to serum where it elevates total levels of serum BGP (Figure 2). Total bone ·levels of BGP change slowly, as the BGP-replete matrix synthesized prior to Warfarin treatment is gradually resorbed by osteoclasts and replaced with BGP deficient matrix.

VITAMIN K COUNTERACTS WARFARIN EFFECTS ON BLOOD BUT NOT ON BONE

The protocol devised to measure the effect of chronic Warfarin administration on bone levels of BGP (Figure 3) employed massive Warfarin dosages (7.7 mg/100 g body weight/day) together with the minimum vitamin K dosage needed to prevent acute problems due to bleeding (10). Animals maintained on this protocol for the long periods needed to observe altered bone structure (8 months) were remarkably free of any bleeding problems even though bone levels of BGP remained at 2% of normal (11).

We have recently discovered that the vitamin K dosage regimen employed in our Warfarin protocol completely counteracts the effect of Warfarin on blood coagulation after approximately 7 days (1) (Figure 4).

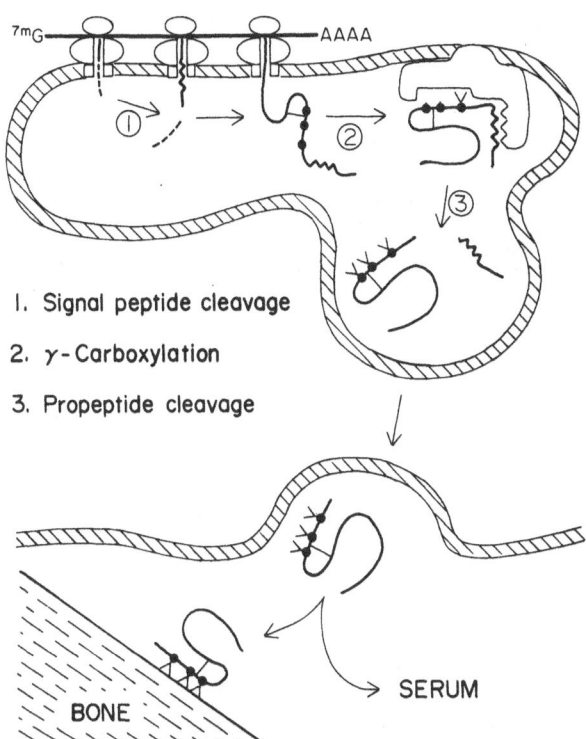

1. Signal peptide cleavage

2. γ-Carboxylation

3. Propeptide cleavage

Fig. 1. Schematic depiction of BGP biosynthesis by a bone cell. Hatched double lines indicate cell membranes: a single intracellular membrane-bound compartment represents the endoplasmic reticulum, golgi apparatus, and secretory vesicles; the lower membrane is the plasma membrane. Portions of the BGP molecule are represented by the following symbols: dotted line, signal peptide; wavy line, putative targeting segment of propeptide; thin line, disulfide bond; solid circle, Glu; solid circle with V attached, Gla.

We had previously failed to recognize this effect because coagulation times were in fact quite elevated at 3 to 4 days of treatment with Warfarin plus vitamin K (Figure 4), the time arbitrarily chosen in the earlier studies to establish the proper vitamin K dosage. Pretreatment for 7 days with the vitamin K dosage used in the protocol reduced the degree to which coagulation times were prolonged after 4 days of Warfarin treatment (Figure 4). The prolonged coagulation time at 4 days of Warfarin treatment could be completely prevented by the administration of a single dose of 40 mg vitamin K per 100 g body weight one day prior to the start of treatment with Warfarin plus vitamin K (1). Surprisingly, the hydroxyapatite binding activity of serum BGP remained at 5 percent of normal regardless of vitamin K pretreatment or the duration of treatment with vitamin K plus Warfarin (1).

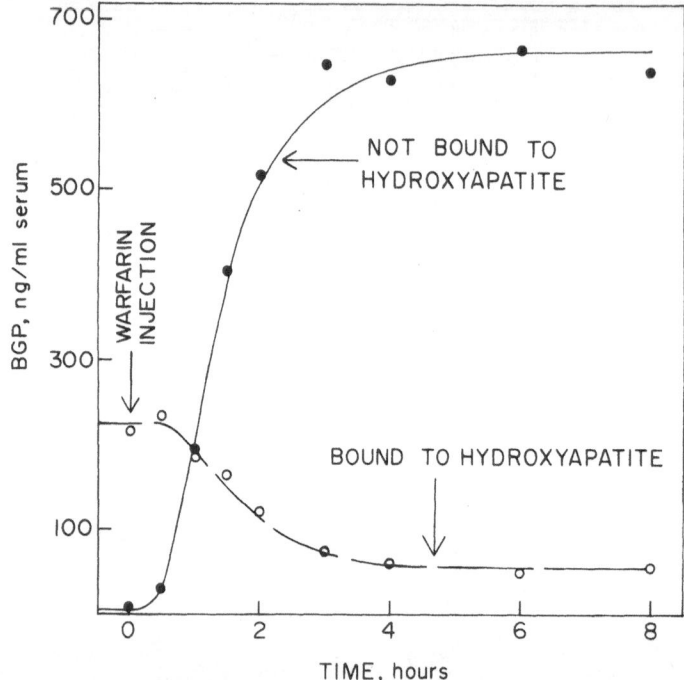

Fig. 2. Effect of Warfarin on the hydroxyapatite binding properties of serum BGP in 1-month-old rats. At time zero, rats received 7.7 mg of Warfarin per 100 g body weight. Serum samples were removed at the indicated times and tested for hydroxyapatite binding as described (8). O, serum BGP not bound to hydroxyapatite; O, serum BGP bound to hydroxyapatite. (From Price, Williamson, and Lothringer (8); used with permission).

To obtain a better measure of the ability of vitamin K to counteract the effect of Warfarin on blood coagulation and on serum BGP, we next evaluated the Warfarin dose dependence of both effects in rats treated with vitamin K compared to rats which did not receive the vitamin (1). As can be seen in Figures 5 and 6, vitamin K treatment completely prevented the ability of high Warfarin doses to prolong blood coagulation times but had essentially no ability to alter the Warfarin dose dependence of the serum BGP response. Since, in the absence of vitamin K treatment, comparable Warfarin dosages were required to double coagulation times (50µg/100g/day) and to reduce the hydroxyapatite binding activity of BGP by 50% (30µg/100g/day), the inherent Warfarin sensitivity of the bone and liver systems are identical. The difference between the two systems is that vitamin K treatment completely counteracts Warfarin effects on blood coagulation but not on BGP.

The ability of high vitamin K dosages to counteract the effect of Warfarin on blood coagulation has been known for many years (12). Present evidence indicates that vitamin K treatment enables a Warfarin-insensitive enzyme to reduce the vitamin K epoxide product of the γ-carboxylation reaction back to the hydroquinone (13,14). Without vitamin K treatment, endogenous levels of vitamin K in the hepatocyte are evidently too low to allow significant reduction of the epoxide by this

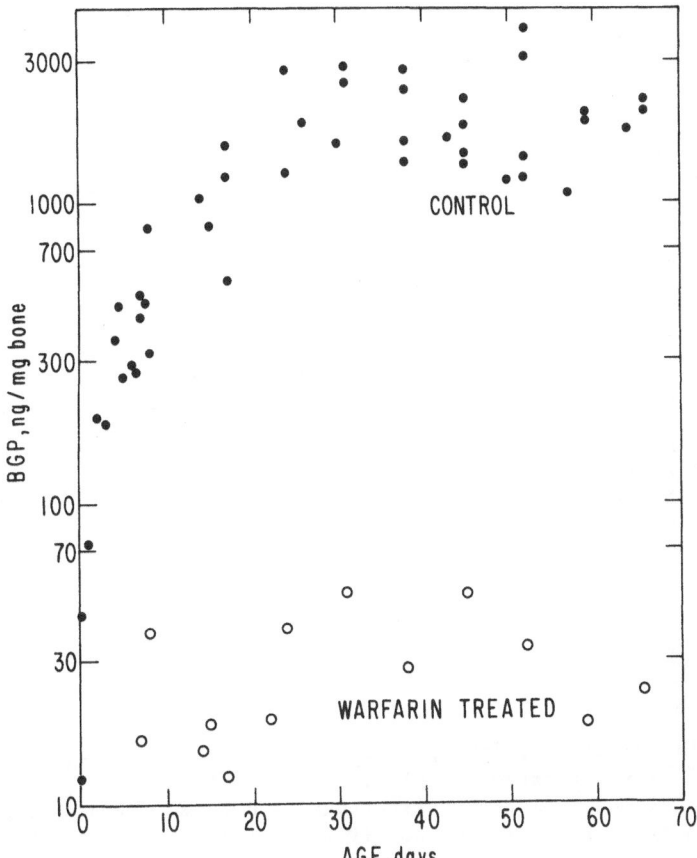

Fig. 3. BGP levels in bone from Warfarin-treated and control rats. Rats were treated daily with (per 100 g body weight) either 7.7 mg Warfarin plus 0.77 mg vitamin K (O) or 0.77 mg vitamin K alone (O). Rats were killed at each indicated age and bone levels of BGP were determined as described (10). It should be noted that the level of BGP in bone normally rises rapidly after birth in rats, and so the effect of Warfarin in this experiment appears as a suppression of the normal developmental increase rather than as an absolute decrease from normal BGP levels. (From Price and Williamson (10); used with permission.)

Warfarin-insensitive pathway and γ-carboxylation ceases. Our results demonstrate that this Warfarin insensitive pathway is not significantly active in the osteoblasts of vitamin K-treated rats. Osteoblasts therefore must either lack the Warfarin insensitive epoxide reductase or are unable to accumulate sufficient vitamin K to enable this enzyme to function at a rate sufficient to support γ-carboxylation of BGP.

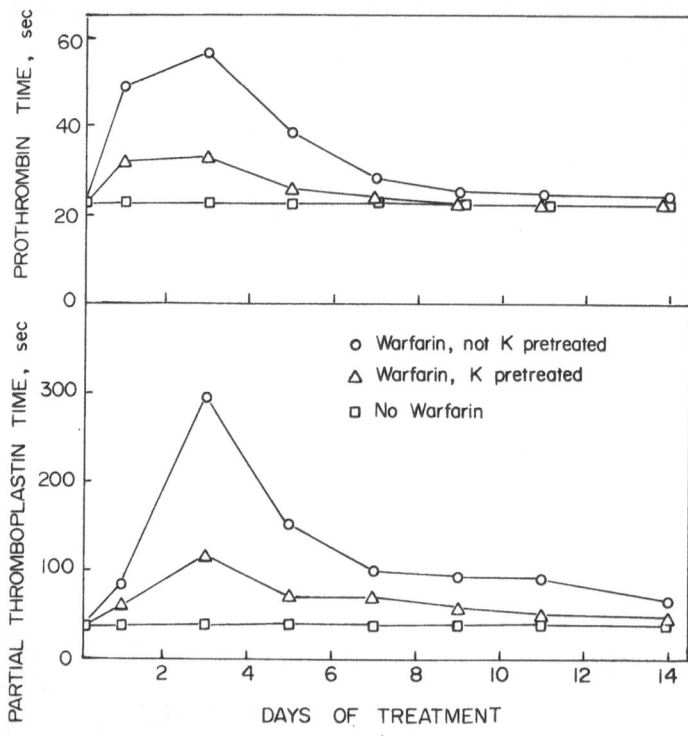

Fig. 4. Effect of vitamin K pre-treatment on the coagulation times of Warfarin-treated weanling rats. Starting at 26 days of age, rats received daily injections of 0.77 mg vitamin K_1 per 100 g body weight (Δ) or no vitamin K (O) for 7 days. Beginning at 33 days of age, both groups then received daily injections of 0.77 mg vitamin K_1 and 7.7 mg Warfarin per 100 g body weight. Age matched control animals ([]) received neither vitamin K_1 nor Warfarin. Prothrombin times (top) and partial thromboplastin times (bottom) are the average values for plasma samples drawn from four animals in each group at the indicated times after the start of Warfarin treatment. (From Price and Kaneda (1); used with permission.)

BIOLOGICAL EFFECTS OF LONG TERM TREATMENT WITH WARFARIN PLUS VITAMIN K

The discovery that vitamin K counteracts the effect of Warfarin on blood coagulation but not on BGP synthesis has enabled us to employ quite large Warfarin doses without any effect on blood coagulation (1). Thus the daily dosage of Warfarin, 7.7 mg/100g/day, was over 150 fold greater than the dose required to lower the hydroxyapatite activity of BGP by 50 percent but blood coagulation times were never greater than normal. Any physiological changes elicited by the Warfarin plus vitamin K protocol must therefore be interpreted as a direct effect of Warfarin on bone, or on any other tissue with similar vitamin K metabolism, rather than as any possible effect on blood coagulation.

The general health of rats maintained from birth to 8 months of age on the Warfarin plus vitamin K protocol was exceptionally good. Weight gain was unimpaired over the 8 months of treatment (10), although there

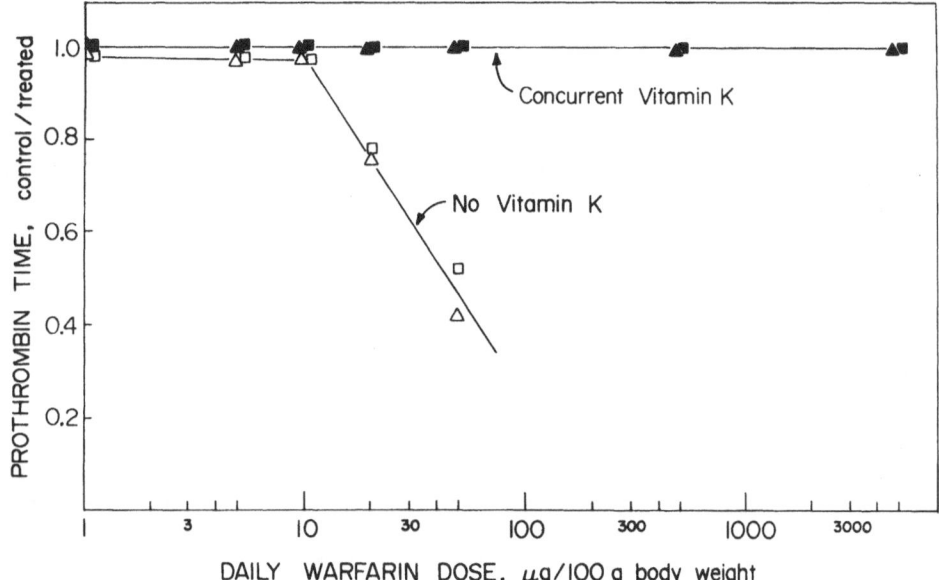

Fig. 5. Comparison of the effect of Warfarin dosage on the coagulation
times of plasma from rats treated with vitamin K_1 to that of
rats that did not receive vitamin K. Solid symbols, rats 22
days of age which received daily injections of 0.77 mg vitamin
K_1 per 100 g body weight for 6 days and then were given this
vitamin K_1 dosage plus daily dosages of the indicated amount of
Warfarin for 7 days (Δ) and for 14 days ([]). Open symbols,
rats 29 days of age which received daily dosages of the indicated amount of Warfarin for 7 days (Δ) and for 14 days ([]).
Each data point is the ratio of the average coagulation time in
4 untreated controls to the average coagulation time in 4
animals from each treatment group. (From Price and Kaneda (1);
used with permission.)

was a slight decrease in bone growth after 3 months of age (see below).
At no time during the 8 months of treatment was a significant difference
noted in any parameter measured in the standard SMAC test of serum from
experimental and control rats. There was also no difference between
experimental and control animals in visual appearance, radiological
analysis of skeletal morphology, dentition, or the general ability to
see and hear. Upon necropsy, rats maintained from birth to 8 months of
age on Warfarin plus vitamin K did have marked subcutaneous fibrosis in
the area of the daily subcutaneous injections. Control rats, which
received daily injections of vitamin K, did not have subcutaneous
fibrosis. This fibrosis could reveal a major vitamin K-dependent role
in inflammation and injury repair. Alternatively, the relatively alka-
line pH of the sodium Warfarin solutions may have irritated tissues at
the site of injection resulting in eventual scarring.

To date, the only effect of long term treatment with Warfarin plus
vitamin K which can be unambiguously related to the direct action of
Warfarin is the excessive mineralization of growth plate cartilage with

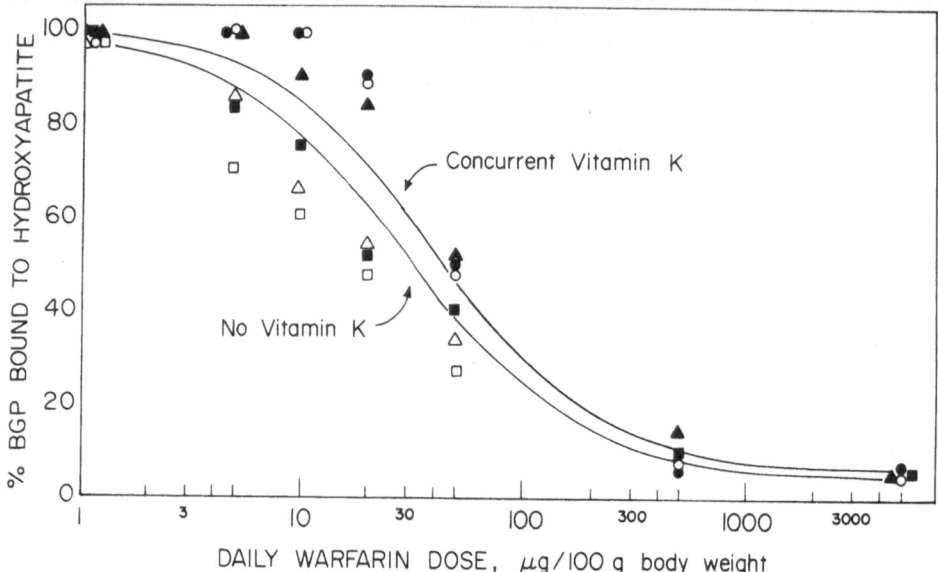

Fig. 6. Comparison of the effect of Warfarin dosage on the hydroxyapatite binding activity of serum BGP from rats treated concurrently with vitamin K_1 to that of rats that did not receive
vitamin K_1. Solid symbols, rats 22 days of age first received
daily injections of 0.77 mg vitamin K_1 per 100 g body weight
for 7 days and then were given this vitamin K_1 dosage plus
daily dosages of the indicated amount of Warfarin for 1 day
(O), 7 days (Δ), and 14 days ([]). Each data point represents
the average percentage of serum BGP which bound to hydroxyapatite in 4 animals from each treatment group. (From Price and
Kaneda (1); used with permission.)

eventual fusion of the growth plate (11). In rats treated from birth to
8 months of age with Warfarin plus vitamin K, growth plates were completely fused and longitudinal growth had ceased. The overall length of
the long bones was accordingly reduced; for example, tibias of experimental animals were 7 percent shorter than the 8 month old control rats.
Subsequent investigations revealed that growth plate mineralization
first becomes apparent at 3 months of age, the time at which rapid
skeletal growth is complete in the rat (2). This pattern of excessive
growth plate mineralization is strikingly similar to the fetal Warfarin
syndrome in humans, a disorder seen in infants whose mothers had
received Warfarin during the first trimester of pregnancy (15). We have
interpreted these observations as evidence that vitamin K-dependent bone
proteins normally inhibit the seeded crystal growth of hydroxyapatite
from the fully mineralized metaphysis into growth plate cartilage. When
the action of vitamin K is antagonized by Warfarin, the under carboxylated bone proteins now secreted are unable to retard seeded crystal
growth and mineralization consequently engulfs the longitudinal septa of
growth cartilage. This eventually causes growth plate fusion. Bone Gla

protein is a good candidate for the vitamin K-dependent protein which normally inhibits growth plate mineralization, since BGP is a potent inhibitor of hydroxyapatite crystallization only if it is γ-carboxylated (16). However, since corresponding tests of the ability of the more recently discovered matrix Gla protein to inhibit hydroxyapatite formation have not yet been carried out, the question as to which of these vitamin K-dependent bone proteins normally function to retard growth cartilage mineralization remains unresolved.

It seems to us probable that many of the extrahepatic tissues known to synthesize Gla-containing proteins will, like bone, remain fully susceptible to the action of Warfarin in the presence of concurrent vitamin K treatment at the dosages used in our protocol. One argument is teleological: since the impaired synthesis of vitamin K-dependent coagulation factors is lethal, the liver must have the ability to store vitamin K in preference to all other tissues in order to ensure survival in times of dietary vitamin K deficiency. Storage of vitamin K by hepatocytes is required before the liver can use the alternate, Warfarin-insensitive pathway for reduction of vitamin K epoxide to the hydroquinone (1,12-14), and so any tissue unable to store the vitamin is unlikely to be able to counteract the effect of Warfarin. It should be noted in this context that liver is the only organ presently known to store vitamin K (17), and that liver is also the site for storage of other lipid soluble vitamins.

One might take the apparent normality of rats maintained on the Warfarin plus vitamin K protocol as evidence that extrahepatic tissues other than bone are not, in fact, affected by Warfarin in the presence of concurrent treatment with vitamin K. While this may be the case, it seems to me more likely that the role of Gla-containing proteins in the various extrahepatic tissues in which they are found is such that abnormal function is only seen in the context of a specific external stress. The rats maintained from birth to 8 months of age on Warfarin plus vitamin K were fed ad libidium a diet replete in all nutrients and fiber, and were given water continuously (10). They had neither incentive nor opportunities for vigorous exercise, and the level of intelligence which they required to feed themselves was minimal. At no point in the 8 months were the rats exposed to any communicable disease, and at no point did the rats receive significant trauma to tissues (other than the subcutaneous injections noted above). In short, the Warfarin plus vitamin K-treated rats were maintained in an environment remarkably free of stress.

We have, in fact, observed a defect in the bone metabolism of animals treated with Warfarin plus vitamin K which was only seen in the context of physiological stress. Rats received pharmacologic dosages of the active metabolite of vitamin D, $1,25(OH)_2D_3$, together with either Warfarin plus vitamin K or vitamin K alone (18). Treatment with $1,25(OH)_2D_3$ led to the accumulation of unmineralized osteoid in the tibial metaphysis, while treatment with $1,25(OH)_2D_3$ plus Warfarin prevented this accumulation. We have interpreted these observations as evidence that $1,25(OH)_2D_3$ stimulated the synthesis of a vitamin K-dependent mineralization inhibitor, which then caused the accumulation of unmineralized osteoid. Treatment with Warfarin caused the putative vitamin K-dependent mineralization inhibitor to be secreted in an inactive, under-carboxylated form and consequently allowed the mineralization of osteoid (18). We further suggested that the vitamin K-dependent mineralization inhibitor is BGP, since the synthesis of BGP is in fact stimulated 6 to 10 fold by $1,25(OH)_2D_3$ (19). With the recent discovery that MGP is similarly stimulated 6 to 10 fold by $1,25(OH)_2D_3$ in osteoblastic cells, either MGP or BGP must now be regarded as candidates for the $1,25(OH)_2D_3$ regulated protein which inhibits osteoid mineralization.

IMPLICATIONS FOR WARFARIN PROPHYLAXIS

The first and most obvious implication of the discovery that vitamin K counteracts Warfarin effects on blood coagulation but not on BGP synthesis is that blood coagulation tests provide a reliable measure only of the effect of Warfarin on the hepatocyte. It is erroneous to infer Warfarin sensitivity on bone from the effect on coagulation times, because dietary levels of vitamin K (from food and intestinal flora) determine the dose of Warfarin required to prolong blood coagulation but not the dose required to inhibit normal BGP synthesis. Thus it is possible to have two individuals, one with a high average daily intake of vitamin K and a correspondingly high Warfarin dose required for prolonged blood coagulation time and another with a low vitamin K intake and a correspondingly far lower Warfarin dose required to increase coagulation times. The first individual, based on our present results, will have far greater impairment of BGP synthesis than the second. This individual will be correspondingly at greater risk for any complication, such as bone metabolic changes noted above, which is attributable to the impaired synthesis of a Gla-containing protein by an extrahepatic tissue whose vitamin K metabolism is similar to bone. When the therapeutic objective is to reduce the activity of the blood coagulation factors synthesized by the liver, it would therefore seem to be advisable to regulate vitamin K intake so as to minimize the Warfarin dosage required.

The second, more intriguing implication to Warfarin prophylaxis is that we can now contemplate an entirely new use for this drug. We can, by selectively counteracting the effect of Warfarin on blood coagulation with vitamin K, stringently suppress the γ-carboxylation of Gla-containing proteins in bone and (as we have argued) other extrahepatic tissues without any concern whatever about bleeding complications.

There is at least one area in which we believe there is sufficient evidence to justify experimental tests of the therapeutic efficacy of the Warfarin plus vitamin K protocol. Over the past seven years numerous studies have established the synthesis of vitamin K-dependent blood coagulation factors by endothelial cells (20,21), monocytes (22,23), and macrophages (24,25,26). Each cell type has the ability, through the action of its endogenous coagulation pathways, to initiate thrombosis. These extrahepatic vitamin-K dependent coagulation systems each should, in our view, be susceptible to inhibition by the Warfarin plus vitamin K protocol. Among the areas where Warfarin has documented activity by a mechanism which could be due to extrahepatic vitamin K-dependent blood coagulation are the suppression of tumor metastasis (27-31) and the suppression of delayed-type hypersensitivity (32). Certain current therapeutic uses of Warfarin may also be better managed with Warfarin plus vitamin K. For example, venous thrombosis may in many cases be due to endothelial cell activation of blood coagulation by a vitamin K dependent mechanism. This could explain the clinical efficacy of Warfarin in this disorder at doses below those which prolong blood coagulation times (33), since on present evidence we would argue that dietary vitamin K could selectively reduce the effective dose of Warfarin on the hepatic system. It is my hope and expectation that the Warfarin plus vitamin K protocol developed in our laboratory will initiate an exciting new phase in Warfarin prophylaxis.

ACKNOWLEDGEMENTS

This work was supported in part by U.S. Public Health Service Grants AM 25921 and AM 27029.

REFERENCES

1. Paul A. Price and Yuri Kaneda, Vitamin K counteracts the effect of Warfarin in liver but not in bone, Thrombosis Research, (Submitted 1986).

2. Paul A. Price, Vitamin K-dependent formation of bone Gla protein (Osteocalcin) and its function, Vitamins and Hormones 42:65-108 (1985).

3. P.A. Price, J.W. Poser, and N. Raman, Primary structure of the γ-carboxyglutamic acid-containing protein from bovine bone, Proc. Natl. Acad. Sci. USA 73:3374-3375 (1976).

4. P.A. Price and M.K. Williamson, Primary structure of bovine matrix Gla protein, a new vitamin K-dependent bone protein, J. Biol. Chem. 260:14971-14975 (1985).

5. Lydia C. Pan and P.A. Price, The propeptide of rat bone γ-carboxyglutamic acid protein shares homology with other vitamin K-dependent protein precursors, Proc. Natl. Acad. Sci. USA 82:6109-6113 (1985).

6. Lydia C. Pan, Matthew K. Williamson, and P.A. Price, Sequence of the precursor to rat bone γ-carboxyglutamic acid protein that accumulates in Warfarin-treated osteosarcoma cells. J. Biol. Chem. 260:13398-13401 (1985).

7. S.K. Nishimoto and P.A. Price, The vitamin K-dependent bone protein is accumulated within cultured osteosarcoma cells in the presence of the vitamin K antagonist Warfarin. J. Biol. Chem. 260:2832-2836 (1985).

8. P.A. Price, M.K. Williamson, and J.W. Lothringer, Origin of the bone γ-carboxyglutamic acid-containing protein found in plasma and its clearance by kidney and bone. J. Biol. Chem. 256:12760-12766 (1981).

9. P.A. Price and S.K. Nishimoto, Radioimmunoassay for the vitamin K-dependent protein of bone and its discovery in plasma, Proc. Natl. Acad. Sci. USA 77:2234-2238 (1980).

10. P.A. Price and M.K. Williamson, Effects of Warfarin on bone, Studies on the vitamin K-dependent protein of rat bone, J. Biol. Chem. 256:12754-12759 (1981).

11. P.A. Price, M.K. Williamson, T. Haba, R.B. Dell, and W.S.S. Jee, Excessive mineralization with growth plate closure in rats on chronic Warfarin treatment, Proc. Natl. Acad. Sci. USA 79:7734-7738 (1982).

12. J. Lowenthal and J.A. MacFarlane, The nature of the antagonism between vitamin K and indirect anticoagulants, J. Pharmacol. Exp. Ther. 143:273-277 (1964).

13. A.K. Willingham and J.T. Matschiner, Changes in phylloquinone epoxidase activity related to prothrombin synthesis and microsomal clotting activity in the rat, Biochem. J. 140:435-441 (1974).

14. R. Wallin, S.D. Patrick, and T.D. Ballard, Vitamin K antagonism of coumarin intoxication in the rat Thromb. Haemost. 55:235-239 (1986).

15. J.G. Hall, R.M. Pauli, K.M. Wilson, Maternal and fetal sequelae of anticoagulation during pregnancy Am. J. Med. 68:122-140 (1980).

16. J.W. Poser and P.A. Price, A method for decarboxylation of γ-carboxyglutamic acid in proteins, J. Biol. Chem. 254:431-436

(1979).

17. M.J. Thierry and J.W. Suttie, Effect of warfarin and the chloro analog of vitamin K_1 Arch. Biochem. Biophys. 147:430-435 (1971).

18. P.A. Price and S.A. Sloper, The effect of Warfarin administration on the bone response to 1,25-dihydroxyvitamin D_3, in: Endocrine Control of Bone and Calcium Metabolism, D.V. Chu, ed., pp. 69-72 (1984).

19. P.A. Price and S.A. Baukol, 1,25-dihydroxyvitamain D_3 increases synthesis of the vitamin K-dependent bone protein by osteosarcoma cells. J. Biol. Chem. 255:11660-11663 (1980).

20. D.M. Stern, P.P. Nawroth, K. Harris, and C.T. Esmon, Cultured bovine aortic endothelial cells promote activated protein C-protein S-mediated inactivation of factor V_a, J. Biol. Chem. 261:713-718 (1986).

21. D.S. Fair, R.A. Marlar, and E.G. Levin, Human endothelial cells synthesize protein S, Blood 67:1168-1171 (1986).

22. B. Østerud and Bjørklid, Human factor VII assqciated with endotoxin stimulated monocytes in whole blood, Biochem. Biophys. Res. Comm. 108:620-626 (1982).

23. B.P. Tsao, D.S. Fair, L.K. Curtiss, and T.S. Edgington, Monocytes can be induced by lipopolysaccharide-triggered T lymphocytes to express functional factor VII/VIIa protease activity, J. Exp. Med. 159:1042-1057 (1984).

24. B. Østerud, U. Lindahl, and R. Seljelid, Macrophages produce blood coagulation factors, FEBS Letters 120:41-43 (1980).

25. U. Lindahl, S.O. Kolset, J. Bøgwald, B. Østerud, and R. Seljelid, Studies, with a luminogenic peptide substrate, on blood coagulation factor X/Xa produced by mouse peritoneal macrophages, Biochem. J. 206:231-237 (1982).

26. H.A. Chapman, Jr., C.L. Allen, and O.L. Stone, Human alveolar macrophages synthesize factor VII in vitro, J. Clin. Invest. 75:2030-2037 (1985).

27. M. Colucci, F. Delaini, G. Vitti DeBellis, D. Locati, A. Poggi, N. Semeraro, and M.B. Donati, Warfarin inhibits both procoagulant activity and metastatic capacity of Lewis Lung carcinoma cells, Role of vitamin K Deficiency, Biochem. Pharm. 32:1689-1691 (1983).

28. B.L. Neubauer, K.G. Bemis, K.L. Best, R.L. Goode, D.M. Hoover, G.F. Smith, L.R. Tanzer, and R.L. Merriman, Inhibitory effect of Warfarin on the metastasis of the PAIII prostatic adenocarcinoma in the rat J. Urol. 135:163-166 (1986).

29. N.L.M. Goeting, G.A. Trotter, and I. Taylor, Effect of warfarin on formation and growth of pre-neoplastic lesions in chemically induced colorectal cancer in the rat, Br. J. Surg. 73:487-489 (1986).

30. P. Hilgard and B. Maat, Mechanism of lung tumour colony reduction caused by coumarin anticoagulation, Europ. J. Cancer 15:183-187 (1979).

31. L.R. Zacharski, W.G. Henderson, F.R. Rickles, W.B. Forman, C.J. Cornell, R.J. Forcier, R.L. Edwrds, E. Headley, S.-H. Kim, J.F. O'Donnell, R. O'Dell, K. Tornyos, and H. Kwaan, Effect of warfarin anticoagulation on survival in carcinoma of the lung, colon, head and neck, and prostate, Final Report of VA cooperative study #75, Cancer 53:2046-2052 (1983).

32. R.L. Edwards and F.R. Rickles, Delayed hypersensitivity in man: Effects of systemic anticoagulation, Science 200:541-543 (1978).

33. M.M. Bern, A. Bothe, B. Bistrian, C.D. Champagne, M.S. Keane, and G.L. Blackburn, Prophylaxis against central vein thrombosis with low-dose warfarin, Surgery 99:216-221 (1985).

HUMAN GENES FOR FACTOR IX AND OTHER VITAMIN K DEPENDENT

BLOOD PROTEINS

Kotoku Kurachi and Shi-Han Chen
Department of Human Genetics, University of Michigan
Medical School, Ann Arbor, Michigan 48109 (K.K) and
Department of Pediatrics, University of Washington
Seattle, Washington 98195 (S-H. C.)

Factor IX is a plasma glycoprotein with m.w. 57,000. It is a single chain precurser to a serine protease which participates in the middle phase of blood coagulation. It is activated by factor XIa (activated factor XI) as well as by a complex of factor VII-tissue factor to a two chain form serine protease, factor IXa. Factor IX is one of the half a dozen blood proteins which require vitamin K for their normal biosynthesis. These proteins include factor VII, factor IX, factor X, prothrombin, protein C, protein S and protein Z. The first four proteins are blood coagulation factors. Protein C functions as an efficient regulator of blood coagulation by inactivating factors VIIIa and Va in the presence of protein S[1]. Protein S also has a possible regulatory role in the complement system by binding to C4b binding protein. The function for protein Z is not known at the present time[2]. The first about ten glutamic acid residues which are located within the amino-terminal about 40 amino acid sequence of these proteins are converted to gamma carboxylglutamic acid residues (gla residues) in a reaction catalyzed by a membrane-bound carboxylase(s) in the presence of vitamin K as a cofactor[3]. These gla residues in the proteins serve as the sites to bind calcium ions which are required for the optimal activities for these proteins. These calcium ions bound at these gla residues, in turn, serve as sites for binding phospholipids on the membrane. The calcium ions bound to some specific gla sites may also trigger significant conformational changes in these proteins [4,5]. Recently the crystallographic three dimensional structure of the fragment 1 of prothrombin which contains gla domain and one of the two kringle structures has been determined at 2.8Å resolution by Park and

Tulinsky[6]. The most of the gla containing region up to the first 35
amino acid residues of the amino terminal portion was found to be highly
disorderd. Recent intensive studies on these proteins by means of
molecular cloning and protein chemistry have provided us a number of
exciting knowledges of their structures, biosyntheses as well as on
their evolutions. In this paper, we will review the recent progress in
this field by primarily focusing on the recent studies on the normal as
well as abnormal genes for factor IX.

Structure of the Normal Gene for Factor IX and its Comparison with the Genes for other Vitamin K Dependent Proteins

As shown in the Figure 1, factor IX is made up by a unique
arrangement of various domain structures defined based on its amino acid
sequence[7]. This overall modular (or multidomain) structure of factor IX
is also common to the other vitamin K dependent proteins including
factor X[10], factor VII[37], and protein C[9]. Besides factor IX, factor X,
factor VII, and prothrombin have preleader sequences (signal peptides)
followed by proleader sequence (probably 17 to about 20 amino acid
residues in length), gla containing regions, two epidermal growth
factor-like domains except for prothrombin which has two kringle
structures instead, linking region (about 15 to 20 amino acid residues
in length), activation peptide sequence, and catalytic subunit (serine
protease subunit). Bovine and human protein S recently reported by
Dahlbäck et al.[1] and by Lundwall et al.[8] also have leader sequences
which apparently composed of pre (signal) and proleader sequences, gla
domain (eleven gla residues contained), and four growth factor-like
domains, however, its carboxyl-terminal half (about 380 amino acid
residues) has no homology to serine proteases. Protein Z also has a
high homology for its overall structure to factor IX and others[2]. It,
however, lacks two of the essential residues for its charge-relay
system, consequently it does not have serine protease activity. The
remarkable homology in the modular structure of these proteins are also
extended to their clear homology in the overall gene organization. The
complete nucleotide sequences of the genes for human factor IX[7], protein .
C[9], prothrombin (S. F. Degen, Personal Communication), factor VII
(P. O'Hara, Personal Communication) have been determined and overall
gene organization and partial nucleotide sequence of factor X have also
been determined[10]. The nucleotide sequence of cDNA for protein S has
recently been published[1,8].

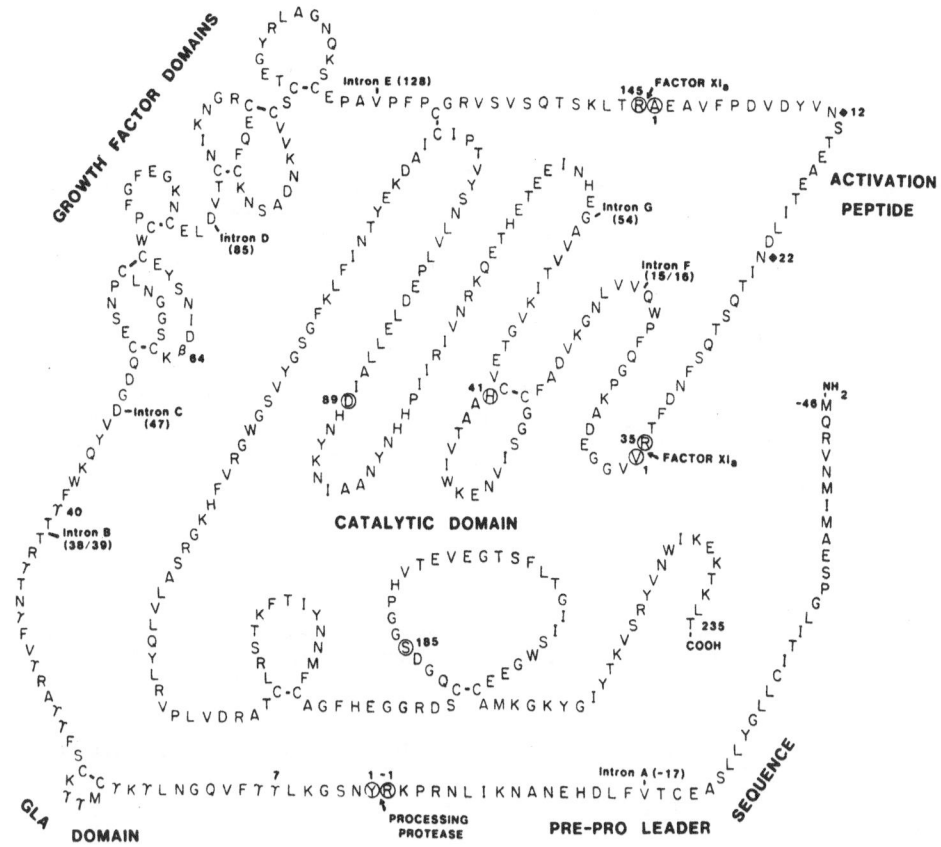

Fig. 1 A tentative domain structure of human prepro factor IX.
Taken from Yoshitake et al., 1985 (reference 7) with
permission.

The gene for factor IX which spans about 33.5 kb has seven introns
in its coding region as shown in Figure 2. It has five Alu repetitive
sequences in some of the introns (see Figure 2) and 3'-flanking region
as shown by arrows in the Figure 2, and a few KpnI and its subfamily
Hind III repetitive sequences in its 5'-flanking region as well as in
the intron D. The positions of these introns in the amino acid sequence
of prepro protein of factor IX is also shown in the Figure 1. The
introns are, in general, located at such positions to separate
structural and functional domains of the protein. The exon I codes the
5'-noncoding region and also signal peptide. It is interesting to note
that the position of the intron A at the amino acid -17 is close but not

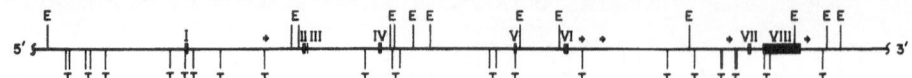

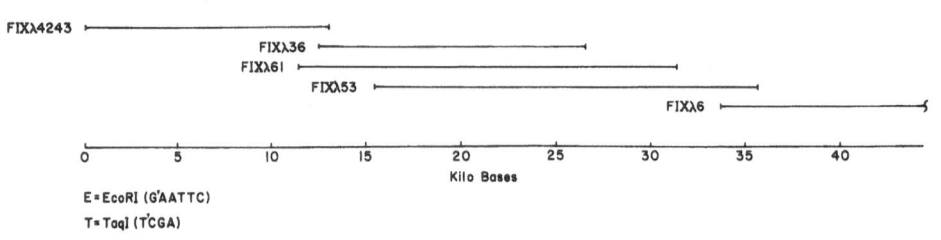

E = EcoRI (G⁀AATTC)
T = TaqI (T⁀CGA)
♦ = Alu sequences

Fig. 2   The organization of the gene for human factor IX. FIXλs
         indicate overlapping genomic clones isolated and sequenced.
         Taken from Yoshitake et al., 1985 (reference 7) with permission.

Table I.   Comparison of locations, phasings and sizes of introns in
           various vitamin K dependent proteins.

INTRON	PROTEIN	LOCATION (amino acid)	SPLICE JUNCTION TYPE	SIZE (bp)
A	FACTOR X	-17	I	?
	FACTOR IX	-17	I	6206
	PROTEIN C	-19	I	1263
	FACTOR VII	-17 (or -39)	I	2600 (1100)
	PROTHROMBIN	-17	I	400
B	FACTOR X	37/38	0	7400
	FACTOR IX	37/38	0	188
	PROTEIN C	37/38	0	1462
	FACTOR VII	37/38	0	1900
	PROTHROMBIN	37/38	0	700
C	FACTOR X	46	I	950
	FACTOR IX	47	I	3689
	PROTEIN C	46	I	92
	FACTOR VII	46	I	100
	PROTHROMBIN	46	I	200
D	FACTOR X	84	I	1800
	FACTOR IX	85	I	7163
	PROTEIN C	92	I	102
	FACTOR VII	84	I	1600
E	FACTOR X	128	I	2900
	FACTOR IX	128	I	2565
	PROTEIN C	137	I	2668
	PROTHROMBIN	131	I	1000
F	FACTOR X	15/16	0	3400
	FACTOR IX	15/16	0	9473
	PROTEIN C	15/16	0	873
	FACTOR VII	15/16	0	600
G	FACTOR X	55	I	1700
	FACTOR IX	54	I	668
	PROTEIN C	55	I	1129
	FACTOR VII	57	I	800

exactly the same site of the cleavage between Thr(-18) and Cys(-19) by signal peptidase[11,12] whereas the factor X gene, the position for intron A, and the cleavage site by signal peptidase appear to coincide to be at val(-17)[13]. The exon II codes for proleader sequence and the gla domain indicating that these two domains are genetically in the same unit. The exon III is the smallest among the exons and code for the link region which contains the thrombin sensitive hydrophobic cluster[6]. The exons IV and V code for each of the two epidermal growth factor-like domains. The exon VI codes for a link region and the activation peptide. The exon VII is coding a domain containing a histidine residue which is involved in the charge relay system of the protease and the exon VIII codes for the rest of the entire catalitic subunit. The gene of factor IX apparently lacks any introns in its 5'-noncoding region since a human cDNA clone extending to the third nucleotide from the estimated cap site[14] was also obtained (unpublished data) and the sequence of this cDNA extended well beyond the corresponding site of an intron found in the 5'-noncoding region at 28 bases upstream of ATG (Met) of the protein C gene[15]. Whether or not the genes for prothrombin, factor X, and factor VIII have an intron in their 5'-noncoding region is not known at the present time. As shown in the Table I, the remarkable conservation for the locations and the splicing phases are observed for all the introns in the coding region of factor IX, factor X, protein C and the first three introns of prothrombin.

The gene for factor VII also has analogous positions for introns and splicing phases to factor X, IX and protein C (P. O'Hara, Personal Communication). These high homologies confirm that these proteins have common ancestral gene and diverted in relatively recent events of gene duplication. The fact that various functional and structural modules such as epidermal growth factor-like structure are still significantly homologous for their amino acid sequences among these proteins and coded by single exons indicates that these structures are acquired by the ancestral gene before its original duplication. After gene duplications, a series of secondary mutations including point mutations could then lead to each specialized properties such as high substrate specificity of each proteins.

A comparison of the overall organizations of the human factor IX gene (FIX) and the human genes for factor X (FX), protein C (PC), and prothrombin (PT) is shown in the Figure 3. In spite of the high conservation of the positions and the phases of the introns, and sizes

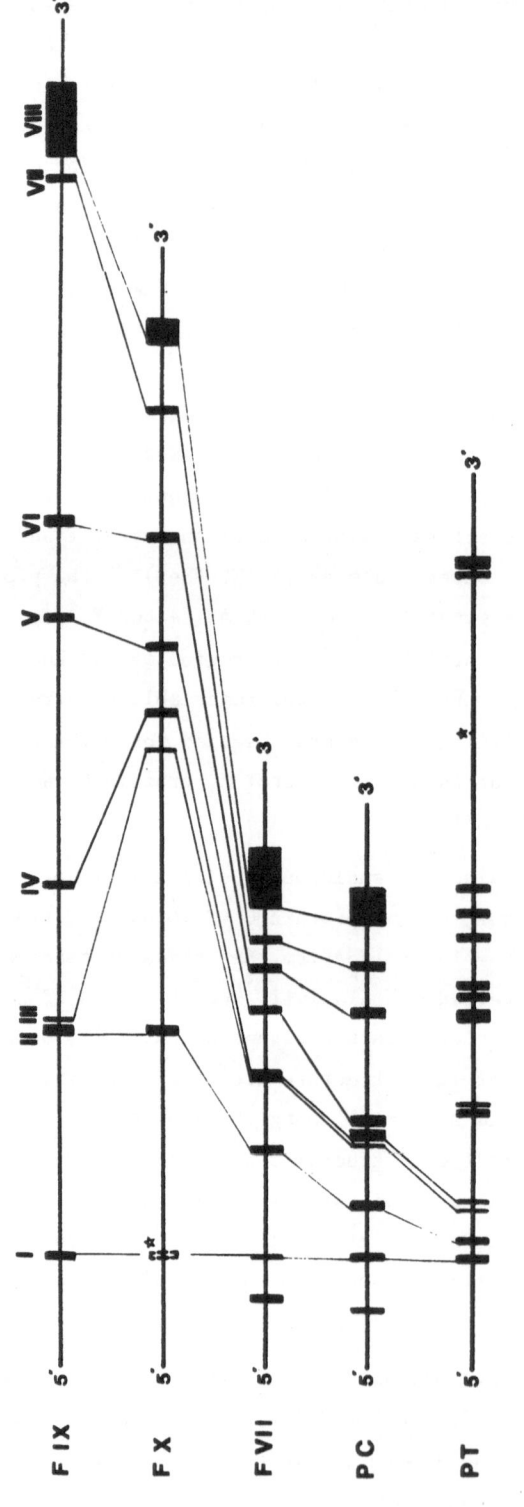
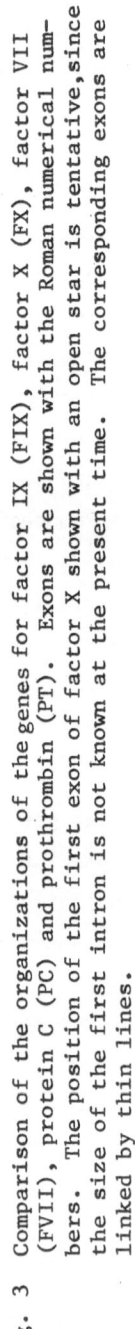

Fig. 3 Comparison of the organizations of the genes for factor IX (FIX), factor X (FX), factor VII (FVII), protein C (PC) and prothrombin (PT). Exons are shown with the Roman numerical numbers. The position of the first exon of factor X shown with an open star is tentative, since the size of the first intron is not known at the present time. The corresponding exons are linked by thin lines.

72

as well as nucleotide sequences of exons, the nucleotide sequences and sizes of the corresponding introns are largely different among the genes for these homologous proteins. The mechanism which generated the large variability of these introns is not known at the present time. One possible explanation is a much weaker genetic constraint on conservation of these intron sequences compared to that applied to the exons. It, however, will not be understood probably until we have precise explanation for the function for introns. The gene organization of prothrombin after the first three introns are quite different from those for factor IX, X and protein C due to the presence of two kringle structures which have little homology to growth factor domains in the amino acid sequence. The gene organization for prothrombin after the first three introns is rather analogous to the gene for TPA which also has two kringle structures[16]. Within the catalytic subunit, prothrombin has three more introns compared to the factor IX gene. Each amino acid residue involved in the charge relay system are coded by a separate exon in prothrombin gene while the only histidine residue is coded by a separate exon in factor IX and other vitamin K dependent protein genes.

The 3' half of the gene for tissue plasminogen activator which contains kringles and catalytic subunit also has a rather analogous, although not exactly the same, organization to the corresponding region of the gene for prothrombin [16]. This strongly indicates that these two genes are evolved from common ancestral gene and further diverged by the gene shuffling events acquiring the different genetic material for their 5' region. It also appears possible that the introns could play some important roles in shuffling of domains since they often appear between domains and in the some relative positions in the amino acid sequence of various proteins.

In the Figure 4, the amino acid sequences of preproleader sequence for vitamin K dependent proteins which are available at the present time are shown. All these proteins apparently have a preproleader sequence which contains a signal peptide region followed by a proleader sequence. In general, the amino terminal half regions (first about 20 to 30 amino acid residues) appear to be typical for a signal peptide which contains hydrophobic sequences. The carboxyl terminal half sequences, however, contain several invariable residues including Phe(-16), Ala(-10), Ile or Val(-7), Leu(-6) and Arg(-1). The latter region is likely in the proleader sequence since the human factor IX preleader (signal) sequence was shown to be possibly cleaved by a signal peptid in between

```
                               -10                                    -30
Human Factor IX    Met Gln Arg Val Asn Met Ile Met Ala Glu Ser Pro Gly Leu Ile Thr Ile Cys Leu Leu Gly Tyr Leu
Human Factor X                     Met Gly Arg Pro Leu His Leu Val Leu Leu Ser Ala Ser Leu Ala Gly Leu
Bovine Factor X                    Met Ala Gly Leu Leu His Leu Val Leu Leu Ser Thr Ala Leu Gly Gly Leu
Human Factor VII                       Met Val Ser Gln Ala Leu Arg Leu Leu Cys Leu Leu Leu Gly Leu
Human Protein C            Met Trp Gln Leu Thr Ser Leu Leu Leu Phe Val Ala Thr Trp Gly Ile Ser Gly Thr
Bovine Protein C                       Thr Ser Leu Leu Leu Phe Val Thr Ile Trp Gly Ile Ser Ser Thr
Human Protein S
Bovine Protein S               Met Arg Val Leu Gly Gly Arg Thr Gly Thr Leu Leu Ala Cys Leu Ala Leu Val
Human Prothrombin              Met Ala Arg Val Arg Gln Leu Pro Gly Cys Leu Ala Leu Ala Ala Leu Cys Ser
Bovine prothrombin     Met Ala Arg Val Arg Gly Pro Arg Leu Pro Gly Cys Leu Ala Leu Ala Ala Leu Phe Ser
```

```
                        -20                              -10                          -1
Human Factor IX    Leu Ser Ala Glu Cys Thr Val |Phe| Leu Asp His Glu Asn |Ala| Asn Lys Ile |Leu| Asn Arg Pro |Lys Arg| Tyr
Human Factor X     Leu Leu Leu Gly Glu Ser Leu |Phe| Ile Arg Arg Glu Gln |Ala| Asn Asn Ile |Leu| Ala Arg Val |Thr| Arg Ala
Bovine Factor X    Leu Arg Pro Ala Gly Ser Val |Phe| Leu Ala Arg Asp Gln |Ala| His Arg Val |Leu| Gln Arg Ala |Arg Arg| Ala
Human Factor VII   Gln Gly Cys Leu Ala Ala Val |Phe| Val Thr Gln Glu Glu |Ala| His Gly Val |Leu| His Arg Arg |Arg Arg| Ala
Human protein C    Pro Ala Pro Leu Asp Ser Val |Phe| Ser Ser Ser Glu Arg |Ala| His Gln Val |Leu| Arg Ile Arg |Lys Arg| Ala
Bovine protein C   Pro Ala Pro Pro Asp Ser Val |Phe| Ser Ser Ser Gln Arg |Ala| His Gln Val |Leu| Arg Ile Arg |Lys Arg| Ala
Human Protein S                            Leu Ser Lys Gln Gln |Ala| Ser Gln Val |Leu| Val Arg Lys |Arg Arg| Ala
Bovine Protein S   Leu Pro Val Leu Glu Ala Asn |Phe| Leu Ser Arg Gln His |Ala| Ser Gln Val |Leu| Ile Arg Arg |Arg Arg| Ala
Human Prothrombin  Leu Val His Ser Gln His Val |Phe| Leu Ala Pro Gln Gln |Ala| Arg Ser Leu |Leu| Gln Arg Val |Arg Arg| Ala
Bovine Prothrombin Leu Val His Ser Gln His Val |Phe| Leu Pro His Gln Gln |Ala| Ser Ser Leu |Leu| Gln Arg Ala |Arg Arg| Ala
```

Fig. 4 Comparison of the amino acid sequences of the preproleader sequences of the various vitamin K dependent proteins. See the text for the various sources of the data compiled in this Figure.

Cys(-19) and Thr(-18). These conserved sequences may have important roles in the co-translational modification, such as gamma carboxylation of glutamic acid residues in the amino terminal region of matured proteins. This was further tested by analyzing various abnormal factor IX genes that have defects in this area and also more systematically by site-directed mutagenesis studies on this region of the genes. A typical dibasic sequence at the carboxyl end of the proleader sequences, is replaced by Thr(-2) Arg(-1) in human factor X [10]. Bovine factor X which contains ArgArg sequence at this position was reported to be cleaved between Ser(-18) and Val(-17) by signal peptidase[13]. Precursor factor X with 17 amino acid long proleader sequence attached is then processed by a processing enzyme to generate mature factor X. The same processing must be taking place for human factor X even with the atypical sequence at the carboxyl end of the proleader sequence since matured factor X with Ala at its amino terminal end is normaly isolated from human plasma.

The amino terminal sequences of vitamin K dependent proteins are also shown in the Figure 5. This region shows almost 50% homology for their amino acid sequences among these proteins. All gla residues within the first 35 amino acid residues are conserved among these proteins which participate in blood coagulation and its regulation.

	+1					+10								+20					
Human Factor IX	Tyr	Asn Ser Gly Lys	Leu Gla Gla	Phe Val Gln Gly Asn	Leu Gla Arg Gla Cys	Met	Gla Gla	Lys	Cys
Human Factor X	Ala	Asn Ser - Phe	Leu Gla Gla	Met Lys Lys Gly His	Leu Gla Arg Gla Cys	Met	Gla Gla	Thr	Cys
Bovine Factor X	Ala	Asn Ser - Phe	Leu Gla Gla	Val Lys Gln Gly Asn	Leu Gla Arg Gla Cys	Leu	Gla Gla	Ala	Cys
Human Factor VII	Ala	Asn Ala - Phe	Leu Gla Gla	Leu Arg Pro Gly Ser	Leu Gla Arg Gla Cys	Lys	Gla Gla	Gln	Cys
Human Protein C	Ala	Asn Ser - Phe	Leu Gla Gla	Leu Arg His Ser Ser	Leu Gla Arg Gla Cys	Ile	Gla Gla	Ile	Cys
Bovine Protein C	Ala	Asn Ser - Phe	Leu Gla Gla	Leu Arg Pro Gly Asn	Val Gla Arg Gla Cys	Ser	Gla Gla	Val	Cys
Human Protein S	Ala	Asn Ser - Leu	Leu Gla Gla	Thr Lys Gln Gly Asn	Leu Gla Arg Gla Cys	Ile	Gla Gla	Leu	Cys
Bovine Protein S	Ala	Asn Thr - Leu	Leu Gla Gla	Thr Lys Lys Gly Asn	Leu Gla Arg Gla Cys	Ile	Gla Gla	Leu	Cys
Human Prothrombin	Ala	Asn Thr - Phe	Leu Gla Gla	Val Arg Lys Gly Asn	Leu Gla Arg Gla Cys	Val	Gla Gla	Thr	Cys
Bovine Prothrombin	Ala	Asn Lys Gly Phe	Leu Gla Gla	Val Arg Lys Gly Asn	Leu Gla Arg Gla Cys	Leu	Gla Gla	Pro	Cys

		+30					+40			
Human Factor IX	Ser Phe	Gla Gla Ala	Arg	Gla Val Phe	Gla Asn Thr Gla Arg	Thr	Thr Gla	Phe Trp	Lys Gln Tyr
Human Factor X	Ser Tyr	Gla Gla Ala	Arg	Gla Val Phe	Gla Asp Ser Asp Lys	Thr	Asn Gla	Phe Trp	Asn Lys Tyr
Bovine Factor X	Ser Leu	Gla Gla Ala	Arg	Gla Val Phe	Gla Asp Ala Gla Gln	Thr	Asp Gla	Phe Trp	Ser Lys Tyr
Human Factor VII	Ser Phe	Gla Gla Ala	Arg	Gla Ile Phe	Lys Asp Ala Gla Arg	Thr	Lys Leu	Phe Trp	Ile Ser Tyr
Human Protein C	Asp Phe	Gla Gla Ala	Lys	Gla Ile Phe	Gln Asn Val Asp Asp	Thr	Leu Ala	Phe Trp	Ser Lys His
Bovine Protein C	Gla Phe	Gla Gla Ala	Arg	Gla Ile Phe	Gln Asn Thr Gla Asp	Thr	Met Ala	Phe Trp	Ser Lys Tyr
Human Protein S	Asn Lys	Gla Gla Ala	Arg	Gla Val Phe	Gla Asn Asp Pro Gla	Thr	Asp Tyr	Phe Tyr	Pro Lys Tyr
Bovine Protein S	Asn Lys	Gla Gla Ala	Arg	Gla Ile Phe	Gla Asn Asn Pro Gla	Thr	Glu Tyr	Phe Tyr	Pro Lys Tyr
Human Prothrombin	Ser Tyr	Gla Gla Ala	Phe	Gla Ala Leu	Gla Ser Ser Thr Ala	Thr	Asp Val	Phe Trp	Ala Lys Tyr
Bovine Prothrombin	Ser Arg	Gla Gla Ala	Phe	Gla Ala Leu	Gla Ser Leu Ser Ala	Thr	Asp Ala	Phe Trp	Ala Lys Tyr

Fig. 5 Comparison of the amino acid sequences of the amino terminal region of the various vitamin K dependent proteins.

In the bone gla protein, however, glutamic acid residues in the amino terminal region are not necessarily all modified (see the article by Dr. Price in this proceeding and also see 36). This difference among these proteins suggest that not only the specific proleader sequences but also some specific amino acid sequence in the amino terminal region of the mature proteins are required to have specific glutamic acid residues in this region properly carboxylated. The conserved amino acid residues including these gla residues are likely to have critical roles in binding calcium ions and also in keeping the critical conformation of this region. The gla residues at +16, +25, and/or +26 of prothrombin were found to be closely correlated to its ability to undergo a calcium-induced conformational change and also its ability to bind to membrane[17]. A loss of the gla residue at -16 is associated with a total loss of the coagulant activity of prothrombin. It is also very interesting to note that the region containing the first 35 amino acid residues of the mature protein is highly disordered for its three dimensional structure in crystals[6]. This suggests that the conformation of this region may have a high flexibility, and upon binding calcium ions this region may be able to undergo a significant conformational change which may be required for factor IX activity.

Polymorphisms in the Gene for Human Factor IX

To date, several polymorphisms linked to factor IX gene have been reported and the precise polymorphic sites for these polymorphisms[7,18,19] except for the Bam HI polymorphism have been identified. The polymorphic site for the Bam HI polymorphism has been estimated to be about 300 bases 5′ upstream to the exon I[20]. These polymorphic restriction sites are summarized in Figure 6. These include polymorphisms which can be easily detected as restriction fragment length polymorphisms employing restriction enzymes such as Taq I, Dde I/ Hinf I, Xmn I, Msp I and Bam HI, and Ala/Thr (G/A) polymorphism at the third amino acid of the activation peptide. These polymorphic sites, however, are in linkage dysequilibrium and the usefulnes of these polymorphisms in the carrier detection is about 67% at the present time. The polymorphism at a Taq 1 site which generates a major allele (1.8 kb) with a frequency of 60% and a minor allele (1.4 kb) with a frequency of 40% has been proved to be particularly useful for the prenatal diagnosis and for the carrier detection. It is interesting to note that these common polymorphisms in European and North American caucasians are

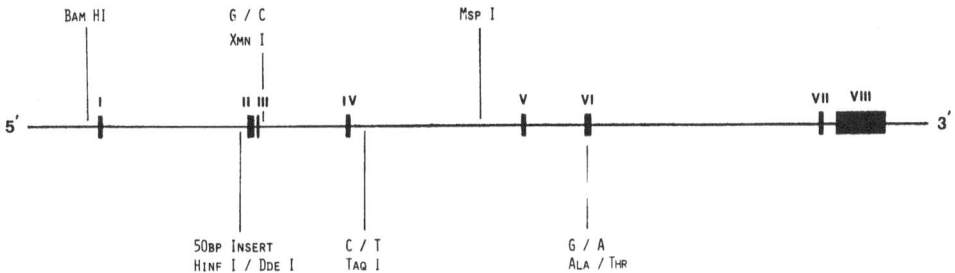

Fig. 6 Intragenic polymorphisms of human factor IX gene. Exons are
shown by solid boxes with Roman numerical numbers.

apparently missing in Asians making a carrier detection employing these
common polymorphisms impossible for Asian populations at the present
time[21,22].

Abnormal Genes for Human Factor IX

More than a dozen abnormal genes for human factor IX have been
characterized and reported to date[23,24]. The mechanisms underlining the
abnormalities of these genes are very heterogeneous including point
mutations, partial and gross deletions as well as insertions. Some of
the well characterized abnormal factor IX genes are summarized in Figure
7. Among these, abnormal factor IX genes[12,13] with mutations in its
leader sequence are particularly interesting because those mutations
apparently prohibit a processing enzyme to cleave off the proleader
sequence. The secreted factor IX polypeptide chain is longer than that
of normal factor IX and the patients have rather mild symptoms. In
factor IX[Chapel Hill], the Arg residue at the activation site is changed
to a His residue thus prohibiting proteolytic activation of factor IX[23].
In one of the abnormal factor IX genes, the donor splicing junction
sequence of the exon VI is changed from GT to TT prohibiting a normal
splicing event resulting in a abnormal factor IX causing a severe
bleeding disorder in the patient[25]. A number of abnormal factor IX
genes with partial and gross deletions have been also found [25-28]. In
our work one of those factor IX[26], factor IX [Seattle], was found to have
about 10 kb intragenic deletion including exons V and VI. These exons
are coding the second growth factor like domain and the connecting
region with activation peptide. In the blood and urine of the patient
carrying this gene, a truncated polypeptide chain which binds to factor
IX specific antibody was detected[29]. This patient does not have any

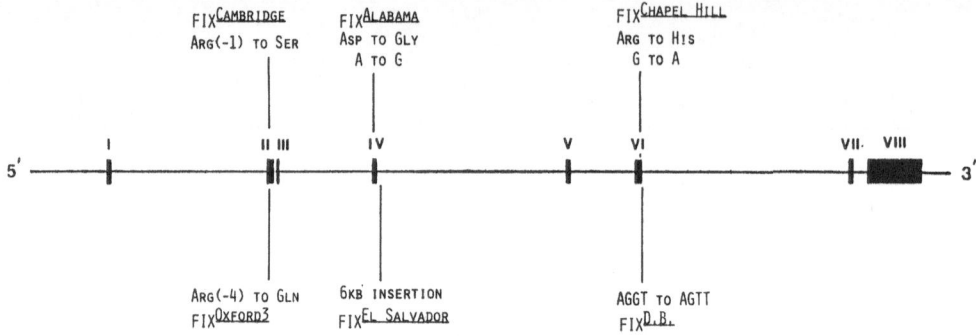

Fig. 7 Various mutations found in abnormal human factor IX genes.
A number of abnormal factor IX genes with partial and gross
deletions are not shown in this Figure.

detectable inhibitor against factor IX in his blood. Giannelli et al.[26]
suggested that individuals with abnormal factor IX genes with various
deletions may be predisposed to inhibitor formations. This attractive
hypothesis, however, has to be further tested. More recently, an
abnormal factor IX gene with an unusual insertion was also found[30]. The
factor IX, called factor IX El Salvador, contains an extra sequence of
about 6 kb in the vicinity of the exon IV. A further analysis of the
DNA sequence of the insert is in progress in our laboratory.

Expression of the Biologically Active Human Factor IX in the Mammalian Cells

Several groups have successfully expressed the factor IX cDNA
hooked to various expression vectors in appropriate mammalian expression
systems including cultured cells as well as a transgenic mouse. We have
produced biologically active human factor IX in the cultured baby
hamster kidney cells employing an adenovirus major late promotor[31].
Salle et al.[32] and Anson et al.[33] have also expressed biologically
active factor IX in Hep G2 cells with vaccinia virus promotor vector and
in rat hepatoma cells with molony murine leukemia virus promoter
respectively. In these expression systems, however, the expression
levels were as low as ng to μg of factor IX per ml of the culture media.
In addition, the proper post-translational modification was not complete
in some experiments. More recently, Kaufman et al.[34] have reported a
significantly high expression of factor IX polypeptide chain in Chinese
hamster ovary cells employing a adenovirus major late promotor with SV40
enhancer sequence. In this expression system almost 100μg of factor IX
polypeptide chain per ml of the culture media was obtained, however,
only a minor fraction (about 1.5μg) was biologically active protein.

This is apparently due to a poor post-translational modification in this system. Based on these data, it is obvious that many different types of mammalian cells have the machinary for the proper post-translation modifications, mainly γ-carboxglation of glutamic acid residues besides other modification such as carbohydration. The efficiency of the modification, however, appears too low in order to use these systems for a large scale production of fully active human factor IX which will be used for clinical purposes. More recently, Choo et al.[35] reported that they succeeded to construct transgenic mice introduced with human factor IX cDNA hooked to a sheep metallothionein Ia promotor. They claim that one of the transgenic mice is producing about 7.5ug/ml of active factor IX of the plasma. In this experiment they employed a full length factor IX cDNA including the entire 3' noncoding sequence. In our experiments, however, factor IX cDNA with its most 3'-noncoding sequence replaced with a corresponding growth hormone sequence did not function in the transgenic mice (unpublished data). These differences will be further studied by means of mutagenesis on the factor IX cDNA cDNA which is employed in the transgenic animal experiments.

Acknowledgements

This work was in part supported by the NIH research grant HL 31511 to K. K.

References

1. B. Dahlbäck, A. Lundwall, and J. Stenflo, Primary structure of bovine vitamin K-dependent protein S, Proc. Natl. Acad. Sci. U.S.A. 83:4199–4203 (1986).
2. P. Hojrup, M. S. Jensen, and T. E. Petersen, Amino acid sequence of bovine protein Z: a vitamin K-dependent serine protease homolog, FEBS Lett. 184:333–338 (1985).
3. T. L. Carlisle and J. W. Suttie, Vitamin K dependent carboxylase: subcellular location of the carboxylase and enzymes involved in vitamin K metabolism in rat liver, Biochem. 19:1161–1167 (1980).
4. S. P. Bajaj, Cooperative C^{2+} binding to human factor IX, J. Biol. Chem. 257:4127–4132 (1982).
5. H. A. Liebman, S. A. Limentani, B. C. Furie, and B. Furie, Immunoaffinity purification of factor IX (christmas factor) by using conformation-specific antibodies directed against the factor IX-metal complex, Proc. Natl. Acad. Sci. U.S.A. 82:3879–3883 (1985).
6. C. H. Park and A. Tulinsky, Three dimensional structure of the kringle sequence: structure of prothrombin fragment 1, Biochem. 25:3977–3982 (1986).
7. S. Yoshitake, B. G. Schach, D. C. Foster, E. W. Davie, and K. Kurachi, Nucleotide sequence of the gene for human factor IX (antihemophilic factor B), Biochem. 24:3736–3750 (1985).

8. A. Lundwall, W. Dackowski, E. Cohen, M. Shaffer, A. Mahr, B. Dahlback, J. Stenflo, and R. Wydro, Isolation and sequence of the cDNA for human protein S, a regulator of blood coagulation, Proc. Natl. Acad. Sci. U.S.A. 83:6716-6720 (1986).

9. D. C. Foster, S. Yoshitake, and E. W. Davie, The nucleotide sequence of the gene for human protein C, Proc. Natl. Acad. Sci. U.S.A. 82:4673-4677 (1985).

10. S. P. Leytus, D. C. Foster, K. Kurachi, and E. W. Davie, Gene for human factor X: a blood coagulation factor whose gene organization is essentially identical with that of factor IX and protein C, Biochem. 25:5098-5102 (1986).

11. D. Diuguid, M. J. Rabiet, H. A. Liebman, B. C. Furie, and B. Furie, Factor IX Cambridge: hemophilia B caused by an unprocessed leader sequence on the factor IX NH_2-terminus, Blood 66:(suppl. 1), 333a (1985).

12. A. K. Bently, D. J. G. Rees, C. Rizza, and G. G. Brownlee, Defective propeptide processing of blood clotting factor IX caused by mutation of arginine to glutamine at position -4, Cell 45:343-348 (1986).

13. R. A. Blanchard, K. L. K. Faye, J. M. Barnet, and W. B. Castle, Isolation and characterization of profactor X from the liver of a steer treated with sodium warfarin, Blood 66:(suppl. 1), 331a (1985).

14. D. S. Anson, K. H. Choo, D. J. G. Rees, F. Giannelli, K. Gould, J. A. Huddleston, and G. G. Brownlee, The gene structure of human anti haemophilic factor IX, EMBO J. 3:1053-1060 (1984).

15. J. Plutzky, J. A. Hoskins, G. L. Long, and G. R. Crabtree, Evolution and organization of the human protein C gene, Proc. Natl. Acad. Sci. U.S.A. 83:546-550 (1986).

16. S. J. F. Degen and E. W. Davie, The prothrombin gene and serine protease evolution, Ann. NY Acad. Sci. in press (1986).

17. M. Borowski, B. C. Furie, and B. Furie, Distribution of γ-carboxyglutamic and residues in partially carboxylated human prothrombins, J. Biol. Chem. 261:1624-1628 (1986).

18. D. L. Freedenberg, S.-H. Chen, K. Kurachi, and C. R. Scott, Factor IX gene: localization of the MSP I polymorphic site, Human Genetics 39:(suppl.), A10 (1986).

19. R. A. McGraw, L. M. Davis, C. M. Noyes, R. L. Lundblad, H. R. Roberts, J. B. Graham, and D. W. Stafford, Structure and function of factor IX: defects in haemophilia B, Proc. Natl. Acad. Sci. U.S.A. 82:2847-2851 (1985).

20. C. W. Hay, K. A. Robertson, S.-L. Yong, A. R. Thompson, G. H. Growe, and R. T. A. MacGillivary, Use of a Bam HI polymorphism in the factor IX gene for the determination of hemophilia B carrier status, Blood 67:1508-1511 (1986).

21. T. Kojima, M. Tanimoto, T. Kamiya, Y. Obata, T. Takahashi, R. Ohno, K. Kurachi, and H. Saito, Possible absence of common polymorphisms in coagulation factor IX gene in Japanese, Blood in press (1986).

22. E. T. Pam, S.-H. Chen, K. Kurachi, and C. R. Scott, Lack of RFLP markers within the factor IX gene in Asian populations, Human Genetics 39:(suppl.), A243 (1986).

23. R. A. McGraw, L. M. Davis, R. L. Lundblad, D. W. Stafford, and H. R. Roberts, Sturcture and function of factor IX: defects in haemophilia B, Clinics in Haematology 14:359 (1985).

24. A. R. Thompson, Structure, function and molecular defects of factor IX, Blood 67:565-572 (1986).

25. D. J. G. Rees, C. R. Rizza, and G. G. Brownlee, Haemophilia B caused by a point mutation in a donor splice junction of the

human factor IX gene, <u>Nature</u> 316:643-645 (1985).

26. F. Giannelli, K. H. Choo, D. J. G. Rees, Y. Boyd, C. R. Rizza, and G. G. Brownlee, Gene deletions in patients with haemophilia B and anti-factor IX antibodies, <u>Nature</u> 303:181-182 (1983).

27. S.-H. Chen, S. Yoshitake, P. G. Chance, G. L. Bray, A. R. Thompson, C. R. Scott, and K. Kurachi, An intragenic deletion of the factor IX gene in a family with hemophilia B, <u>J. Clin. Inv.</u> 76:2161-2164 (1985).

28. H. J. Hassan, A. Leonardi, R. Guerriero, C. Chelucci, L. Cianetti, N. Ciavarella, P. Raniezi, D. Pilolli, and C. Peschle, Hemophilia B with inhibitor : molecular analysis of the subtotal deletion of the factor IX gene, <u>Blood</u> 66:728-730 (1985).

29. G. L. Bray and A. R. Thompson, Partial factor IX protein in a pedigree with hemophilia B due to a partial gene deletion, <u>J. clin. Inv.</u> 77:1194-1200 (1986).

30. S.-H. Chen, C. R. Scott, R. Edson, and K. Kurachi, An insertion within the factor IX gene of hemophilia B El Salvador, <u>Human Genetics</u> submitted, (1986).

31. S. Busby, A. Kumar, M. J. Joseph, L. Halfpap, M. Insley, K. Berkner, K. Kurachi, and R. Woodbury, Expression of active human factor IX in transfected cells, <u>Nature</u> 316:271 (1985).

32. H. D. L. Salle, W. Altenburger, R. Elkain, K. Dott, A. Dieterle, R. Drillien, J.-P. Cazenave, R. Tolstoshev, and J.-P. Lecocq, Active γ-carboxylated human factor IX expressed using recombinant DNA techniques, <u>Nature</u> 316;268 (1985).

33. D. S. Anson, D. E. G. Austen, and G. G. Brownlee, Expression of active human clotting factor IX from recombinant DNA clones in mammalian cells, <u>Nature</u> 315:683 (1985).

34. R. J. Kaufman, L. C. Wasley, B. C. Furie, B. Furie, and C. B. Shoemaker , Expression, purification, and characterization of recombinant γ-carboxylated factor IX synthesized in Chinese hamster ovary cells, <u>J. Biol. Chem.</u> 261:9622-9628 (1986).

35. K. H. Choo, K. Raphael, W. McAdam, and M. G. Peterson, Expression of active human blood clotting factor IX in transgenic mice, <u>Human Genetics</u> 39:(suppl. 3), A192 (1986).

36. L. C. Pan and P. A. Price, The propeptide of rat bone γ-carboxyglutamic acid protein shares homology with other vitamin K-dependent protein precursors, <u>Proc. Natl. Acad. Sci. U.S.A.</u> 82:6109-6113 (1985).

37. F. S. Hagen, C. L. Gray, P. O'Hara, F. J. Grant, G. C. Saari, R. G. Woodbury, C. E. Hart, M. Insley, W. Kisiel, K. Kurachi, and E. W. Davie, Characterization of a cDNA coding for human factor VII, <u>Proc. Natl. Acad. Sci. U.S.A.</u> 83:2412-2416 (1986).

TISSUE FACTOR AND THE INITIATION OF BLOOD COAGULATION

Yale Nemerson

Departments of Medicine and Biochemistry
Mount Sinai School of Medicine
New York, N.Y.

INTRODUCTION: In the two decades since the introduction of the cascade and waterfall models of blood coagulation [1,2], the investigative emphasis has been on the "intrinsic" system of coagulation. In this system, coagulation is initiated by Hageman factor, which is presumably activated by virtue of an interaction with a "surface", and proceeds by way of several intermediate steps to form thrombin. Although each of these papers explicitly recognized that tissue factor and factor VII markedly accelerated clotting, neither included this step in the coagulation scheme. Put differently, neither model included a step in which the interaction of blood with damaged tissues was viewed as a stimulus for initiating coagulation.

Much of the theory of coagulation has been derived from studying patients lacking specific clotting factors. Although the addition of tissue extracts was known to accelerate coagulation, little credence was given to its physiological role mainly because the extracts completely corrected the defect in hemophiliac plasma whereas the latter clotted in a remarkably prolonged manner in glass. Further, it was known that tissue factor/factor VII directly activated factor X, thus apparently obviating the need for factors VIII and IX. Accordingly, tissue factor, the active procoagulant in fixed tissues, was assigned a negligible role in coagulation. It is noteworthy that the "tissue factor" used for these clinical studies consisted of brain or lung homogenates. An interesting fact relating to these measurements is that when "dilute" tissue factor was utilized, hemophiliacs had abnormally prolonged "prothrombin times". However, the unspoken but prevailing view was that long prothrombin times were somehow artifactual; inasmuch as clotting times as short as 12 seconds were obtainable with "optimal" concentrations of tissue factor and dilute preparation yielded clotting times 2-3 fold longer, the latter data were essentially ignored.

The now classical views of the coagulation system derived from hypotheses proposed both by MacFarlane [1] and by Davie and Ratnoff[2] and were essential to future research inasmuch as they introduced the concept of sequential proteolytic zymogen activations as the fundamental mechanism regulating coagulation. However, at the time all the known clotting factors were considered zymogens; the resulting schemes were as follows:

```
    XII
  XI------->XIa
      IX------->IXa
         VIII------->VIIIa
             X--------->Xa
                 V------->Va
                     II---------->thrombin
```

thrombin then catalyzed the proteolytic conversion of fibrinogen to fibrin.

In contrast, as early as 1886, Woolridge induced coagulation in dogs by injection of various fractions of calf tissues [3]. Woolridge deduced that the active compound contained (and required) protein and lipid: extraction with ether plus alcohol, which removed the lipids, or incubation with pepsin, a proteolytic enzyme abolished the activity of the preparations. By 1912, Howell was fractionating tissue preparations by organic solvent extraction and confirmed that the aqueous tissue extract, "thromboplastin", was much more active than the lipid "partial thromboplastin" in in vitro assays [4]. These experiments laid the groundwork for the reconstitution of tissue factor from lipid and protein moieties by Chargaff and co-workers [5]. A lipoprotein fraction was suspended in sodium deoxycholate which solubilized the lipid and protein moieties of tissue factor. Following dialysis, the product was a powerful procoagulant. Thus Chargaff most likely succeeded in reassociating the two components of tissue factor. In the same paper, Chargaff also demonstrated the catalytic nature of tissue factor by demonstrating that tissue factor was not "consumed" during prothrombin activation.

Some 25 years later, systematic studies of the lipid and protein components of tissue factor were initiated. In the 1980s the protein component of tissue factor was isolated from bovine [6] and human tissues [7,8]. Tissue factor from both species has an apparent mol wt of 44,000. Tissue factor is rich in carbohydrates, but it is not clear whether they are required for coagulant activity. In its delipidated state, tissue factor has at most 0.01% of its potential activity [6]. However, exploiting the techniques introduced by Chargaff, recombination with lipid, and hence reactivation, is readily accomplished [9,10,11,12]. Recently, we found octyl glucoside to be the detergent of choice owing to the fact that it is readily dialyzable. Using this technique, the reassociation results in large lipid vesicles (ca. 150 nm) of fairly narrow size distribution [13]. The tissue factor molecules are randomly inserted into the vesicles so that about half the molecules face outward and are accessible to factor VII whereas the other half face inward and are kinetically silent.

THE MECHANISM OF ACTION OF TISSUE FACTOR: Tissue factor functions as an essential activator of factors VII and VIIa. Perhaps the best way to conceptualize this mechanism is to view the tissue factor/factor VII complex as a holoenzyme consisting of a catalytic subunit, factor VII (VIIa), and a regulatory subunit, tissue factor. Thus, in the absence of either component, there is no catalytic activity. This phenomenon is of particular importance inasmuch as factor VII uniquely appears to have catalytic activity. Thus, if factor VII were proteolytically active in the absence of tissue factor continuous in vivo coagulation would ensue.

FACTOR VII, AN ACTIVE ZYMOGEN: Factor VII is a single chain gla-containing protein of about 50 kilodaltons. As isolated from bovine plasma, it has an apparent activity of about 2% of its proteolytically cleaved derivative, 2-chain factor VIIa [14]. Similarly, the human protein has some 4% of the apparent activity of human factor VIIa [15]. Further, when the active site-directed irreversible enzyme inhibitor, diisopropyl-fluorophosphate (DFP), is added to bovine plasma, factor VII activity is reduced to zero whereas all other clotting factors were unaffected [16]. Thus, it seemed likely that factor VII had coagulant activity, but the presence of factor VIIa in both pure preparations and plasma could not be ruled out. Parenthetically, it should be noted that no plasma inhibitor of factor VIIa has been described.

Experimentally, it is difficult to distinguish between a zymogen preparation that has 2% of the activity of its derivative enzyme and a zymogen that has endogenous activity equal to 2% of the enzyme. This problem was approached by first determining the rate of incorporation of radiolabelled DFP into the zymogen and enzyme [17]. Under these conditions, a 2% contamination would introduce only a minimal error as the rate constants are fairly similar and each species binds DFP with a stoichiometry of 1:1.

Inasmuch as DFP is used in vast excess over the proteins, the reaction may be treated as pseudo-first order. The incorporation of DFP into each species is simply determined as a function of time. Then using appropriate curve fitting techniques (or simply a semi-log plot) the constants can be estimated. Using this approach, we found the rate of incorporation into pure bovine factor VIIa to be $0.130 +/- 0.001$ min^{-1}, whereas the rate into the zymogen was $0.032 +/- 0.001$ min^{-1}. When the decay of factor VIIa activity was measured, it had a rate constant of $0.0127 +/- 0.004$ min^{-1}. The agreement between the incorporation and inactivation rates for factor VIIa indicate the validity of this strategy. When the decay of the activity of the zymogen was studied, it was curvilinear, immediately indicating that the activity could not be due to contamination with factor VIIa (the decay of which was linear on a first order plot). Knowing the incorporation rates for both species, we could then solve for the activity of the zymogen by fitting the following equation to the data describing the activity of the zymogen preparation following the addition of DFP:

$$Y = c_1 e^{-k_1 t} + c_2 e^{-k_2 t}$$

where Y is the remaining activity at time t; k1 and k2 are the first order rate constants for incorporation of DFP into the zymogen and enzyme, respectively, and C1 and C2 describe the contribution of the zymogen and enzyme to the overall activity. The analysis showed that in a zymogen preparation which was 35-fold activatable, about one-third of the activity was directly attributable to the activity of the zymogen, the remainder being due to contamination with a small amount of enzyme. From these data we calculated that zymogen factor VII had 0.8% of the coagulant activity of factor VIIa. Put differently, the enzyme was only 120-fold more active than the zymogen. This is in marked contrast with other enzyme-zymogen pairs. For example, the clotting time of thrombin-free prothrombin and fibrinogen shows prothrombin to be an inert zymogen with respect to proteolysis.

Similar studies have not yet been reported for the human protein, although the fact that the zymogen is inhibited by DFP at about one quarter the rate of the enzyme [15] certainly suggests that human factor VII is also coagulant-active. This being the case, it follows that coagulation can be initiated by complex formation between factor VII and tissue factor. That is, a purely physical event <u>not</u> <u>requiring</u> <u>the</u> <u>scission</u> <u>of</u> <u>a</u> <u>peptide</u> <u>bond</u> is sufficient to promote clot formation. Because the enzyme, factor VIIa, has 120-fold the activity of the zymogen, the potential for enormous acceleration of the initiating event is evident. Indeed, one product of the initial reaction, factor Xa, is evidently the most potent enzyme that can catalyze this conversion, although factor IXa and thrombin possess lesser activities [14,18]. While the events leading to the conversion of zymogen VII to factor VIIa <u>in</u> <u>vivo</u> certainly are not known, it is of potential interest that the Xa-catalyzed conversion of the zymogen is tissue factor-dependent [19]. In effect, then, one can imagine that tissue factor combines with the zymogen producing a catalytically active complex. One product of the subsequent reactions is activated factor X; the latter then cleaves factor VII thus increasing the initiating burst over 100-fold. An obvious advantage to this hypothetical scenario is that the burst of coagulant activity arising from tissue injury would be proportional to the tissue factor content of the injured tissues and perhaps, therefore, to the extent of that injury. Tissue factor thus may act as a high fidelity transducer of physical injury into clot formation.

KINETICS OF THE TISSUE FACTOR PATHWAY: A thorough understanding of the tissue factor pathway rests, in the end, on an adequate kinetic model of these reactions. For such modelling studies it would be desirable to use zymogen factor VII as well as VIIa. However, due to the instability of the former (it gets cleaved during the course of the reactions), all experiments have been performed using the 2-chain enzyme.

When the reaction is studied using purified components and tissue factor reconstituted with phosphatidyl choline (PC), no activity is detectable in the absence of either tissue factor or factor VII. Further, when tissue factor and factor VIIa are varied in a systematic manner, the resultant activity is always proportional to the concentration of the lesser ligand. This is consistent with a model in which the catalytic complex consists of tissue factor and factor VIIa in equimolar amounts [20]. This conclusion is consistent with equilibrium measurements which show that these components interact with a stoichiometry of 1:1 [13]. These data indicate that tissue factor may be viewed as an essential enzyme activator. Assuming that the product-forming complex contains three components, tissue factor, factor VIIa and substrate (either factor IX or factor X), the following pertains:

$$\text{[Tissue factor:VIIa:factor X]} \xrightarrow{\text{kcat}} \text{factor Xa + TF:VIIa}$$

where kcat is the catalytic rate constant which describes the rate at which the above complex breaks down into product and the TF:VIIa species. Alternatively, the complex could break down into product and free tissue factor and factor VIIa. However, this mechanism proved to be untenable as it is inconsistent with our experimental data.

Given this mechanism, and assuming the product-forming complex consists of the above species with a stoichiometry of 1:1:1, there are three ways the components may assemble, each yielding different kinetic consequences. First, the assembly may be entirely random with the complex resulting from the following species: tissue factor:VIIa, tissue factor:substrate and VIIa:substrate, as well as free tissue factor, factor VIIa and substrate. It is readily demonstrable that this mechanism results in obligatory substrate inhibition. The underlying mechanism of this phenomenon is that as substrate is added, substrate:VIIa and substrate:tissue factor complexes are formed at the ultimate expense of the ternary, product-forming species. As this inhibition is contrary to experimental data, the fully random model may be readily excluded.

If tissue factor bound both enzyme and substrate (but free enzyme and substrate did not form complexes) then the mechanism is deemed partial random. The equations describing this model have been derived [20]; again, this mechanism predicts certain quantitative parameters which do not agree with experimental data. Accordingly, it was possible to reject this model. What remains is an essential activation, fully ordered model for the tissue factor dependent-reactions:

$$\text{TF + VIIa} \overset{K1}{\longleftrightarrow} \text{TF:VIIa + S} \overset{K2}{\longleftrightarrow} \text{TF:VIIa:S} \overset{\text{kcat}}{\longrightarrow} \text{P + TF:VIIa}$$

where S is either factor X or IX and P is either Xa or IXa. K1 and K2 are equilibrium binding constants and kcat is the catalytic rate constant as defined above. The equation describing this mechanism was fit to a data set consisting of 246 determinations of the reaction velocity of a system consisting of multiple concentrations of tissue factor, factor VIIa and factor X. The fit yielded the following parameters:

$$K1 = 0.09 \; +/- \; 0.001 \; nM$$
$$K2 = 283.8 \; +/- \; 20.1 \quad nM$$
$$kcat = 210.0 \; +/- \; 4.5 \quad min^{-1}$$

The extraordinarily small error bars indicate a very good fit of the equation to the experimental data. However, this model also was not acceptable because K1 was found to be 4.54 +/- 1.37 nM when determined under true equilibrium conditions. Owing to this extraordinary discrepancy, and to the fact that the alternative models were readily rejected, we postulated a novel variation of the essential activation, ordered addition model. Our reasoning was as follows: the fundamental problem lay in the fact that K1 determined directly was two orders of magnitude greater than K1 determined kinetically. All the alternative essential activation models, as discussed above, were rejected for various reasons and none necessarily led to tighter binding of the enzyme to tissue factor. Accordingly, we postulated a mechanism in which factor VIIa underwent a conformational change upon complexation with tissue factor thus enabling the enzyme to recognize and bind its natural substrates. Upon substrate binding, yet another conformational change is imposed upon the enzyme leading to a tighter association with tissue factor. The resulting scheme, modified from [20] to show all the unidirectional rate constants is:

In essence, all the starred species are substrate-induced kinetic transients. In order for this model to accommodate the discrepancy in K1, we found that the spontaneous formation of AE^* must be minimal; i.e., k10 (and hence k6) must be very small. The reason for this is that for the apparent binding constant to be some much tighter, species must exist in the presence of substrate which are not present when just enzyme and tissue factor interact. In proteolytic reactions, the back reaction forming peptide bonds is generally vanishingly small; hence k12 may be ignored.

Is the true substrate for the Tissue Factor Pathway Lipid-Bound?
    Most investigators have assumed that for coagulation to function,

acidic lipids must be present. In a sense this is absolutely true as the prothrombinase complex will not assemble on neutral vesicles because factor V (at least) will not bind [21]. However, as cell surfaces contain little or no acidic lipids, it is not clear that cell systems exhibit the same requirements. It is possible, for example, that platelets and perhaps other cells have specific receptors for this essential cofactor. Further, because factors II,VII,IX and X are not gamma-carboxylated in the absence of vitamin K and they do not bind to acidic vesicles nor do they exhibit biological activity. Thus, it has generally been assumed that lipid binding of the vitamin k-dependent proteins is an essential requirement for their activation.

Unlike other procoagulant proteins, tissue factor is inserted into vesicles (rather than simply being bound) and is biologically active in this milieu. We therefore had the opportunity to approach directly the problem of substrate localization [22].

The logic of the experiments was as follows: 1) Use vesicles composed of phosphatidyl serine and phosphatidyl choline (PS:PC, 30:70), and employ sufficient lipid (500 mM) so that some 85% of the substrate (factor X) was bound to lipid. Under these conditions, displacement of any significant fraction of bound substrate would be reflected in a large increase in the concentration of free substrate. 2) Utilize a substance which competes with factor X for available sites on the vesicles, thus allowing manipulation of the two pools; 3) Demonstrate that the substance has no other effect on the catalytic apparatus, _per se_. 4) Finally, correlate the velocity measurements with the concentration of bound and free substrates. Clearly the substrate pool that correlates best with the velocities will be the controlling pool.

Recent experiments performed in our laboratory utilized prothrombin fragment 1 as the displacing ligand. It was readily shown that fragment 1 had no effect on catalysis because there was no effect on a reaction in which tissue factor was reconstituted with PC. Under these circumstances, the substrate was entirely free and the velocities in the presence and absence of fragment 1 were indistinguishable. Conversely, when the same experiment was performed utilizing PS:PC (30:70) vesicles the addition of fragment 1 resulted in large increases in velocity. As fragment 1 decreased the concentration of bound substrate and increased the concentration free in solution, we concluded that free substrate was preferentially hydrolyzed in this system. A corollary to this statement is that binding to phospholipids renders the substrates inaccessible to the tissue factor/factor VIIa complex. As both the complex and the substrates reside on the same lipid vesicles, this was an unexpected finding.

THE TISSUE FACTOR PATHWAY OF COAGULATION: For many years it was thought that tissue factor/factor VII catalyzed only the activation of factor X. Because factors VIII and IX are clearly required for normal hemostasis and inasmuch as this pathway was thought to bypass these factors, the tissue factor pathway was thought not to be hemostatically essential. However, Osterud and Rapaport [23] made the very important observation that this system also activated factor IX. Thus, the following pathway of coagulation became feasible:

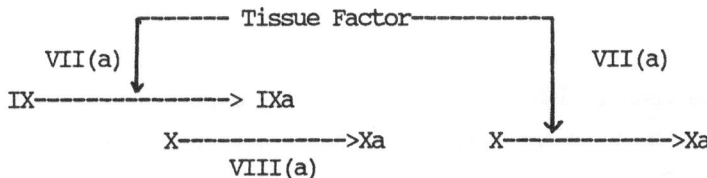

The sum of Xa produced by these two reactions would then form catalytic component of the prothrombinase complex, thus leading to thrombin production. We have studied the efficiency of factor IX activation and factor X activation by tissue factor and factor VIIa. In these studies we varied the lipid composition of the vesicles from pure PC to PS:PC (30:70). Under all conditions, the efficiency of factor X activation, expressed as kcat/Km, was about 35-fold greater than that for factor IX activation. Even allowing for substantial amplification by the action of factors IXa and VIII in producing activated factor X, the role of factor IX activation via tissue factor was unclear. On this basis, we postulated the existence of a substance which modulated the substrate specificity of tissue factor/factor VII.

In our laboratory, the examination of many plasma fractions for this activity was fruitless. We consequently turned to cell surface components reasoning that tissue factor is known to be on cell surfaces and hence that tissue factor-initiated coagulation might well occur in contact with these compounds. In experiments yet to be published we have found that heparin, dextran sulfate and heparan sulfate stimulate the activation of factor IX without affecting the rate of activation of factor X. Our initial experiments with heparin and dextran sulfate showed that the acceleration was due to a decrease in the Km as well as an increase in the kcat. The effect was most dramatic when pure PC vesicles were employed, the kcat/Km being 17-fold more efficient in the presence of optimal quantities of these polysaccharides. There was essentially no kinetic difference between heparin and dextran sulfate. While heparan sulfate stimulates to the same degree, much larger quantities are required to achieve equal effects. Inasmuch as tissue factor and heparan sulfate probably are in close approximation to each other on the cell surface, the meaning of fluid phase experiments is not clear. It is possible that on the cell surface tissue factor and heparan sulfate are complexed, thus rendering the meaning of a dissociation constant ambiguous. It is also possible that the observed stimulations are purely in vitro artifacts. However, evidence that the tissue factor pathway dominates in cell-surface mediated coagulation comes from the studies of Stern and his colleagues [24] who showed that endothelial cells have tissue factor as judged by their ability to activate factor X in a factor VII-dependent manner. The activation was readily inhibited by an antibody directed against bovine tissue factor. Most importantly, the rate of activation of factor X was enhanced some 10-fold when factors VIIIa and IX were included in the reaction [25]. A conclusion that may be drawn from these experiments is that endothelial cell-surface tissue factor rapidly activates factor IX which, in the presence of factor VIIIa, generates much more Xa than the direct activation via factor tissue factor and factor VIIa. Our current view, which is under active investigation in our laboratory, is that the cell surface proteoglycans modulate the activity of tissue factor which results in very rapid activation of factor X.

THE BIOLOGICAL SIGNIFICANCE OF THE TISSUE FACTOR PATHWAY: It is readily apparent from the above considerations that the relative contributions of the extrinsic and intrinsic pathways to hemostasis and thrombosis is a most complex question. It is clear that when trying to evaluate the activation of factor IX by factor XIa vs. the tissue factor pathway, much needs to be known. For example, is tissue factor biologically available in membranes consisting of mostly phosphatidyl choline or are the inner phosphatidyl serine-containing membrane leaflets the initiators of coagulation? Are the true substrates free in solution or lipid-bound? Should the tissue factor dependent activation of factor IX be evaluated in the presence of acidic polysaccharides? The ultimate answers will require much ingenious experimentation to determine the site and chemical milieu of the tissue factor dependent initiation of coagulation.

REFERENCES

1. MacFarlane, R.G., An Enzyme Cascade in the Blood Clotting. Mechanism and its Function as a Biological Amolifier. Nature 202:498 (1964).

2. Davie, E.W. and Ratnoff, O.D., Waterfall Sequence for Intrinsic Blood Clotting. Science 145:1310 (1964).

3. Woolridge, L.C. "On the Chemistry of the Blood and Other Scientfic Papers," KeganPaul, Trench, Trubner & Co., Ltd. London, pp. 135-137.

4. Howell, W.H., The Nature and Action of the Thromboplastin (zymoplastic) Substance of the Tissues. Am. J. Physiol. 31:1 (1912).

5. Chargaff, E. Studies on the Mechanism of the Thromboplastic Effect. J. Biol. Chem. 173:253 (1948).

6. Bach, R.R., Nemrson, Y., and Konigsberg, W.K.,Purification and Characterization of Bovine Tissue Factor. J. Biol. Chem 256:8324 (1981).

7. Broze, G.J., Leykam,J.E., Schwartz, B.D. and Miletich, J.P., Purification of Human Brain Tissue Factor. J. Biol. Chem. 260:10917 (1985).

8. Guha, A., Bach, R.R., Konigsberg, W.K. and Nemerson, Y., Affinity Purification of Human Tissue Factor: Interaction of Factor VII and Tissue Factor in Detergent Micelles, Proc. Nat. Acad. Sci. 83:299 (1986).

9. Studer, A. Contribution a L'etude de la Thrombokinase, in "Jubilee Volume Dedicated to Emile Cristophe Barell," The Roche Companies, Basel, (1946).

10. Kuhn, R. and Klesse, P.C., Zur Chemischen Konstitution des Lipoids der Thrombokinase, Naturwissenschaften 44:352, (1957).

11. Nemrson, Y., The Phospholipid Requirement of Tissue Factor in Blood Coagulation, J. Clin. Invest. 47:72 (1968).

12. Hvatum M. and Prydz, H., Studies on Tissue Thromboplastin. I. Solubilization with sodium deoxycholate, Biochim. Biophys. Acta 130:92 (1966).

13. Bach, R.R., Gentry, R. and Nemerson, Y., Factor VII Binding to Tissue Factor in Reconstituted Phospholipid Vesicles: Induction of Cooperativity by Phosphatidylserine, Biochem. 25:4007 (1986).

14. Radcliffe, R. and Nemerson, Y., The Activation and Control of Factor VII by Activated Factor X and Thrombin, J. Biol. Chem. 250:388 (1975).

15. Broze, G.J. and Majerus, P.W., Purification and Characterization of Human Coagulation Factor VII. J. Biol. Chem. 255:1242 (1980).

16. Nemerson, Y. and Esnouf, M.P., Activation of a Proteolytic System by a Membrane Lipoprotein: The Mechanism of Action of Tissue Factor, Proc. Natl. Acad. Sci. 70:310 (1973).

17. Zur, M., Radcliffe, R.D., Oberdick, J. and Nemerson, Y., The Dual Role of Factor VII in Blood Coagulation. Initiation of a Proteolytic system by a Zymogen, J. Biol. Chem. 257:5623 (1982).

18. Seligsohn, U., Osterud, B., Brown, S.F., Griffin, J.H. and Rapaport, S.I., Activation of Human Factor VII in Plasma and Purified Systems, J. Clin. Invest. 64:1056 (1979).

19. Nemerson, Y. and Repke, D., Tissue Factor Accelerates the Activation of Factor VII: The Role of a Bifunctional Coagulation Cofactor, Thrombosis Research 40:351 (1986).

20. Nemerson, Y. and Gentry, R., An Ordered Addition, Essential Activation Model of the Tissue Factor Pathway of Coagulation: Evidence for a Conformational Cage, Biochemistry 25:4020 (1986).

21. van de Waart, P., Bruls, H., Hemker, H.C. and Lindhout,T., Interaction of Bovine Blood Clotting Factor Va and its Subunits with Phospholipid Vesicles, Biochemistry 22:2427 (1983).

22. Forman, S. and Nemerson, Y., A Membrane-Dependent Coagulation Reaction is Independent of the Concentration of Phospholipid-Bound Substrate: Fluid Phase Factor X Regulates the Extrinsic System, Proc. Natl. Acad. Sci. 83:4675 (1986).

23. Osterud, B. and Rapaport, S.I., Activation of Factor IX by the Reaction Product of tissue factor and factor VII: Additional Pathway for Inititating Blood Coagulation. Proc. Natl. Acad. Sci. 74:5260 (1977).

24. Nawroth, P., Stern, D., Kisiel, W. and Bach, R., Cellular Requirements for Tissue Factor Generation by Bovine Aortic Endothelial Cells in Culture. Thrombosis Research 40:677 (1985).

25. Stern, D., Nawroth, P., Handley,D. and Kisiel,W., An Endothelial Cell-Dependent Pathway of Coagulation. Proc. Natl. Acad. Sci. 82:2523 (1985).

INR – CALIBRATION OF THE THERAPEUTIC RANGE

Leon Poller

UK Reference Laboratory for Anticoagulant Reagents
& Control, Withington Hospital, Manchester M20 8LR, U.K.

THE NEED TO DEVELOP THE INTERNATIONAL NORMALISED RATIO (INR) SYSTEM

The prothrombin time (PT) is the most important coagulation test. After many years of disagreement, an international system of standardisation has been accepted. Fifty years after Quick[1] described the PT to detect coagulation defects, the control of oral anticoagulant therapy is still largely dependent on the test. Many modifications to the original technique have been introduced, and new methods have been developed specifically, e.g. the prothrombin and proconvertin test (P and P test),[2] and the Thrombotest,[3] but their application has been limited in comparison. Clinical reports of anticoagulant trials, giving no details of the PT method are still published.[(e.g.4)]

An international survey has shown how the lack of standardisation particularly of tissue extract thromboplastin reagents has contributed to undesirable differences in the intensity of anticoagulant treatment at different centres.[5] Consequently, the PT result of a patient may indicate overdosage at one hospital, but underdosage at another, dependent entirely on the laboratory methodology. An example of the variation in dosage at different centres is given in Fig.I. Hospitals using relatively insensitive thromboplastins of rabbit origin gave a higher mean warfarin dose than those using a PT method based on a human brain thromboplastin. An approximately fourfold difference can be seen in the extremes of the mean dose of the different groups.

STEPS TOWARDS STANDARDISATION

The first large-scale attempt to standardise the PT began in Manchester in 1962 with the development of a procedure for producing thromboplastin showing uniformity between batches for hospitals covering a population of 5 million.[6] Over the next decade this local standardisation scheme evolved into the British System for anticoagulant control, with batches of Manchester Comparative Reagent (MCR) designated British Comparative Thromboplastin (BCT). In 1965, Biggs,[7] then demonstrated that a dilution curve could be expressed linearly by plotting the prothrombin ratio against the reciprocal of the concentration of plasma. A national system of PT reporting was introduced in the United Kingdom in 1969 based on the ratio obtained with

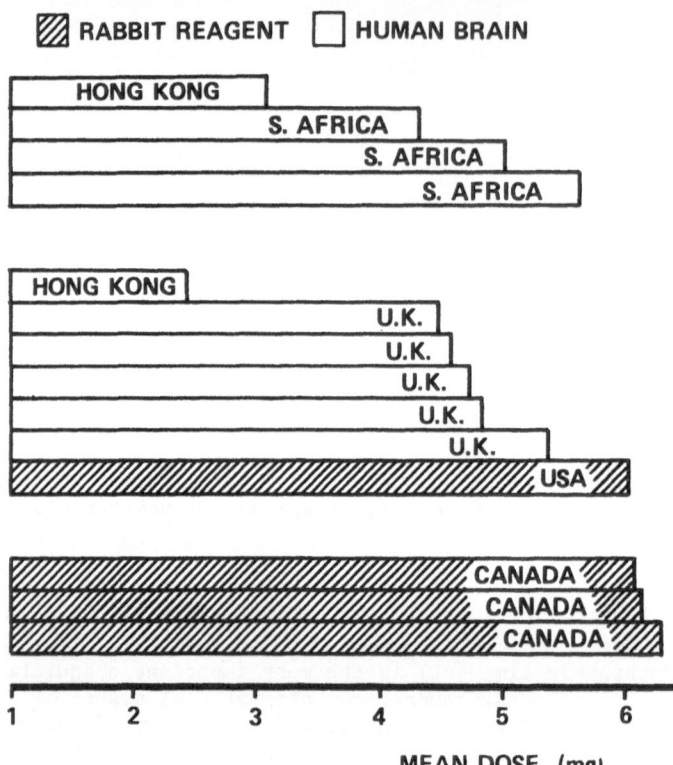

Fig.I. Differences in the warfarin dosages in different countries in relation to the type of animal tissue extract used.

BCT.[8] These were termed British Ratios and provided a common basis for testing, reporting and dosage. The introduction of BCT as a reference reagent has also been influential in establishing similar standardisation schemes in other countries. An alternative scheme was proposed in the United States by the College of American Pathologists, which was based on reference plasmas artificially depleted of the vitamin K-dependent clotting factors.[9]

THE WHO SCHEME FOR THROMBOPLASTIN CALIBRATION

Between 1967 and 1970 a series of lyophilised thromboplastin preparations were prepared for the International Committee on Thrombosis and Haemostasis (ICTH) as reference reagents. In 1977 WHO designated a batch of thromboplastin (67/40) as the primary International Reference Preparation (IRP). Other thromboplastins were to be assigned a value after calibration with 67/40. The IRP (67/40) was defined as 1.0. Secondary reference thromboplastins were also introduced because the supply of the primary IRP was limited.

The first WHO scheme had little impact. There was no evidence concerning the stability of 67/40 thromboplastin which was the lynch-pin of the scheme. The statistical method was a problem e.g. the relationship between results with two reagents had to pass through the (I,I) origin. In many instances, this theoretical relationship does not hold. A noticeable curve was also apparent when dissimilar combined and plain preparations were compared. Kirkwood,[10] pointed out that the original WHO scheme did not meet requirements for biological standardisation.

THE INR SYSTEM

A revised WHO calibration procedure emerged from a collaborative study performed under the European Community Bureau Commun de Référence (BCR).[11] This procedure was confirmed in a larger international study from the United Kingdom Reference Laboratory to calibrate the replacement 2nd primary WHO IRP.[12] Three secondary reference thromboplastins were developed by the BCR and designated human plain, bovine combined and rabbit plain.

The logarithms of PT's with different thromboplastins were shown to have a linear relationship and this was used to calibrate the reagents. The new formula also embraces the PT of the normal group on the correlation line. The linear relationship between the logarithms of PT's was estimated by a procedure which is referred to as the "least squares estimation of a functional relationship" also described as orthogonal regression. This procedure allows for the biological and experimental variation from the calibration line of PT's of individual patients. The revised calibration procedure was adopted by WHO in 1983.

A batch of British Comparative Thromboplastin, BCT/253 was adopted in 1983 by WHO as a replacement for the 1st primary International Reference Thromboplastin (human plain). WHO also replaced the two secondary IRP's, WHO rabbit reference thromboplastin 70/178 and 68/434, with new reference materials designated RBT/79 (rabbit) and a bovine reference thromboplastin (OBT/79). The relationship of the reference preparations is illustrated in Fig.2.

INTERNATIONAL COMMITTEE FOR STANDARDISATION IN HAEMATOLOGY (ICSH) REFERENCE THROMBOPLASTIN

The limited availability of the WHO IRP led to the production of the secondary IRP. For many reasons, mainly currency regulations, the BCR preparations, for which there is a charge, have not been available to many Eastern European and developing countries. As a result, an international reference preparation (BCT/441) was prepared for the International Committee for Standardisation in Haematology (ICSH) and calibrated in 1985.[13] This is available, without charge, to designated national control laboratories.

Nomenclature:

The INR is the prothrombin ratio it is calculated would have been obtained if the 1st WHO primary IRP had been used in the test. It is based on the International Sensitivity Index (ISI). This is the slope of the calibration line for any thromboplastin. It is obtained with logarithms of the PT's of the primary IRP plotted on the vertical axis against the logarithms of the PT's obtained with the secondary thromboplastin on the same set of normal and anticoagulated patient plasmas. A secondary IRP or a manufacturer's house standard which has been calibrated against a secondary IRP is used in practice and not the primary IRP.

Calibration is based on parallel testing of the local reagent and a designated reference thromboplastin with a known ISI. For a full calibration, 20 normal plasmas and 60 coumarin treated patients' plasma must be tested with both reagents. Patient selection is important and the coumarin

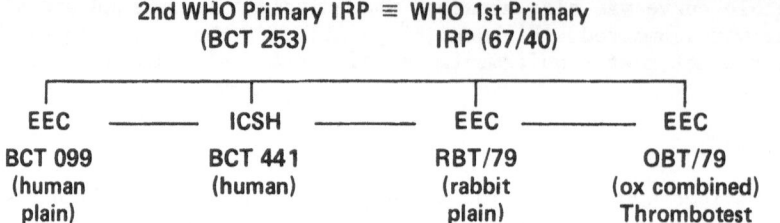

Fig.2. The hierarchical structure of thromboplastin calibration.

plasmas should cover a good range of values between 1.5 and 5.0 ratios with
the IRP. Only samples from patients stabilized on long-term treatment can
be included.

The method for calculating ISI's and INR's is as follows. The PT in
seconds of all plasma specimens (20 normal subjects and 60 patients) are
converted to the corresponding logarithms. Let z be the logarithm of a PT
per second determined with the reference material (RM) and x be the logarithm of PT per second determined with the House Standard or local preparation to be calibrated. The relationship $z = a_1 + b_1 x$ is calculated by
the following formulas, in which a_1 and b_1 are the orthogonal regression
line parameters:

$$b_1 = m + \sqrt{m^2 + 1}$$

$$m = \frac{\Sigma(x - \bar{x})^2 - \Sigma(z - \bar{z})^2}{2\Sigma(x - \bar{x})(z - \bar{z})} = \frac{1}{2r}\left[\frac{s_z}{s_x} - \frac{s_x}{s_z}\right]$$

$$\text{and } a_1 = \bar{z} - b_1\bar{x};$$

where $\bar{x}$ is the arithmetical mean of x, and $\bar{z}$ the mean of z, s_x and s_z are
the standard deviations of the x and z values and r the correlation
coefficient.

Calibration lines from the multicentre exercise to determine the ISI
of the replacement primary WHO IRP (BCT/253) are given in Fig.3. A modification of the calibration is required if the normal values and the coumarin
patients' results do not lie on the same orthogonal regression line. If the
normal line is significantly different ($d \neq o$) a correction is recommended
by Tomenson.[14] A test is made of the hypothesis that the mean logarithms of
the prothrombin times of normal subjects lie on the orthogonal regression
line of patients' plasmas. If this hypothesis is rejected the vertical
distance of the mean logarithms of the normal prothrombin times from the
line is incorporated in the conversion formula for prothrombin ratios as
follows $y = 10^d \times b$.

With the certified parameters a and b of the calibration line of the
RM against WHO preparation 67/40, the intercept and slope of the House
Standard in relation to WHO preparation 67/40 are as follows:

Intercept: $a + b.a_1$

Slope: $b.b_1$

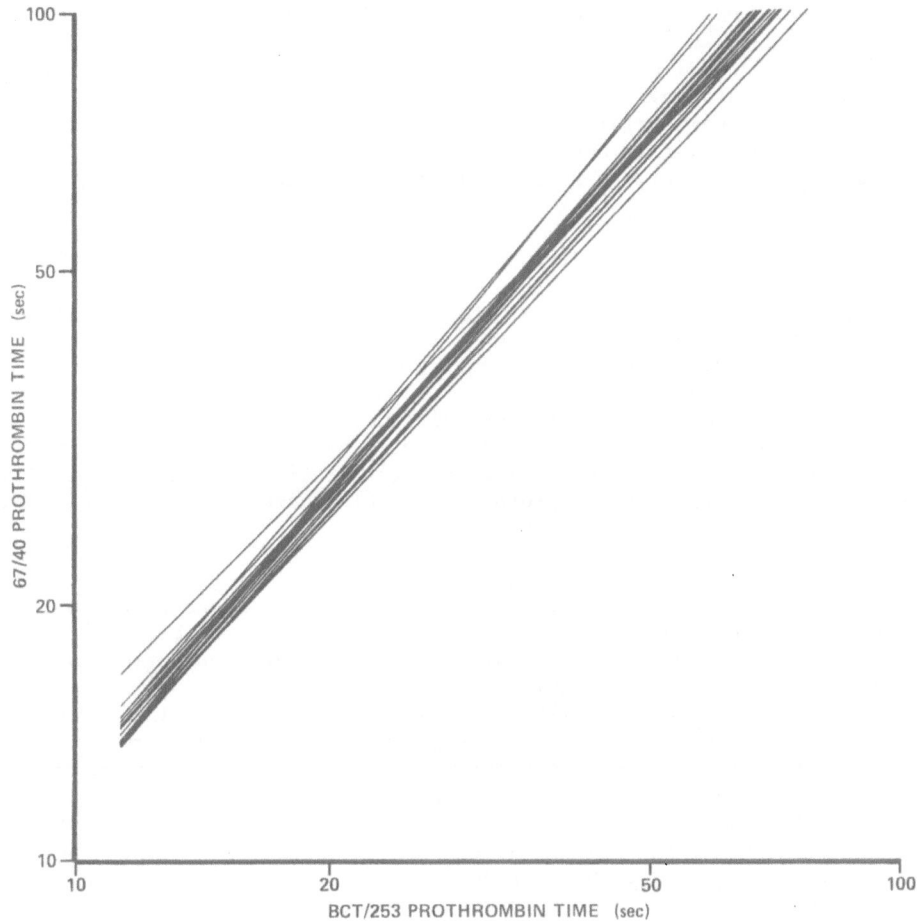

Fig.3.   Calibration of BCT/253 orthogonal regression lines from
         multicentre exercise.

To transform the logarithmic value into the value that would have been
obtained with 67/40, the following equation is used:

$$PT_{67/40} + antilog(a + b.a_1 + b.b_1 .x)$$

The calculation is much simpler, however, if PT ratios are used instead of
PT's. The a values are no longer needed. The conversion of the PT ratio
with a House Standard (R_{HS}) into a ratio that would have been obtained with
67/40 ($R_{67/40}$) is easily done by the formula

$$R_{67/40} = R_{HS}^{b. b^1}$$

The principle is illustrated in Fig.2. Example: RBT with a stated ISI of
I.4I3, a ratio of 2.5 corresponds to $(2.5)^{1.413} = 3.65$.

It is reassuring that very few laboratories will ever have to perform
a calibration. Laboratories using either a nationally recognized thromboplastin reagent or a commercial reagent will have no need to do so, since
the ISI or INR table should be provided by the manufacturer or a national
control laboratory.

The human brain WHO 2nd primary IRP (BCT/253) has an ISI of I.085 (I.I ascribed by WHO). The EEC (BCR) secondary reference preparation of BCT (099) has an ISI of I.048 and the International Committee for Standard-isation in Haematology (ICSH) international reference preparation BCT/44I an ISI of I.04.[13] Commercial thromboplastin reagents are invariably much less sensitive. The majority have an ISI between 2.0 and 2.5. The range of values of representative thromboplastin reagents is given in Fig.4.

THE LIMITATIONS OF THE INR SYSTEM

With the introduction of the INR system does the sensitivity of a thromboplastin matter as long as an ISI is provided? The INR system provides a reasonable guide to therapeutic equivalents particularly in the long term patients but unfortunately it is not always a reliable guide to the intensity of anticoagulation in an individual patient and particularly in the early stages of treatment as exemplified by the results of the pros-pective trial from Hamilton (Hull et al.).[15] Patients were randomised into groups and controlled by the prothrombin ratios based on the prothrombin time test incorporating either Simplastin reagent or by MCR.

A PT of 57 seconds with MCR gives an INR of 4.7. Figure 4 illustrates the scatter of results obtained with Simplastin corresponding to an INR of 4.7 with MCR. Figure 5 illustrates the reduction in reliability of the prothrombin time test with increasing ISI of the thromboplastin. As the ISI increases the width of the therapeutic range in ratios corresponding to the therapeutic range in INR progressively diminishes. The lower limit of the therapeutic range also progressively approaches the normal values i.e. the discrimination of the therapeutic prothrombin ratio from the normal range became progressively less. Furthermore, as the coefficient of variation (CV) has been shown to be constant and similar with the various widely used thromboplastins by US CAP surveys (Koepke),[16] and the UK surveys (in the region of 5-6 per cent irrespective of thromboplastin used), the effect of laboratory error in measurement becomes proportionately greater with increasing ISI.

There are limits to the reliability of the INR with some thrombo-plastins in the early days of coumarin treatment and in unstable patients. ISI calibrations are performed on long-term stabilised patients when the coumarin dependent clotting factors have been depressed to a steady level. Typical INR values in three patients during the induction phase of treatment obtained with a group of different thromboplastin reagents are seen in Figs.6 & 7. An INR was derived directly from the results with the 2nd WHO primary human brain IRP and the values with the other reagents were as far as possible derived from the manufacturers' tables. Two major facts emerge. Unlike the situation in long-term stabilised patients, during the induction phase of therapy the INR values of the various reagents are less dependable. Some reagents furthermore display a consistent trend to under or over-estimate the INR which suggests calibration errors by the manufacturer. Simple advice to rely on the INR values irrespective of the sensitivity (ISI) of the thromboplastin extracts used, although partly solving the problem of the gross variations in results with different reagents cannot therefore be regarded as a suffic-iently reliable guide to dosage. During the induction phase of treatment, during the first days or weeks of coumarin administration and in non-stabilised patients the reliability of the INR result will be greatly influenced by the type of thromboplastin supplied by the manufacturer. The INR system should however encourage manufacturers to produce reagents of improved sensitivity (low ISI) and thus reduce the difficulties. Examples of the differences with the various reagents with long-term patients in the UK have been obtained from the National External Quality

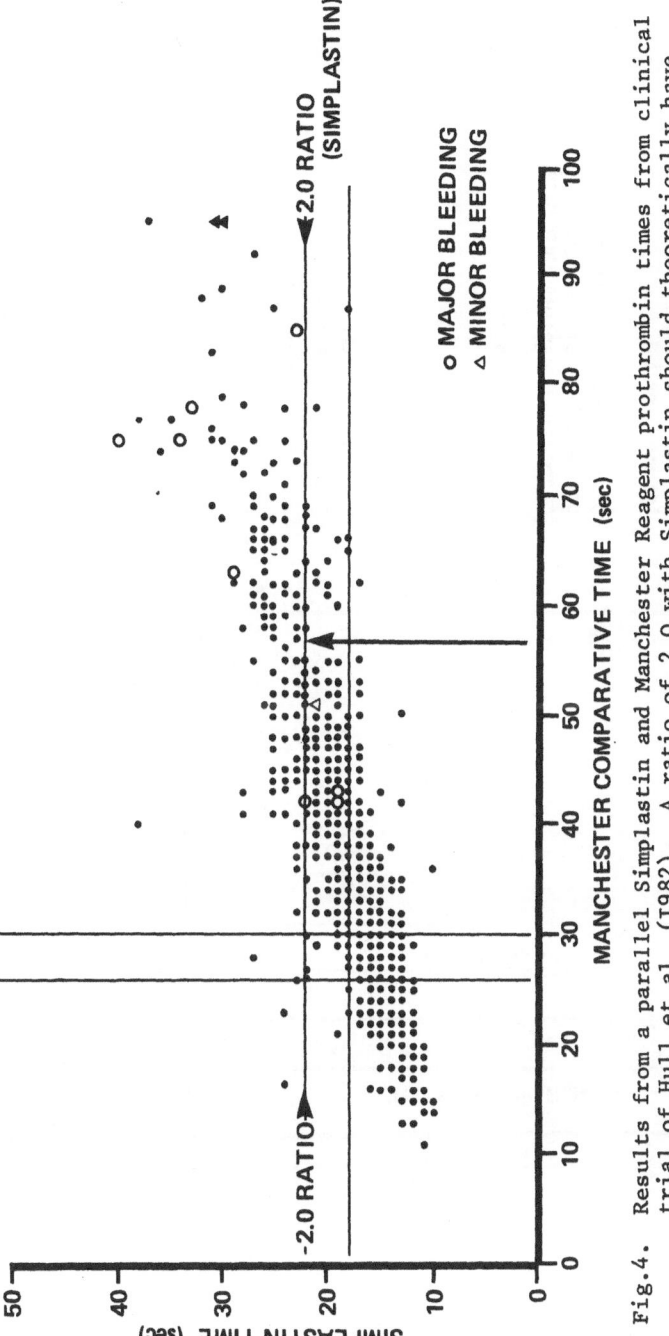

Fig. 4. Results from a parallel Simplastin and Manchester Reagent prothrombin times from clinical trial of Hull et al. (1982). A ratio of 2.0 with Simplastin should theoretically have provided a value of 4.7 ratio (INR) with Manchester Reagent. The scatter of values obtained is an indication of the error of the method comparing these two unlike reagents.

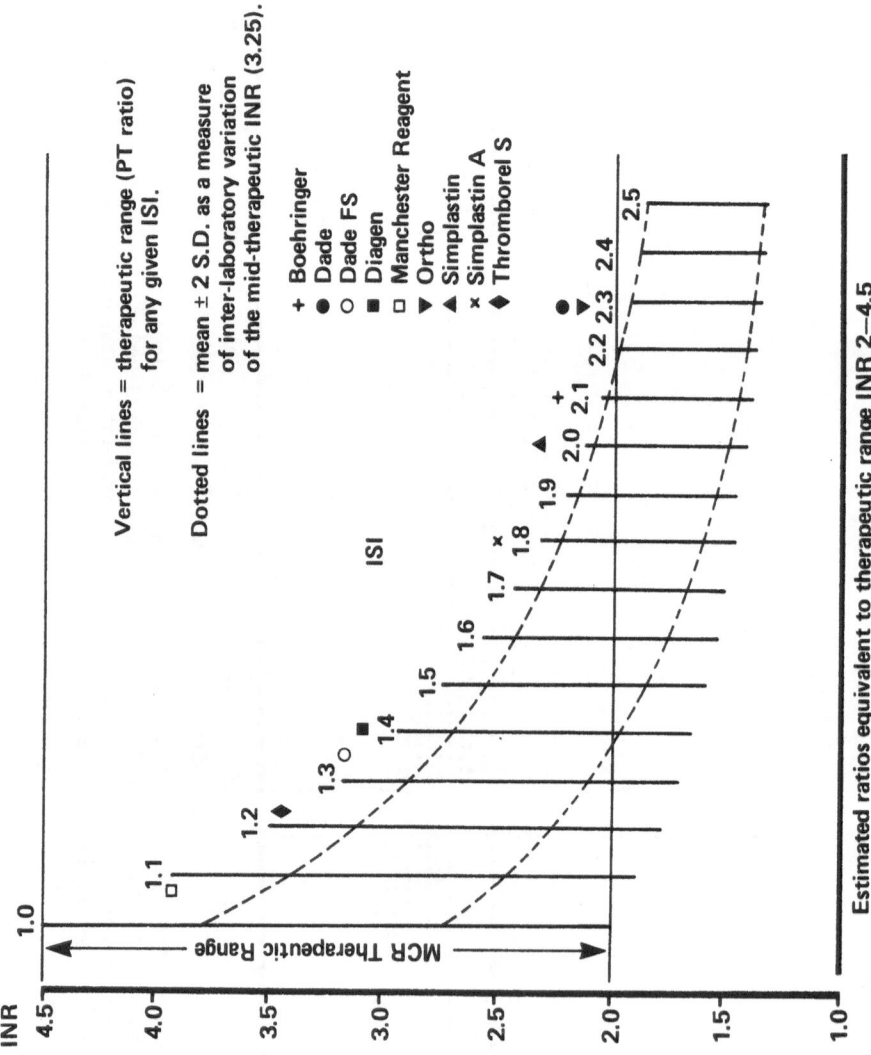

Fig.5. The ISI values of thromboplastins and the effect of ISI
with the therapeutic range and discrimination of
therapeutic ratios from normal with individual reagents.

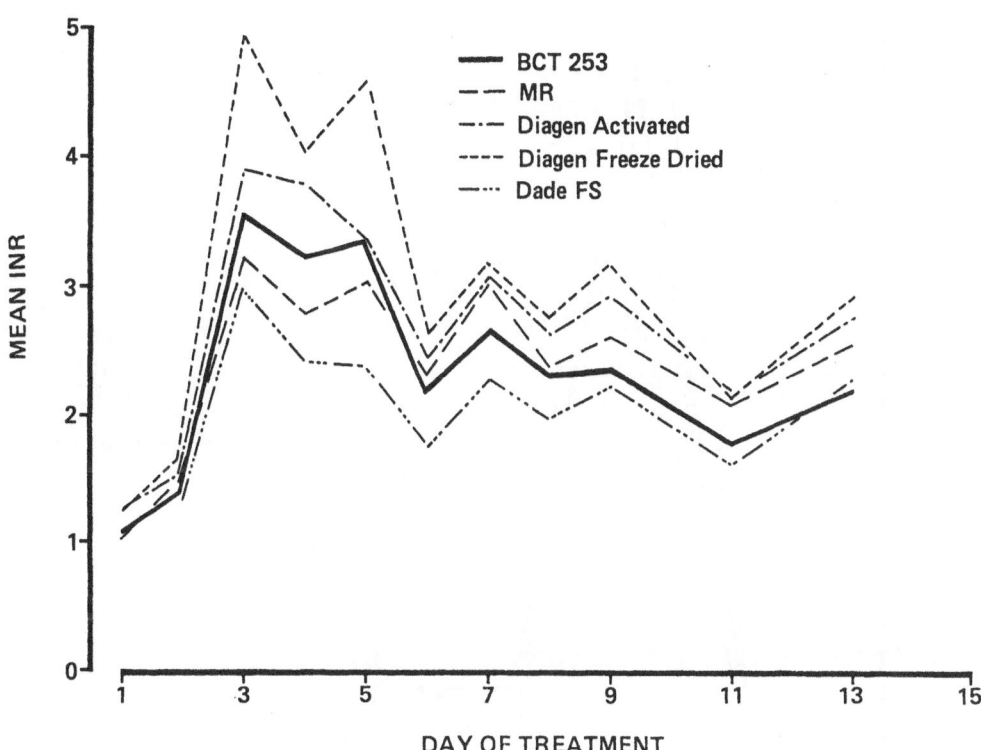

Fig.6. INR responses with different thromboplastin preparations
during induction phase of oral anticoagulant treatment.

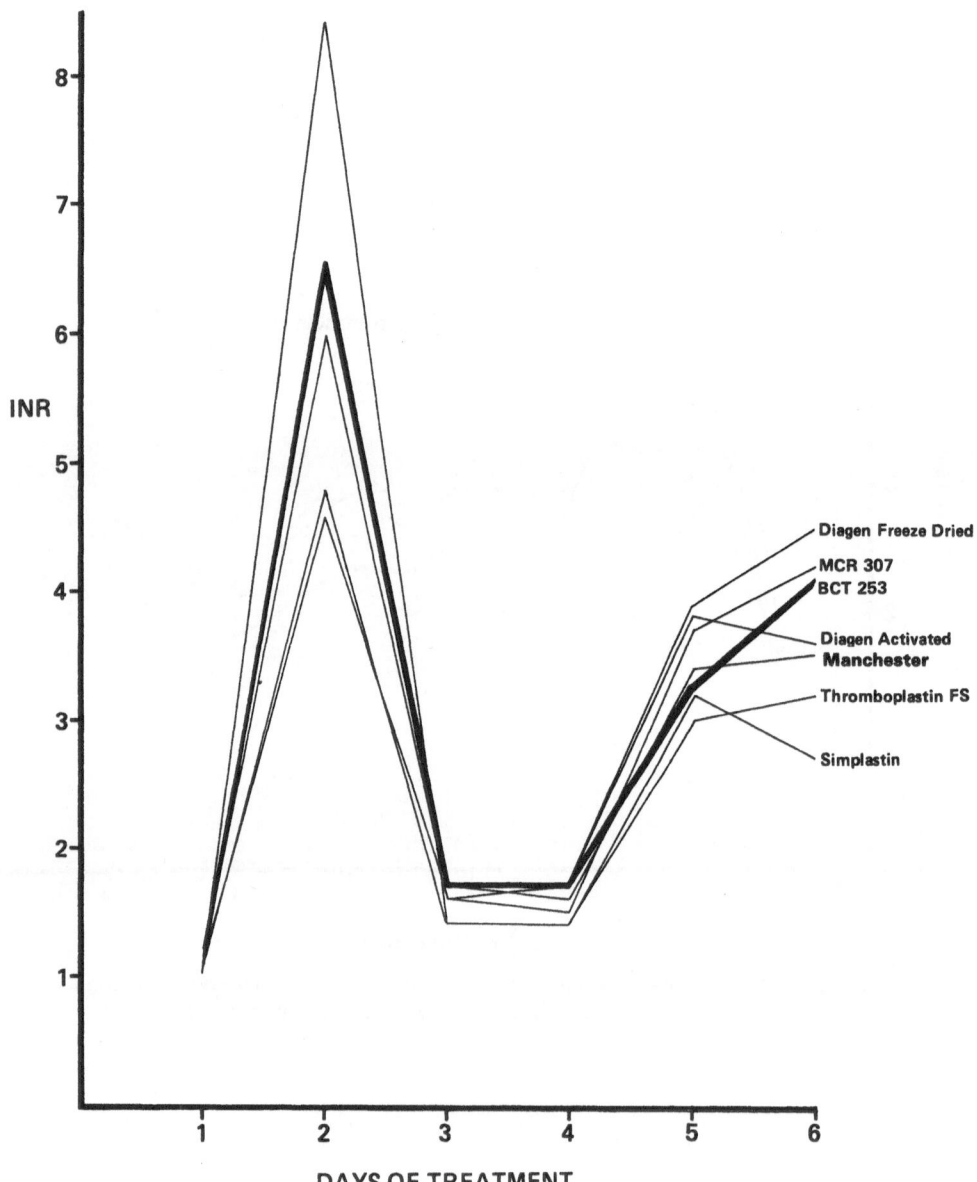

Fig.7. INR responses with different thromboplastin preparations
during induction phase of oral anticoagulant treatment.

TABLE 1

Diagen Activated.	Mean INR (3 plasmas)
Coag-a-Mate x 2 (5), Coag-a-Pet (dual)(3)	2.56
Burkard/S & G (4)	2.69
KC IO (8), Manual (26)	3.00
Biomatic 2000 (3)	3.36

Manchester.	Mean INR (3 plasmas)
Biodata (9)	2.45
Coag-a-Pet (dual)(II)	2.49
Coag-a-Mate x 2 (I5)	2.5I
Fibrometer (5), Hyland Clotek (3), Lancer (8)	2.56
Cobas Fibro Roche (3), Burkard/S & G	2.59
KC IO (20)	2.62
Fibrintimer (I8)	2.63
Manual (I9I)	2.64
Biomatic BIO (5)	2.67
Biomatic 2000 (9)	2.7I

(figures in parenthesis = number of users)

I986 Series (8 plasmas)	Mean INR
Thromboplastin FS	2.39
Thromborel S	2.54
Manchester	2.76
Diagen Activated	2.95
Diagen FD	3.2I

Assessment scheme in blood coagulation. (see Table I) Automation is seen to cause additional problems as some coagulometers are seen to give results which diverge considerably from the overall mean and from the manual method.

The implementation of the INR system is by no means a simple task however. There has been a great improvement in the performance of national control laboratories represented in the WHO International programme conducted from the UK Reference Laboratory. Their performance in reporting INR with their local reagent is now comparable with that one result with the BCT reference preparation in the same laboratories which is a dramatic improvement from the situation of two years ago when the system was first applied.

ERRORS IN CALIBRATION BY MANUFACTURERS

A good deal of work remains to improve the manufacturers' calibrations of their own reagents.

INR values in clinical practice are largely derived from calibrations undertaken by commercial manufacturers. That these are not yet being adequately performed is suggested by the previous results and confirmed by the independent calibration by two UK laboratories (UK Reference Laboratory and Welsh National School of Medicine) of those manufacturers' products where an ISI is provided. (see Table 2) The data from the Welsh School of Medicine is provided by permission of Dr. J.C. Giddings. The true INR of a plasma with a stated INR of 4.0 according to manufacturers' INR tables as given in Table 3.

TABLE 2

Reagent	Stated ISI (manufacturer)	Observed ISI lab.I.	lab.2.
Dade FS	I.18	I.36	I.3I
Diagen A	I.4	I.5I	I.67
Manchester	I.12	-	I.I3
Thromborel S	I.07	I.23	I.24

TABLE 3

True INR values for a stated INR of 4.0 from manufacturer's tables.

Dade FS	4.9
Diagen A	4.5
Manchester	4.0
Thromborel S	4.9

The limitations of this scheme in long-term stabilised patients are reflected in the results from the UK National External Quality Assessment Scheme in Blood Coagulation. (see Table 4) The results are derived from samples of long-term stabilised patients and show the extent of the divergence in mean INR with thromboplastin used in the UK. These reflect

TABLE 4

Survey No.53 (1986)

Plasma No: Reagent/Method	No. of users	I1 Mean INR	I2 Mean INR	I3 Mean INR
Diagen Activated	56	2.98	2.64	3.I5
Diagen Freeze-dried	9	3.I2	2.8I	3.I3
Manchester	3I6	2.90	2.28	2.67
Thromboplastin FS	8	2.38	2.02	2.28
Thromborel S	3	2.33	I.93	2.I3
All reagents	392	2.90	2.33	2.74

the accuracy of manufacturers' calibrations.

It may be concluded that it is desirable to employ a reagent of optimum sensitivity (low ISI) for control of oral anticoagulant dosage. As the prothrombin time is used not only for control of anticoagulant dosage but also to screen coagulation disorders and to assess liver function, ability to detect individual defects of extrinsic clotting factors is important. Screening for liver disease and monitoring its progress demands good sensitivity to factor VII.

To summarise the present position on PT standardisation it can be stated that the introduction of the INR system is a considerable advance. It should pave the way to safer and more effective anticoagulant treatment and the development of safer methods of laboratory control as well as providing a common scale for dosage and clinical trials. It should provide manufacturers with a procedure for assessing the relative sensitivity of their reagents to depression of vitamin K-dependent clotting factors and perhaps promote improved reagents. Not until manufacturers produce high sensitivity reagents and accurately calibrate their reagents will the situation improve. The INR/ISI system should now provide a mechanism to achieve this goal and improve standards of clinical oral anticoagulant dose administration.

THERAPEUTIC RANGES

Therapeutic ranges of anticoagulation can be established only by planned randomised clinical trials in the prevention or treatment of the relevant thrombotic disorder. These must be of sufficient size and duration to assess the clinically relevant end-point.

Oral anticoagulant treatment is very dependent for its effectiveness and safety on laboratory control by the PT test. The lower limit of a therapeutic range should be the minimum coagulation defect necessary for the prevention of recurrence or extension of an established thrombotic episode. There is no virtue in choosing a coagulation defect which is safe from haemorrhage if it does not protect against thrombosis. The upper limit should be the coagulation defect which prevents thrombosis but in normal circumstances does not cause either spontaneous bleeding or excessive bleeding in response to haemostatic challenge. The greater the target coagulation defect inevitably the higher must be the risk of haemorrhage.

Table 5 gives the recommendations on treatment ranges of the British Society for Haematology (BSH).

The BSH based its proposals on clinical trial reports (e.g. Sevitt and Gallagher,[17] Poller and Taberner,[5] and Hull et al.[16]), cumulative experience in the British system for anticoagulant control, and a UK national survey of current practice in 1983. Whereas the limits for the prophylaxis and the treatment of venous thrombosis have been clearly defined, they are less clear for arterial thrombosis.

Before the introduction of the INR system it was not possible to make valid comparisons between the intensity of anticoagulation in clinical trials at individual centres using different laboratory methodology or reagents. It is now even possible to reassess some of the major clinical trials on the basis of the INR values. This is because MCR thromboplastin, because of its rigid programme of standardisation, has been unchanged over the years with relatively unchanged ISI values. During this time MCR has been used to calibrate the respective local thromboplastin reagents in the trials which reference will be made in this presentation. Thus the target INR values can be determined with reasonable accuracy retrospectively.

MYOCARDIAL INFARCTION

When oral anticoagulants were first introduced the claims were exaggerated; but, as Mitchell,[18] commented, the discipline required for sound clinical trials had not been developed at that time.

The introduction of new laboratory methods (such as the "P + P test",[2] and Thrombotest,[3]) specifically designed for control or oral anticoagulants led organisers of trials in the 1960's - unsuspectingly - to provide a less intense coagulation defect than previously. Dosage in an important Danish study,[19] was based on the "P and P" test and aimed at 10-25% activity, which is equivalent to only 1.2 and 1.5 INR. The British Medical Research Council's short term study published in 1969,[20] was regarded as a model of trial design but regrettably used a homoeopathic target coagulation defect of 15% Thrombotest activity (1.6 International Normalised Ratio approx.) in place of the more intense defect in its previous, more favourable long term studies. The mean anticoagulant dose differed considerably in the two trials (71.6 mg. phenindione in the second study against the higher dose of 108 mg. in the first). Anticoagulants in myocardial infarction fell out of favour in the 60's and 70's.

The report of the Sixty-plus Reinfarction Group of the Netherlands Thrombosis Service revived the issue.[21] This was a randomised double blind study of 878 patients (mean age 61.6 years with 85% men) based on sound clinical and laboratory control. The target therapeutic range of 5% to 10% Thrombotest activity (INR 2.0 to 4.5) was achieved in 72% of tests. The mortality was 13.4% in a two year follow-up in the placebo group but 7.6% in those treated with coumarin. The cynic could reasonably argue that the only conclusion to be drawn from the Sixty-plus study is that once oral anticoagulant treatment has been established for six months it is dangerous to stop. The reported low incidence of severe haemorrhagic events (one in 25 treatment years) in the Dutch study would be unlikely to be matched in countries where more intense anticoagulation is still practised.

TABLE 5. - Proposed therapeutic ranges (British Society for Haematology guidelines on oral anticoagulants, 1984).

British ratio (INR)*	Clinical state
2.0–2.5	Prophylaxis of deep vein thrombosis including high risk surgery 2.0–3.0 for hip surgery and operations for fractured femur.
2.0–3.0	Treatment of deep vein thrombosis, pulmonary embolism, transient ischaemic attacks.
3.0–4.5	Recurrent deep vein thrombosis and pulmonary embolism; arterial disease including myocardial infarction; arterial grafts; cardiac prosthetic valves and grafts.

* British ratios and international normalised ratios (INR) are virtually identical within the therapeutic range.

Administration of oral anticoagulants to patients after deep vein thrombosis with or without associated pulmonary embolism has been accepted clinical practice since the early 1940's.

The only controlled prospective randomised trial among the early studies was reported from Britain, but it has been criticised because of the small numbers.[22] Since that time on ethical grounds no investigators have felt justified in including untreated controls in clinical trials of anticoagulants in deep vein thrombosis.

Studies at McMaster University have clarified the value of warfarin in deep vein thrombosis. Warfarin was given to patients with acute deep vein thrombosis after 14 days of administration of heparin. In the first study the patients were randomised into two groups given warfarin and low dose subcutaneous heparin (5000 units three times a day).[23] There were nine recurrences of deep vein thrombosis in 35 patients given low dose heparin but no recurrence in the 33 patients given warfarin. In this study and the follow-up study using the same target prothrombin ratios with Simplastin, 1.5 to 2.0 (INR equivalent 3.0-4.5), the incidence of bleeding with oral anticoagulants was 21% to 22%.[24] Bleeding complications are, however, relatively uncommon using the therapeutic ranges usual in Britain. In the third randomised study,[16] a less intense, British type of range based on a 2.0 to 2.5 ratio range with Manchester Comparative Reagent (INR 2.0-2.5) was compared with the 1.5 to 2.0 Simplastin ratio range. The incidence of bleeding was 22.4% with Simplastin control but only 4.3% with the Manchester Comparative Reagent control (p = 0.015), though both regimens were equally successful in preventing rethrombosis. The mean doses of warfarin were 5.8 mg. and 4.9 mg. respectively. The McMaster trials have convincingly shown not only the value of warfarin in the treatment of deep vein thrombosis but also the greater safety from haemorrhage that comes from a combination of a sensitive control technique with an International Normalised Ratio range of 2.0 to 2.5. Unfortunately, with most of the present commercial reagents overdosage may still occur even with this low range, particularly in the early days of treatment, owing to their relative insensitivity to the coumarin induced defect at this stage.

PROPHYLAXIS AGAINST DEEP VEIN THROMBOSIS

Oral anticoagulants are still regarded as the most certain protection against deep vein thrombosis, though they have not proved popular with surgeons because of their fear of bleeding. Low dose heparin and some non-invasive procedures have therefore been preferred - despite their failures in high risk patients.

The first controlled study of oral anticoagulants was at the Birmingham Accident Hospital.[17] Three hundred patients with recent hip fractures were allocated to oral anticoagulant or control groups according to day of admission. The target for anticoagulant control was a ratio of 2.0 to 3.0 using a Quick test thromboplastin matched against Manchester Comparative Reagent (INR equivalent 2.0 to 3.0). The incidence of clinical deep vein thrombosis was reduced from 28.7% to 2.7% by oral anticoagulants; the more reliable necropsy data indicated a reduction of deep vein thrombosis from 83% to 14%. In a further controlled necropsy study Sevitt and Innes,[25] found that a 10-25% Thrombotest range of activity was inadequate to protect against deep vein thrombosis but ratios (INR) greater than 2.0 with the Quick test calibrated against Manchester Comparative Reagent did give protection.

Taberner et al.,[26] carried out a controlled randomised study which showed the effectiveness of oral anticoagulation in prophylaxis in a group of patients at moderate risk undergoing surgery for gynaecological disorders. The therapeutic range target of 2.0 to 2.5 with Manchester Comparative Reagent (INR 2.0 to 2.5) was achieved preoperatively. This reduced the incidence of deep vein thrombosis without increasing operative bleeding.

PROSTHETIC HEART VALVES

Oral anticoagulants are given long term, usually on a lifelong basis, for patients with prosthetic heart valves. The indications are strong for patients with mitral valve prostheses, whereas tissue valves are safer, particularly in the aortic position, and may not need anticoagulant protection. The therapeutic range of 3.0 to 4.5 British ratios (INR) given in Table I represents current practice based on the 1983 survey from 270 major British centres.

REFERENCES

I.   A. J. Quick, The prothrombin in haemophilia and in obstructive jaundice, J. Biol. Chem. I09:73-74 (I935).
2.   P. A. Owren and K. Aas, The control of dicoumarol therapy and the quantitative determination of prothrombin and proconvertin, Scand. J. Clin. Lab. Invest. 3:20I-208 (I95I).
3.   P. A. Owren, Thrombotest: a new method for controlling anticoagulant therapy, Lancet ii:754-758 (I959).
4.   C. W. Francis, V. J. Marder, E. C. McCollister, and S. Yankoolbodi, Two step warfarin therapy, J. Am. Med. Assoc. 249:374-378 (I983).
5.   L. Poller and D. A. Taberner, Dosage and Control of oral anticoagulants, An international survey, Br. J. Haematol. 5I:479 (I982).
6.   L. Poller, Standardisation of anticoagulant treatment: The Manchester Regional Thromboplastin Scheme, Br. Med. J. 2:565-566 (I964).
7.   R. Biggs, Report on the standardisation of the one stage prothrombin time for the control of anticoagulant therapy, in: "Genetics and the interaction of blood clotting factors," R. B. Hunter, I. S. Wright and F. Koller, eds., Thrombosis et Diathesis Haemorrhagica Supplement I7:303-327 (I965).
8.   L. Poller, The British Comparative Thromboplastin: the use of the national thromboplastin reagent for uniformity of laboratory control of oral anticoagulants and expression of results, Assoc. Clin. Pathol., Broadsheet No.7I (I970).
9.   J. B. Miale and J. W. Kent, Standardisation of the therapeutic range for oral anticoagulants based on standard reference plasmas, Am. J. Clin. Pathol., 60:453-457 (I972).
I0. T. B. L. Kirkwood, Calibration of reference thromboplastins, Thromb. Haemost. (Stuttgart) 49:238-244 (I983).
II. J. Hermans, A. M. P. H. van den Besselaar, E. A. Loeliger, and E. A. van der Veld, A collaborative calibration study of reference materials for thromboplastins, Thromb. Haemost. (Stuttgart) 50:3: 7I2-7I7 (I983).
I2. J. M. Thomson, J. A. Tomenson, and L. Poller, The calibration of the Second Primary International Reference Preparation for Thromboplastin (Thromboplastin, human, plain, coded BCT/253), Thromb. Haemost. (Stuttgart) 52:336-342 (I984).
I3. J. M. Thomson, K. V. Darby, and L. Poller, Calibration of BCT/44I the ICSH Reference Preparation for Thromboplastin, Thromb. Haemost. (Stuttgart) 55:379-382 (I986).

14. J. A. Tomenson, A statistician's independent evaluation, in: "Thromboplastin calibration and oral anticoagulant control," A. M. H. P. van den Besselaar, H. R. Gralnick, and S. M. Lewis, eds., Martinus Nijhoff, The Hague (1984).

15. R. Hull, J. Hirsh, R. Jay, C. Carter, C. England, M. Gent, A. G. Turpie, D. McLaughlin, P. Dodd, M. Thomas, G. Rascob, and P. Ockelford, Different intensities of anticoagulation in the long-term treatment of proximal venous thrombosis, N. Eng. J. Med. 307:1676-1681 (1982).

16. J. Koepke, Use of survey validated plasma as a means of prothrombin time standardisation, in: "Standardisation of coagulation assays," D. Triplett, ed., College of Clinical Pathologists, Skokie, Illinois (1982).

17. S. Sevitt and N. G. Gallagher, Prevention of venous thrombosis and pulmonary embolism in injured patients, Lancet ii:974-980 (1959).

18. J. R. A. Mitchell, Anticoagulants in coronary heart disease, Lancet i: 257-262 (1981).

19. J. Hilden, K. Iverson, F. Rasschon, and M. Schwarz, Anticoagulants in acute myocardial infarction, Lancet ii:327-331 (1961).

20. Medical Research Council, Assessment of short-term anticoagulant administration after cardiac infarction, Br. Med. J. 1:335-342 (1969).

21. Sixty-Plus Reinfarction Group, A double-blind trial to assess long-term oral anticoagulant therapy in elderly patients with myocardial infarction, Lancet ii:989-994 (1981).

22. D. W. Barrit and S. C. Jordan, Anticoagulant drugs in the treatment of thromboembolism, Lancet i:1309-1312 (1962).

23. R. Hull, T. Delmore, E. Genton, J. Hirsh, M. Gent, D. Sackett, D. McLoughlin, and P. Armstrong, Warfarin sodium versus low-dose heparin in the long-term treatment of venous thrombosis, N. Eng. J. Med. 301:855-858 (1979).

24. R. Hull, T. Delmore, C. Carter, J. Hirst, E. Genton, M. Gent, J. Turpie, and D. McLoughlin, Adjusted subcutaneous heparin versus warfarin sodium in the long-term treatment of venous thrombosis, N. Eng. J. Med. 306:189-194 (1982).

25. S. Sevitt and D. Innes, Prothrombin time and Thrombotest in injured patients on prophylactic anticoagulant therapy, Lancet i:124-130 (1964).

26. D. A. Taberner, L. Poller, R. W. Burslem, and J. B. Jones, Oral anticoagulants controlled by British Comparative Thromboplastin versus low-dose heparin prophylaxis of deep vein thrombosis, Br. Med. J. 1:272-274 (1978).

COLD-PROMOTED ACTIVATION OF FACTOR VII AND

SHORTENING OF THE PROTHROMBIN TIME

Harvey R. Gralnick and Olga J. Wilson

Hematology Service, Clinical Pathology Department
Clinical Center, National Institutes of Health
Building 10, Room 2C390, Bethesda, MD 20892

INTRODUCTION

The previous speakers have summarized our knowledge concerning the biochemistry, function, synthesis and molecular biology of the coagulation factors II, VII, IX, X, and protein C and S. In particular, they have highlighted the role of the gamma carboxyglutamic acid, the biosynthetic rates and the specific steps in the activation of these proteins. This has led to a clear understanding of the biologic effect of the vitamin K antagonists. The studies of tissue factor have elucidated various aspects of this apoprotein and its function. Yet with this great body of knowledge, there is still a great deal of consternation about the test most commonly utilized to clinically monitor the effects of vitamin K antagonists, the prothrombin time.

As you have just heard, the calibration of therapeutic range by the International Normalized Ratio has been proposed so that the intensity of the anticoagulation can be better standardized throughout the world. Recent difficulties have been recognized in interpreting the blood test which monitors the potency of the anticoagulation. A variety of the important aspects which affect the prothrombin time must be considered in the decision-making process of the clinician in administering this drug to patients and maintaining a safe level of anticoagulation.

The prothrombin time is the most common coagulation procedure performed in the hemostasis laboratory. It is used as a measure of the extrinsic coagulation system to monitor warfarin anticoagulant therapy, as an indicator of hepatic disease, to detect inhibitors of blood coagula-tion and as a general screening test for blood coagulation. It is important in all blood coagulation assays that the sample be obtained without inducing cellular activation, coagulation factor activation or activation of other systems which may modify hemostasis, i.e., fibrinolysis, prekallikrein-bradykinin, etc. It is hoped that the sample collected for blood coagulation analysis is a reflection of the blood circulating in the patient, i.e, neither in-vitro activation nor other artifacts have occurred in the sample. In an attempt to standardize the pretest variables, the National Committee on Clinical Laboratory Standards (NCCLS) has provided a guideline for the collection, transport and preparation of blood specimens for coagulation testing and performance of coagulation assays,[1] and a second document on the proposed guideline for the one-stage prothrombin time.[2] These two guidelines are intended to increase the uniformity in the collection, storage and preparation of blood or plasma before and during coagulation testing. Adherence to these guidelines should reduce the number of potential artifacts in the pretest and testing period.

Some of the major areas of concern which have been examined are the concentration of sodium citrate anticoagulant most efficacious for performing the prothrombin time, the type of collection system most suited for reducing or eliminating in vitro activation of blood, and the processing and storage of plasma or whole blood to maintain the blood as near as possible to its in-vivo state.

Studies of the sodium citrate anticoagulant at 109 and 129 mM (3.2% and 3.8%, respectively) have indicated no major differences in the prothrombin time in normal individuals or in those individuals who were receiving oral anticoagulants.[3]

Four collection systems for analyzing the prothrombin time, a borosilicate evacuated system, a siliconized borosilicate evacuated system, a new generation of siliconized borosilicate evacuated tubes and the use of polypropylene or polystyrene tubes were examined. The prothrombin time of blood collected in the borosilicate or the siliconized borosilicate tubes had a progressive shortening of the prothrombin time.[3-5] In general, by 2 hours the prothrombin time of normal or anticoagulated blood had shortened by 12-15% and by 4 hours was shortened by 22-28% (Figure 1). The blood collected in the new generation of siliconized borosilicate tubes showed a marked improvement in the in-vitro shortening of the prothrombin time. Normal blood showed insignificant amounts of shortening over a 4- to 6-hour incubation period, and the blood from the majority of anticoagulated patients (60%) showed no significant activation when held at $4^{\circ}C$ for 4 hours.[6] At 4 hours 40% of the patients had a 10-27% shortening of the prothrombin time (Figure 2). At 6 hours this decrease in the prothrombin time varied between 12-42%. When blood was collected in polypropylene tubes and the prothrombin time analyzed, less than 10% shortening of the prothrombin time was seen in patients receiving oral anticoagulants and in normal individuals. All samples are stable for at least 6 hours either as plasma separated from cells or whole blood in polypropylene tubes.

The Dutch group and the group from Manchester, England, have shown similar results when the blood of normal individuals or patients receiving oral anticoagulant therapy had been analyzed in an evacuated tube system.[4,7] van den Besselaar and Loeliger found that the prothrombin time was shortened when the blood was collected and maintained at ambient temperatures.[4] Their results are very similar to our results in that polystyrene tubes showed minimal activation while either glass or a variety of siliconized borosilicate evacuated tubes showed significant shortening of the prothrombin time. They showed that acid treatment of siliconized glass markedly reduced the in-vitro shortening of the prothrombin time. The glass tubes had to be acid treated for 12 days.

van den Besselaar et al. have stated that the new siliconized process of the evacuated tube system is suitable for long-term storage of blood for the determination of the prothrombin time.[8] These results seem to be in disagreement with those mentioned above,[6] and this may be due to the fact that pooled plasma was used in their studies to determine the stability of plasma. It is not stated how many individual patients were studied over a time course, and the paper describes only 2 patients studied in this manner. These data, then, may not be much different from our observations since approximately 1 out of 3 patients will have a marked shortening of their prothrombin time in blood collected in these evacuated tubes.

Thomson, who has similar data concerning borosilicate or siliconized borosilicate tubes, has indicated that there is not sufficient evidence on the reliability of the evacuated tube system. She has suggested that it might be worthwhile, if possible, to employee the system most commonly used in Europe and the United Kingdom, i.e., a syringe and a specially prepared tube for coagulation studies.[7]

THE PERCENTAGE SHORTENING OF THE PROTHROMBIN TIME

Effects of Whole Blood Storage

Incubation Temperature	Collection Tube	Normal			
		0'	1'	2'	4'
4°C	Borosilicate	3.4 ± 3.1*	10.3 ± 3.9	17.2 ± 3.5	23.3 ± 2.8
	Silicone Borosilicate	0 ± 2.3	3.4 ± 4.0	11.8 ± 3.6	16.9 ± 1.9
	Polypropylene	0 ± 3.4	1.7 ± 3.6	2.6 ± 2.3	1.7 ± 2.5

*Values are mean percent shortening ± the coefficient of variation.

Figure 1A: The effect of whole blood storage on the thrombin time of blood from a normal individual. The results are expressed as the mean percent decrease in seconds ± the coefficient of variation.

THE PERCENTAGE SHORTENING OF THE PROTHROMBIN TIME

Effects of Whole Blood Storage

Incubation Temperature	Collection Tube	Patient A				Patient B				Patient C			
		0'	1'	2'	4'	0'	1'	2'	4'	0'	1'	2'	4'
4°C	Borosilicate	1.0	11.1	12.6	14.4	7.8	18.6	25.6	29.5	19.4	23.4	29.2	38.5
	Silicone Borosilicate	0	2.6	0	1.5	0.7	6.6	12.4	19.4	8.0	18.6	24.8	35.4
	Polypropylene	0	4.8	5.5	5.5	0	1.6	7.7	5.4	0	0.9	0	2.7

Figure 1B: Similar studies employing the blood from three patients on chronic oral anticoagulant therapy.

Palmer and Gralnick and van den Besselaar and Loeliger have shown that the in vitro shortening of the prothrombin time is not dependent upon any cellular elements.[3,4] When blood is collected and the plasma immediately spun, then separated from the cellular elements, and the plasma stored in borosilicate or siliconized borosilicate tubes, the same degree of shortening of the prothrombin time is seen as when the plamsa is left in contact with the cellular elements (Figure 3).

The in-vitro shortening of the prothrombin time is a major problem in attempting to determine the efficacy of oral anticoagulant therapy as a anti-thrombotic agent. The number of patients who receive oral anticoagulant therapy who will have a marked shortening of the prothrombin time when blood is collected into the new generation of siliconized tubes remains unknown. But clearly, there is a number of patients who will have significant amounts of coagulation activation and shortening of the prothrombin time. Yet this is an improvement since in the studies with the borosilicate and the older generation of siliconized borosilicate tubes, almost all individuals had a shortening of their prothrombin time when their blood was collected in these tubes.

A large collection of investigators have studied the mechanism of the glass activation of coagulation and its effect(s) on coagulation factors. The glass activation of coagulation and resultant increase in factor VII can be traced from approximately 1935 to the present time. In 1935[8], Lenggenhager postulated that blood thromboplastic activity arose after contact of an inactive plasma precursor with a foreign substance.[9] Subsequently, several investigators presented evidence of the glass activation of a plasma thromboplastin precursor. It was considered that this precursor was anti-hemophilic B factor or factor IX. Alexander et al.[10] showed that factor VII activity of serum from blood clotted in silicone-coated tubes was less than that from the serum of blood clotted in contact with glass. They also showed that the addition of tissue factor to the blood increased the factor VII activity of the resultant serum. Rapaport and coworkers[11] showed that the exposure of platelet-poor plasma to glass increased the activity of factor IX and factor VII with no change in factors II, V or VIII. When glass powder was added to plasma, the factor VII activity rose at least three-fold. When this was performed with plasma from patients taking a warfarin derivative, it masked the reductions in the factor VII content of the plasma as the factor VII rose to normal levels. The authors struggled with the possible mechanism for the glass activation of factor IX, only to discover later that activated factor VII or the factor VII tissue factor complex can activate factor IX. In 1955, Hageman factor (factor XII) was first described, and in 1958 it was clear that Hageman factor played an important role in the initiation of blood coagulation induced by glass.[12,13] This series of seemingly unrelated experiments has set forth the basis for discovery during the 1970's of the interaction between the intrinsic and extrinsic pathway of blood coagulation, in particular, the role of activated factor XII on factor VII. This interaction of the contact phase of blood coagulation described during the 1970's is the basis for the cold-promoted activation of the prothrombin time activation and of factor VII seen in patients receiving oral anticoagulant therapy.

Gjonnaess[14] described the cold-promoted shortening of the thrombotest in the plasmas of women on oral contraceptives or in the third trimester of pregnancy. The explanation given for this shortening was an activation of factor VII and activation of the intrinsic coagulation system. Subsequently, this author thought that the activating factor of factor VII was linked to the activation of the kallikrein system, and that the activator was plasma kallikrein.[15] His studies showed that activators of prekallikrein could induce generation of factor VII activator activity which directed his attention towards plasma kallikrein as the activator.[16] Very little attention was given to the possible implications

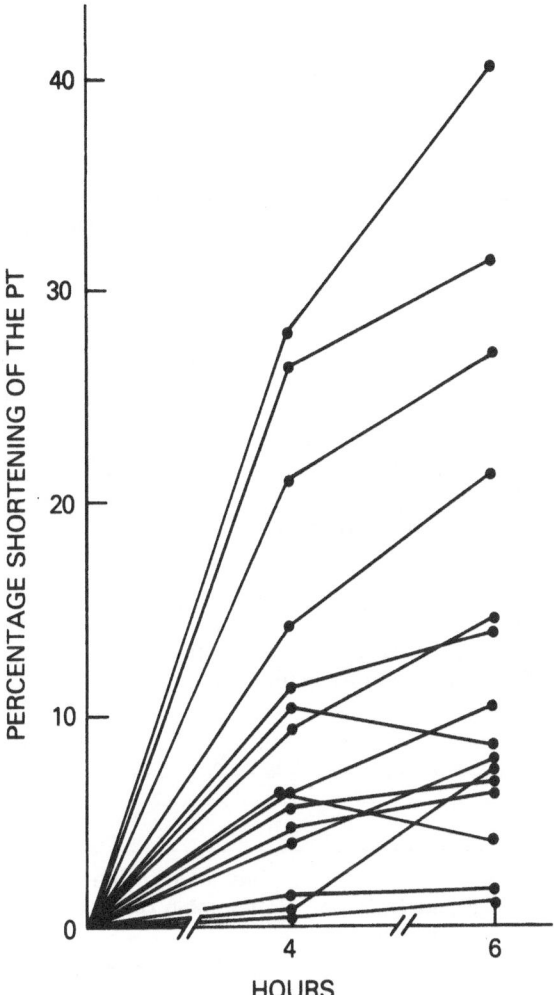

Figure 2: The shortening of the prothrombin time of 15 patients receiving chronic oral anticoagulant therapy. When the blood was collected in the new siliconized borosilicate tubes at 4 and 6 hours, 6 of the 15 patients (40%) have greater than 10% shortening of the prothrombin time. Blood from normal individuals tested in an identical manner showed a 3-4% shortening of the prothrombin time at 6 hours.

of these findings in relation to the prothrombin time or thrombotest in the monitoring of oral anticoagulation therapy.

We and others demonstrated that the prothrombin time in normal individuals and patients receiving warfarin therapy had marked shortening when blood was collected in any type of tube other than polypropylene.[3,5] Studies of the coagulation factors involved in the cold-induced activation of prothrombin time revealed the importance of factors XII, IX and VII, prekallikrein and high molecular weight kininogen (Figure 4).[17] Studies with purified coagulation proteins had previously shown that factor VII activation could be mediated by activated factor XII or factor XII fragments.[18-22] Factor IX also played a role in the activation of factor VII. It was thought that the IX activation was dependent, in part, on the activation of prekallikrein. The activated factor VII resulted in the

THE PERCENTAGE SHORTENING OF THE PROTHROMBIN TIME

Effects of Plasma Storage

Collection Tube	Plasma Tube	Normal			
		30″	1′	2′	4′
BOROSILICATE	Borosilicate	3.7	8.3	16.7	22.2
	Polypropylene	1.0	1.0	1.0	4.5
POLYPROPYLENE	Borosilicate	3.7	6.5	17.5	26.8
	Polypropylene	0	0	1.0	2.8

Figure 3: This depicts the effect of plasma storage in borosilicate or polypropylene tubes. Regardless of the collection tube system, the extent of the plasma activation in the borosilicate tubes was independent of the presence of other cellular elements.

Factor Deficient in Blood	Shortening of the Prothrombin Time (%)	
	2 Hr	4 Hr
None	13.6	21.4
Factor XII	3.0	2.7
HMW Kininogen	<0.5	0.5
Prekallikrein	5.0	6.5
Factor XI	11.0	18.3
Factor IX	8.8	10.9
C̄Ī INH	23.4	39.0

Figure 4: The effect of coagulation factor-deficient blood on the cold-promoted decrease in the prothrombin time. None is blood without any coagulation deficiency, i.e., control. Factor XII-deficient, high molecular weight kininogen-deficient and prekallikrein-deficient blood showed minimal in vitro shortening of the prothrombin time. Factor IX-deficient blood had approximately 50% decrease in the prothrombin time compared to normal blood, while factor XI-deficient blood could not be distinguished from normal. Blood deficient in the C1 INH had the largest decrease in the prothrombin time.

shortening of the prothrombin time. These data were substantiated in whole blood by examining the effect of single coagulation factor deficiency on cold-promoted factor VII activation and shortening of the prothrombin time. Blood deficient in factor XII (Hageman factor) demonstrated little or no cold-induced factor VII activation or shortening of the prothrombin time.[17,23] However, the absence of factor XI did not affect the contact activation of factor VII and the prothrombin time while deficiency of factor IX resulted in an approximately 50% reduction in the degree of cold activation (Figure 4). Plasma deficient in high molecular weight kininogen or plasma deficient in pre-kallikrein had very little cold-promoted activation indicating the important role these two factors play in the enhancement of factor XII activation and ensuing factor VII activation.[17,24]

Our data and that of Miller et al.[25] appear to be in complete agreement that the contact phase of blood coagulation and the intrinsic pathway were the most important aspects of the cold-promoted activation of factor VII and shortening of the prothrombin time. However, recently, Muller et al.[26] have shown that thrombin may also play a role in the cold-promoted activation of factor VII. The differences in the results are difficult to discern. Muller et al used extremely large doses of hirudin, and it appeared that over time the hirudin lost its inhibitory activity. Thus, it is not clear at this time what, if any, role thrombin plays in the cold-promoted activation of factor VII.

We studied the effect of cold activation on blood from normal individuals or patients taking chronic oral anticoagulant drugs and examined the changes in the various coagulation factors. We found that factor VII was the only factor which was consistently elevated with levels varying between 140-320% of baseline value (Figures 5 and 6).[17] There was an excellent correlation of the increase in factor VII activity and the shortening of the prothrombin time (Figure 6). We found that there were no changes in factor X, prekallikrein or factor XII. Also, factors V and IX showed no significant changes over a 4-hour incubation period. It is possible that with longer periods of incubation many of these factors will be modified, however, the longer the incubation period the more likely that results of studies will depend upon the activation as well as the decay of these coagulation proteins.

Studies with purified coagulation proteins have revealed that factor XIIa and factor XII fragments activate factor VII (Figure 7).[18-22] The activation of factor VII is directly proportional to the concentration of the factor XII fragments, and after initial rapid activation of factor VII a plateau is reached. The cause for this plateau has not been elucidated, however, in plasma systems it may be related to the effect of plasma inhibitors such as C1 INH, antithrombin III or the depletion of the pro-enzyme factor VII molecule. In purified systems, this is probably related to depletion of the proenzyme factor VII. Activated factor XII or its fragments are potent activators of the conversion of prekallikrein to kallikrein which then in turn catalyzes the activation of factor XII.[27,28] In purified systems, kallikrein does not directly activate factor VII but probably does indirectly activate factor VII by activating factor IX. Another possibility is that small amounts of factor VII and tissue factor activate factor IX which in turn closes the loop by activating more factor VII.[20-22,29]

In an effort to better understand the mechanism(s) of the cold-activation of factor VII in the prothrombin time, a variety of inhibitors to coagulation factors have been studied (Figure 8). The importance of C1 INH, a naturally-occurring inhibitor, to various aspects of the contact phase of blood coagulation was demonstrated by the addition of semi-purified C1 INH to the collection tube prior to venipuncture.[17] The C1 INH resulted in a concentration-dependent inhibition of the cold activation of the prothrombin time and factor VII. We felt that this was primarily due to the inhibition of the activation of factor XII and factor XII

COAGULATION FACTOR (%)

Tube		VII-X	VII	V	XII	P.T. % Shortening
Siliconized	0	115	84	104	119	+2
	1'	125	113	110	109	-2
	2'	147	138	111	108	-9
	4'	191	259	115	114	-17
Borosilicate	0	103	83	91	-	+2
	1'	143	155	102	90	-9
	2'	161	198	109	97	-16
	4'	238	353	129	95	-25
Polypropylene	0	116	87	110	116	-
	1'	117	84	113	114	+2
	2'	120	82	106	100	+2
	4'	113	84	107	117	+2

Figure 5: The effect of cold-promoted activation of the prothrombin time on coagulation factors.

fragments. Others had previously shown that C1 INH inhibited factor XII fragments, plasmin, kallikrein and the esterase activity of the complement system.[28,30-32] Recently, Weiss et al. have shown that C1 INH also acts upon the autoactivation of Hageman factor by inhibiting fragment formation.[33] They showed that the rate of auto-activation was decreased at $4^{\circ}C$ but that C1 INH activity was inhibited to an even greater degree. Other studies[32,34,35] have demonstrated that cold inhibits the activity of the C1 INH, and that although the functional activity does not change, the amount of biologic activity is significantly reduced. Part of this reduction in activity may be due to the formation of kallikrein or factor XII C1 INH complexes.

Hojima et al.[36] purified a Hageman factor inhibitor from sweet corn seeds (CHFI) and found that it inhibited Hageman factor fragments in a 1:1 M complex. The CHFI did not inhibit human plasma or urinary kallikrein, plasmin, alpha thrombin, bovine factor Xa or alpha chymotrypsin. They found that this inhibitor also blocked the hypotensive action of plasma protein fraction and activated Hageman factor in experimental animals.[37] We employed the purified CHFI in studies to inhibit the cold-promoted activation in siliconized or borosilicate tubes of the prothrombin time in factor VII.[38] We found a dose-dependent inhibition of this reaction. Total inhibition was observed at a final whole blood concentration of 10 µg/ml (Figure 8). The CHFI also prolonged the activated partial thromboplastin time of the same plasma samples.

Work by Nossel et al had shown that a variety of positively-charged substances inhibited the initial phase of the contact stages of coagulation and the inhibition of factor XII activation.[39] One of these substance, cytochrome C, resulted in a dose-dependent inhibition of the activation of factor VII and shortening of the prothrombin time (Figure 8).[38] At approximately 3-6 mg/ml final concentration, cytochrome C reduced the percent shortening of the prothrombin time to approximately 3-4% and the percent increase of factor VII to approximately 15-20%. The addition of aprotinin at relatively high concentrations prevented the cold activation

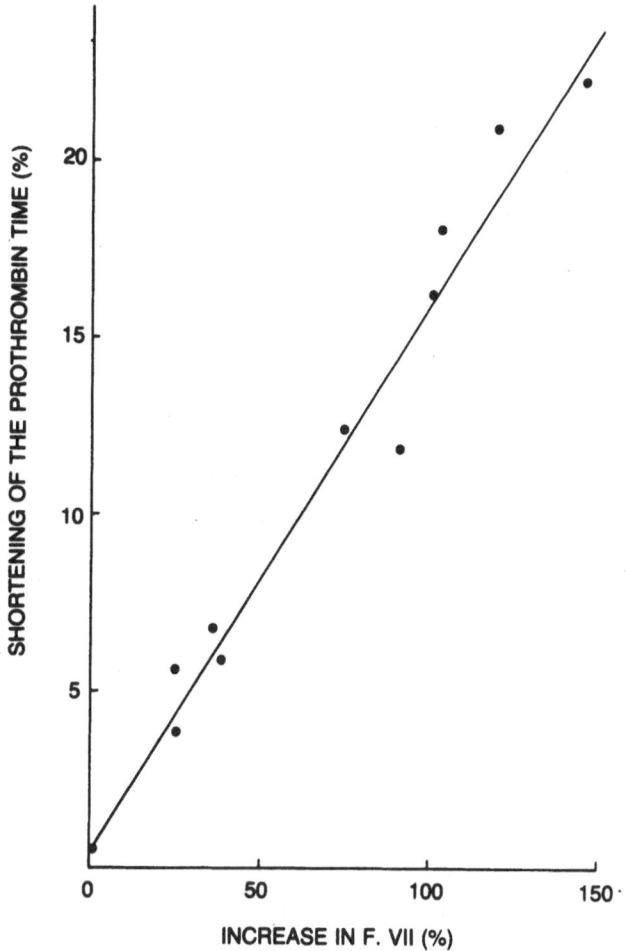

Figure 6: Relationship of the percent decrease in the prothrombin time to the percent increase in factor VII. Factor VII was measured in a one-stage assay with congenital deficient plasma. There was an excellent correlation between the rise in factor VII and the decrease in the prothrombin time.

of factor VII and shortening of the prothrombin time (Figure 9).[37] Aprotinin is a potent inhibitor of the activation of prekallikrein and plasminogen.

When the blood from patients who are congenitally deficient in the C1 INH is studied, the greatest degree of time-dependent cold activation of factor VII and shortening of the prothrombin time is observed.[17] Plasma from these patients also demonstrate the greatest increase in the factor VII activation. When C1 INH antigenic levels were studied over time in normal blood, despite the presence of cold activation and shortening of the prothrombin time, the antigenic C1 INH did not change. However, other investigators using amidolytic and immunologic assays have shown that the C1 INH antigen does not change, but the activity is decreased.[34,35] All of the factor VII cold-promoted activation and inhibition data are summarized in Figure 10.

From the aforementioned problems in obtaining a valid prothrombin time, new methods for measuring the potency of anticoagulation have been suggested. Included among these are the use of chromogenic substrates and

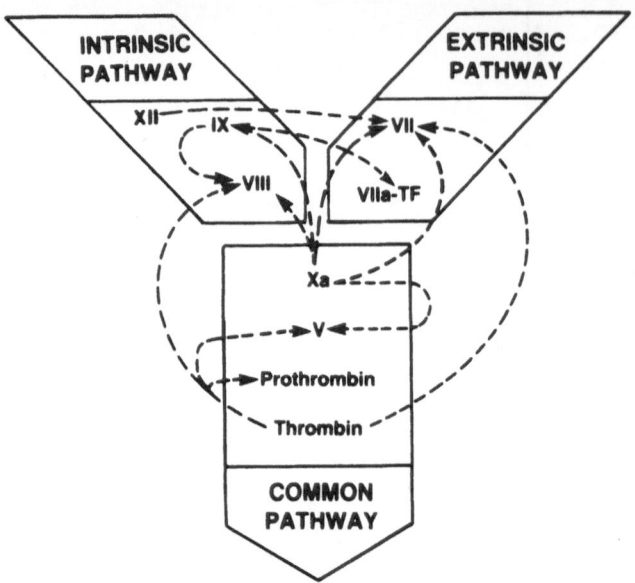

<u>Figure 7</u>: Synopsis of the evidence for coagulation factor activation
in the intrinsic and extrinsic pathway.

monospecific antibodies directed against factors II, VII, IX or X to
measure antigenic levels of these vitamin K-dependent coagulation
proteins.[40-48] The amidolytic assay appears to have a fairly good
correlation with the prothrombin time or thrombotest.[40,41] It does not
appear to be markedly influenced by cold activation, however, the
acarboxylated factor VII may be partially active in the amidolytic
assay.[39]

     The use of the monospecific antibody directed against specific
coagulation proteins have revealed a moderate reduction in the antigenic
level of the vitamin K-dependent coagulation proteins in anticoagulated
individuals, and there is a reasonable correlation with the prothrombin
time assay. However, the antigenic levels do not appear to be as useful or
as rapidly performed as the prothrombin time assay; thus, at the present
time, these assays do not play a significant role in the monitoring of oral
anticoagulation therapy.

     Recently, Furie et al. have described the use of two monospecific
antibodies, one directed against factor II which has a full complement of
gammacarboxyglutamic acid and a second antibody directed against the
agammacarboxyglutamic acid factor II protein.[43] Utilizing immunoassays for
both forms of factor II, the authors found they could not correlate the
level of anticoagulation or bleeding or thrombotic complications and the
level of the abnormal prothrombin. In contrast, they found an excellent
correlation with the level of normal factor II antigen. In 13 individuals
who had bleeding, the authors found that the level of the native
prothrombin antigen was always less than 12 µg/ml (normal range 108 ± 19
µg/ml), and that in those individuals who had thrombotic disorders, 6 of 7
had a native prothrombin antigen level of greater than 24 µg/ml. These
appear to be very specific levels under which and above which there are
complications with oral anticoagulant therapy. The large number of
patients who fell into the under and over categories with no hemorrhagic or
thromboembolic complications would suggest that the high degree of

sensitivity does not parallel the specificity of these assays in defining those individuals who will have bleeding or thromboembolic complications.

It has been reported that bovine thromboplastin does not react to the activated factor VII in cold-activated plasmas as compared to human thromboplastin.[49,50] It has been suggested that the use of these two thromboplastins together give an index of the degree of cold activation. Whether this would be useful in attempting to monitor oral anticoagulant therapy has not been elucidated.

Inhibitor	Prothrombin Time Decrease (%)	Factor VII Increase (%)
None	19.8	140
C̄1 INH		
0.5 u/ml	10.4	70
1.0 u/ml	7.3	60
1.0 u/ml	2.5	20
CHFI		
2.5 μg/ml	10.2	74
5.0 μg/ml	6.1	50
7.5 μg/ml	3.6	16
10 μg/ml	<0.5	<1.0
Cytochrome C		
1.0 mg/ml	7.0	40
3.0 mg/ml	4.0	22
6.0 mg/ml	3.0	14

Figure 8: Inhibitors of cold activation of factor VII. The inhibitors were added to the anticoagulant prior to the venipuncture. Blood was drawn into each tube, maintained at 4 C and at 2 and 4 hours the prothrombin time and factor VII assayed. C1 INH, CHFI and cytochrome C markedly reduced the increase in factor VII and decrease in the prothrombin time in a dose-dependent manner.

The addition of inhibitors such as C1 INH, cytochrome C or the CHFI to the blood sample would surely prevent cold-promoted activation. However, these samples of blood could only be utilized for the determination of the prothrombin time and the measurement of coagulation factors of the extrinsic pathway. They could not be utilized for measurement of the activated partial thromboplastin time or coagulation factors involved in the intrinsic pathway.[38]

Thus, despite our increasing knowledge of the problem of determining the potency of oral anticoagulation, many problems still remain to be overcome. These present challenges to us to insure the safety of patients receiving oral anticoagulants.

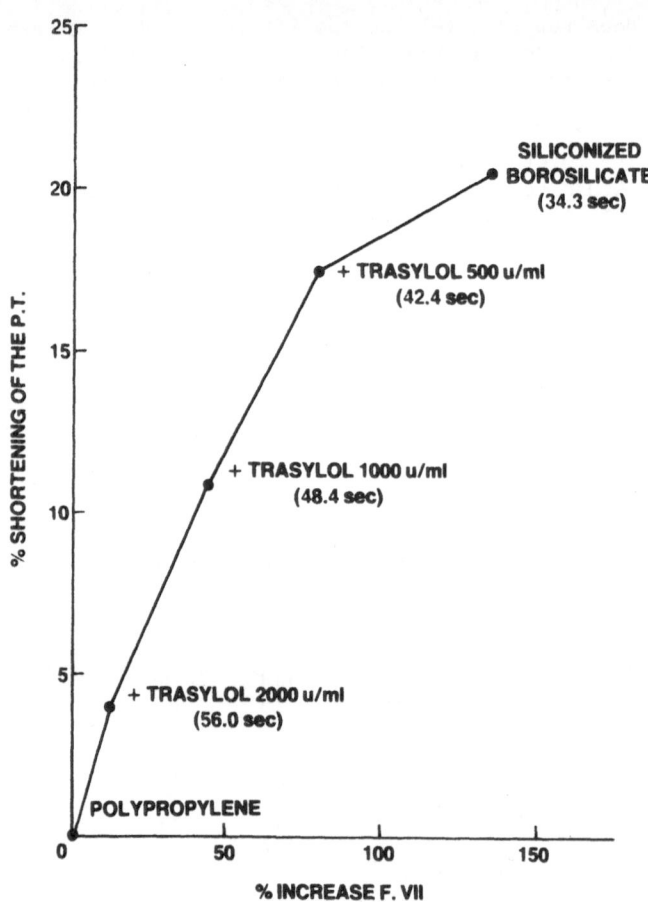

Figure 9: The effect of aprotinin at various concentrations on the cold-activation of factor VII and shortening of the prothrombin time. The figures in parentheses are the activated partial thromboplastin times at each concentration of the inhibitor.

Are there any clinical implications of cold-promoted factor VII activation and increased plasma factor VII levels? In a large epidemiologic study from the Norwick Park study of 1510 white men, it was found that the levels of factors VII:C and VIII:C and fibrinogen were significantly higher in those who died of cardiovascular disease than in those who survived.[51] The association of the elevated factor VII was as strong as the association with elevated blood cholesterol. Further studies from this group suggested that factor VII clotting activity was associated with increased plasma lipid concentrations, and that as the lipid concentrations were reduced by medication the factor VII declined.[52] Subsequent studies from the same group demonstrated that there was an increased conversion of factor VII to factor VIIa in hyperlipidemia.[53] They suggested that this increase in the level of factor VIIa was a measure of activation within the coagulation system and could be used as a measure of increased coaguability in hyperlipidemia and possibly other states. Carvalho et al.[54] found that in type II beta lipoproteinemia there was activation of the contact phase of blood coagulation. They further suggested that there was activation of intrinsic pathway involving prekallikrein and the kallikrein inhibitor. They did not study the prothrombin time, but it would seem likely that in these patients the contact phase of blood coagulation is primed and would result in cold-promoted factor VII activation and they might have baseline elevations of their factor VII.

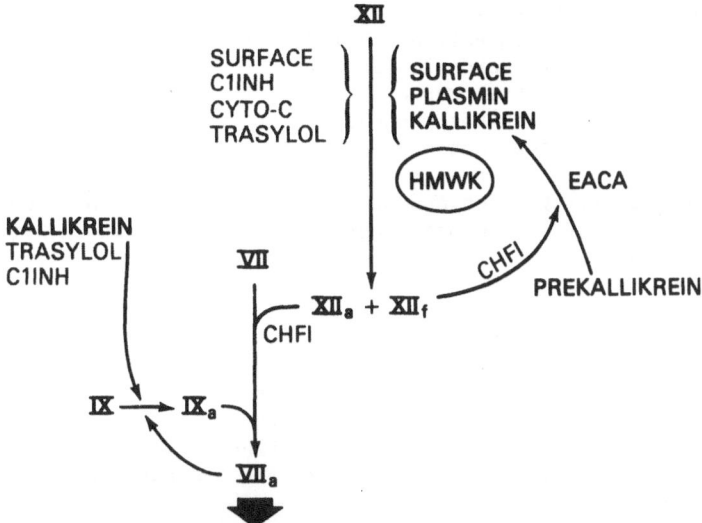

"IN VITRO" ACTIVATION OF PROTHROMBIN TIME

Figure 10: Summary of the mechanisms of in vitro activation of the prothrombin time. Factor XII, either by auto-activation or due to interaction with a negatively-charged surface, activates itself and also activates prekallikrein. Prekallikrein enhances the factor XII activation. Activated factor XII and XII fragments activate factor VII to VIIa. The kallikrein also interacts through factor XI to activate factor IX, and it then activates factor VII. It appears that the contact phase of blood coagulation is most pivotal. In the absence of factor XII, prekallikrein or high molecular weight kininogen, there is virtually no cold activation of the prothrombin time. The kallikrein/factor IXa appeared to contribute approximately 50% in vitro activation of the prothrombin time through activated factor VII. The inhibitors which retard factor XII activation include the type of surface, the C1 INH, cytochrome C (Cyto-C) and aprotinin. The aprotonin and the C1 INH also interfere with the conversion of prekallikrein to kallikrein. The CHFI appears to primarily act on the activated factor XII and the XII fragments by inhibiting the activation of prekallikrein by factor XIIa and inhibiting the activation of factor VII to VIIa by factor XIIa and XII fragments.

Dalaker et al. confirmed the elevated factor VII levels in male patients at high risk for cardiovascular disease and suggested that this increase in factor VII was due to a phospholipid-factor VII complex in their plasma which increased the specific activity of factor VII.[55] Meade described other associated characteristics with increased factor VII such as increasing age, diabetes, obesity, the occurrence of menopause and the use of oral contraceptives, each being associated with increased factor VII levels as well as an increased risk for cardiovascular disease.[56]

van Deijk et al. have found increased levels of activated factor VII in patients with metastatic prostatic carcinoma as compared those individuals who have prostatic carcinoma without metastases or simple benign prostatic hypertrophy.[57] They studied a small number of patients and formulated a working hypothesis that the finding in patients of factor VIIa levels of more than 100% was suggestive of a metastases.

Both pregnancy and the use of oral contraceptives in women has been associated with an increased risk of thromboembolic disorder and increased cardiovascular mortality in premenopausal women. Dalaker and Prydz have shown that the hypercoaguable state in pregnancy is, in part, caused by increased activity of factor VII in plasma.[58] It was believed that the increased factor VII level was due to a circulating complex of factor VII and a phospholipid which was phopholipase C sensitive. They thought this was a form of activated factor VII. In individuals taking oral contraceptives there has been an association of increased levels of factor VII biologic activity which appears to be, in younger individuals, due directly to the use of the oral contraceptives while in individuals not on oral contraceptives, the factor VII appears to rise with age.[59] Gordon et al have shown a marked increase in the cold-promoted activation of factor VII and shortening of the prothrombin time in women using oral contraceptives.[60] This was related to the augmented Hageman factor (factor XII) titers in these patients' plasma. They believe that the high levels of Hageman factor found in the women taking oral contraceptives is needed for the spontaneous cold-promoted activation of factor VII. This group had previously shown high procoagulant and antigenic titers of Hageman factor in these women accompanied by a simultaneous decrease in the plasma C1 INH concentration.[34]

Seligsohn et al.[61] identified a potential problem associated with cold-promoted activation of factor VII. Although they could easily identify individuals who had cold-promoted activation of factor VII in the laboratory, when the blood from these individuals was collected in the blood bank bags, cold-promoted activation of factor VII was not seen. A large number of variables were tested and it appeared that the major reason there was no cold-promoted activation seen in the blood bank plastic bag was related primarily to the different ratio of plasma volume to surface area; the ratio was much smaller in the plasma unit stored in the blood bank versus the laboratory tubes. Thus, this did not allow for an adequate surface for the activation of the contact phase of blood coagulation.

In conclusion, there appears to be a growing body of data which suggests that factor VII in plasma, its total activity or the activated form, may be predictive in long-term epidemiologic studies in defining those individuals who will have cardiovascular events. It also may be associated with or an epiphenomena in the increased incidence of thromboembolic and cardiovascular events in pregnant women or in women taking oral contraceptive medication.

REFERENCES

1. National Committee for Clinical Laboratory Standards. Collection, transport and preparation of blood specimens for coagulation testing and performance of coagulation assays; Approved Guideline. NCCLS Document H21-A, Villanova, PA: NCCLS, (1986).
2. National Committee for Clinical Laboratory Standards. Proposed guidelines for the one-stage prothrombin time test (PT). NCCLS Document H28-P 2:362-380, Villanova, PA: NCCLS (1982).
3. R.N. Palmer, C.M. Kessler, and H.R. Gralnick, Warfarin anticoagulation: Difficulties in interpretation of the prothrombin time, Thromb. Res. 25:125 (1982).
4. A.M.H.P. van den Besselaar and E.A. Loeliger, The effect of contact activation on the prothrombin time with special reference to theuse of evacuated tubes, in: "Standardization of Coagulation Assays: An Overview," D.A. Triplett, ed., College of American Pathologists, Skokie, IL (1982).
5. H.R. Gralnick, C.R. Kessler, and R. Palmer, The prothrombin time: Variables affecting results, in: "Standardization of Coagulation Assays: An Overview," D.A. Triplett, ed., College of American Pathologists, Skokie, IL (1982).

6. R.N. Palmer and H.R. Gralnick, Inhibition of cold-promoted activation of the prothrombin time studies of new siliconized borosilicate collection tubes in normals and patients receiving warfarin, Am. J. Clin. Path. 83:492 (1985).

7. J.A. Thomson, "Blood Coagulation and Haemostasis: A Practical Guide," Churchill Livingstone, London (1985).

8. A.M.H.P. van den Besselaar, L.P. van Halem-Visser, and E.A. Loeliger, The use of evacuated tubes for blood collection in oral anticoagulant control, Thromb. Haemost. 50:676 (1983).

9. K. Lenggenhager, quoted in: "The Coagulation of Blood: Investigations on a New Clotting Factor," P.A. Owren, ed., J. Chr. Gundersen, Oslo, p 53 (1947).

10. B. Alexander, A. DeVries, and R. Goldstein, A factor in serum which accelerated the conversion of prothrombin to thrombin. II. Its evaluation with special reference to the influence of conditions which affect blood coagulation, Blood 4:739 (1949).

11. S.I. Rapaport, K Aas, and P.A. Owren, The effect of glass upon the activity of the various plasma clotting factors, J. Clin. Invest. 34:9 (1954).

12. O.D. Ratnoff and J.E. Colopy, A familial hemorrhagic trait associated with a deficiency of a clot-promoting fraction of plasma. J. Clin. Invest. 34:102 (1955).

13. O.D. Ratnoff and J.M. Rosenblum, Role of Hageman factor in the initiation of clotting by glass: Evidence that glass frees Hageman factor from inhibition, Am. J. Med. 25:160 (1958).

14. H. Gjonnaess, Cold promoted activation of factor VII. I. Evidence for the existence of an activator, Thromb. Diath. Haemorrh. 28:155 (1972).

15. H. Gjonnaess, Cold promoted activation of factor VII. II. Identification of the activator, Thromb. Diathes. Haemorrh. 28:169 (1972).

16. H. Gjonnaess, Cold promoted activation of factor VII. III. Relation to the kallikrein system, Thromb. Diath. Haemorrh. 28:182 (1972).

17. R.N. Palmer and H.R. Gralnick, Cold-induced contact surface activation of the prothrombin time in whole blood, Blood 59:38 (1982).

18. R. Radcliffe, A. Bagdasarian, R. Colman, and Y. Nemerson, Activation of bovein factor VII by Hageman factor fragments, Blood 50:611 (1977).

19. W. Kisiel, K. Fujikawa, and E.W. Davie, Activation of bovine factor VII (proconvertin) by factor XIIa (activated Hageman factor), Biochemistry 16:4189 (1977).

20. K. Laake and B. Osterud, Activation of purified plasma factor VII by human plasmin, plasma kallikrein and activated components of the human intrinsic blood coagulation system, Thromb. Res. 5:759 (1974).

21. U. Seligsohn, B. Sterud, F. Brown, J.H. Griffin, and S.I. Rapaport, Activation of human factor VII in plasma and in purified systems, J. Clin. Invest. 64:1056 (1979).

22. U. Seligsohn, B. Osterud, J. Griffin, and S.I. Rapaport, Evidence for the participation of both activated factor XII and activated factor IX in cold-promoted activaiton of factor VII, Thromb. Res. 13:1049 (1978).

23. H. Gjonnaess, Cold promoted activation of factor VII. IV. Relation to the coagulation system, Thromb. Diath. Haemorrh. 28:194 (1972).

24. H. Saito and O. Ratnoff, Alteration of factor VII activity by activated Fletcher factor (a plasma kallikrein): A potential link between the intrinsic and extrinsic blood clotting system, J. Lab. Clin. Med. 85:405 (1975).

25. G.J. Miller, M.J. Seghatchian, S.J. Walter, D.J. Howarth, S.G. Thompson, M.P. Esnouf, and T.W. Meade, An association between the factor VII coagulant activity and thrombin activity induced by surface/cold exposure of normal human plasma, Brit. J. Haematol. 62:379 (1986).

26. A.D. Muller, W.A. van Deijk, P.P. Devilee, M.S.C. van Dam—Mieras, and H.C. Hemker, The activity state of factor VII in plasma: two pathways for the cold promoted activation of factor VII, Brit. J. Haematol. 62:367 (1986).
27. C. Cochrane and J. Griffin, Molecular assembly in the contact phase of Hageman factor system, Am. J. Med. 67:657 (1979).
28. A. Kaplan, The Hageman factor dependent pathways of human plasma, Microvasc. Res. 8:97 (1974).
29. M. Zur and Y. Nemerson, Kinetics of factor IX activation via the extrinsic pathway: dependence of Km on tissue factor, J. Biol. Chem. 255:5703 (1980).
30. E.A. van Royen, S. Lohman, M. Voss, and K.W. Pondman, C1 inactivator and cold—promoted activation of factor VII, J. Lab. Clin. Med. 92:152 (1978).
31. O.D. Ratnoff, J. Pensky, D. Ogston, and G. Naff, The inhibition of plasmin, plasma kallikrein, plasma permeability factor and the C'1r subcomponent inhibitor, J. Exp. Med. 129:315 (1969).
32. B. Bouma, D. Kerbiriou, R. Vlooswijk, and J. Griffin, Immunological studies of perkallikrein, kallikrein and high—molecular—weight kininogen in normal and deficient plasmas and in normal plasma after cold—promoted activation. J. Lab. Clin. Med. 96:693 (1980).
33. R. Weiss, M. Silverberg, and A.P. Kaplan, The effect of C1 inhibitor upon Hageman factor autoactivation, Blood 68:239 (1986).
34. E.M. Gordon, O.D. Ratnoff, H. Saito, V.H. Donaldson, J. Pensky and P.K. Jones, Rapid fibrinolysis, augmented Hageman factor (factor XII) titers, and decreased C1 esterase inhibitor titers in women taking oral contraceptives, J. Lab. Clin. Med. 96:762 (1980).
35. C. Czendlik, B. Lammie, and F. Duckert, Cold promoted activation and factor XII, prekallikrein and C1—inhibitor, Thromb. Haemost. 53:242 (1985).
36. Y. Hojima, J.V. Pierce, and J.J. Pisano, Hageman factor fragment inhibitor in corn seeds: purification and characterization, Thromb. Res. 20:149 (1980).
37. E. Marks, Y. Hojima, M.E. Frech, H. Keiser, and J.J. Pisano, An inhibitor form corn blocks the hypotensive action of plasma protein fraction and active Hageman factor, Thromb. Res. 23:97 (1981).
38. R.N. Palmer, and H.R. Gralnick, Inhibition of the cold activation of factor VII and the prothrombin time, Am. J. Clin. Path. 81:618 (1984).
39. H. Nossel, H. Rubin, M. Drillings, and R. Hsieh, Inhibition of Hageman factor activation, J. Clin. Invest. 47:1172 (1968).
40. U. Seligsohn, B. Osterud, and S.I. Rapaport, Coupled amidolytic assay for factor VII: Its use with a clotting assay to determine the activity state of factor VII, Blood 52:978 (1978).
41. G. Avvisati, J.W. Ten Cate, E.M. van Wijk, L.H. Kahle, and G. Mariani, Evaluation of a new chromogenic assay for factor VII and its application in patients on oral anticoagulant treatment, Brit. J. Haematol. 45:343 (1980).
42. R.A. Blanchard, B.C. Furie, S.F. Kruger, G. Waneck, M.J. Jorgensen, and B. Furie, Immunoassays of human prothrombin species which correlate with functional coagulant activities. J. Lab. Clin. Med. 101:242 (1983).
43. B. Furie, H.A. Liebman, R.A. Blanchard, M.S. Coleman, S.F. Kruger, and B.C. Furie, Comparison of the native prothrombin antigen and the prothrombin time for monitoring oral anticoagulant therapy, Blood 64:445 (1984).
44. D.J. Howarth, M. Brozovic, Y. Stirling, and M. Reed, Factor VII during warfarin treatment, Scand. J. Haematol. 12:346 (1974).
45. D.S. Fair, Quantitation of factor VII in the plasma of normal and warfarin—treated individuals by radioimmunoassay, Blood 62:784 (1983).

46. A.R. Thompson, Factor IX antigen by radioimmunoassay: Abnormal factor IX protein in patients on warfarin therapy and with hemophilia B, J. Clin. Invest. 59:900 (1977).
47. K.H. Orstavik, and K. Laake, Factor IX in warfarin treated patients, Thromb. Res. 13:207 (1978).
48. D.S. Fair, and T.S. Edgington, Heterogeneity of hereditary and acquired factor X deficiencies by combined immunochemical and functional analyses, Brit. J. Haematol. 59:235 (1985).
49. B. Osterud, How to measure factor VII and factor VII activation, Haemostasis 13:161 (1983).
50. W.A. van Deijk, M.C.E. van Dam-Mieras, A.D. Muller and H.C. Hemker, Evaluation of a coagulation assay determining the activity state of factor VII in plasma, Haemostasis 13:192 (1983).
51. T.W. Meade, R. Chakrabarti, A.P. Haines, W.R.S. North, Y. Stirling, S.G. Thompson, and M. Brozovic, Haemostatic function and cardiovascular death: Early results of a prospective study, Lancet , May 17:1050 (1980).
52. T.W. Meade, A.P. Haines, J.D. Imeson, Y. Stirling, and S.G. Thompson, Menopausal status and haemostatic variables, Lancet i:22 (1983).
53. G.J. Miller, S.J. Walter, Y. Stirling, S.G. Thompson, M.P. Esnouf, and T.W. Meade, Assay of factor VII activity by two techniques: evidence for increased conversion of VII to alpha-VIIa in hyperlipidaemia, with possible implications for ischaemic heart disease, Brit. J. Haematol. 59:249 (1985).
54. A.C.A. Carvalho, R.S. Lees, R.A. Vaillancourt, R.B. Cabral, and R.W. Colman, Activation of the kallikrein system in hyperbetalipoproteinemia, J. Lab. Clin. Med. 91:117 (1978).
55. K. Dalaker, I. Hjermann, and H. Prydz, A novel form of factor VII in plasma from men at risk for cardiovascular disease, Brit. J. Haematol. 61:315 (1985).
56. T.W. Meade, Factor VII and ischaemic heart disease: Epidemiological evidence, Haemostasis 13:178 (1983).
57. W.A. van Deijk, M.C.E. van Dam-Mieras, and A.D. Muller, Activation of factor VII in patients with carcinoma of the prostate: A preliminary report, Haemostasis 13:198 (1983).
58. K. Dalaker, and H. Prydz, The coagulation factor VII in pregnancy, Brit. J. Haematol. 56:233 (1984).
59. T.W. Meade, M. Brozovic, R. Chakrabarti, D.J. Howarth, W.R.S. North, and Y. Stirling, An epidemiological study of the haemostatic and other effect of oral contraceptive, Brit. J. Haematol. 34:353 (1976).
60. E.M. Gordon, O.D. Ratnoff, and P.K. Jones, The role of augmented Hageman factor (factor XII) titers in the cold-promoted activition of factor VII and spontaneous shortening of the prothrombin time in women using oral contraceptives, J. Lab. Clin. Med. 99:363 (1982).
61. U. Seligsohn, A. Zivelin, and S. Bar-Shani, Cold-promoted activation of factor VII: Is it a problem under blood bank conditions? Haemostasis 13:186 (1983).

IMMUNOLOGIC ASPECTS OF VESSEL INJURY AND THROMBOSIS

Carl G. Becker

Professor of Pathology
Cornell University Medical College
New York, New York

INTRODUCTION

Cardiovascular diseases account for over one-half of all deaths in the United States and contribute similarly to the number of deaths in other developed Western countries. More than 80% of these deaths can be attributed to complications of atherosclerosis.

Arteriosclerosis begins in childhood and in its initial stages is characterized by the accumulation in the arterial intima of monocytes[1,2] cells with important recognition and effector functions in the immune system, lipid laden macrophages derived from these monocytes, and by lipid accumulation in and proliferation of vascular smooth muscle cells, perhaps in response to monocyte and platelet derived mitogens[3,4] and proteases[5] derived from these cells and/or plasma.

Following decades of plaque growth and arterial narrowing, thrombotic occlusion may occur leading to myocardial infarction or ischemic necrosis of other organs. The mechanisms most immediately associated with thrombus formation may include plaque ulceration, hemorrhage into a plaque, the effects of changes in flow on vascular endothelium, and more recently described changes in the surface of endothelial cells that may include expression or suppression of molecules, usually proteins or glycoproteins, that favor the occurrence of a thrombotic event. This modulation of endothelial function involves a number of cells and cell products that have previously been studied in connection with their rôle in immune or inflammatory mechanisms and will be discussed in some detail below.

Further, heart attack, presenting as arrhymthia and sudden death, can also occur in the absence of demonstrable occlusion of a major vessel. Experimentally, cardiac dysrrhythmia can be induced by release of inflammatory mediators following allergenic challenge[6]. This may have a counterpart in fatal arrhythmias that have been described in humans following allergic challenge[7]

Epidemiologic studies of heart attack have identified a number of risk factors associated with the external or internal environment including cigarette smoking, hypercholesterolemia, diabetes, hypertension, age and being male. However, in autopsy based, epidemiologic studies of atherosclerosis when cases were stratified according to race, sex, age and disease there remained much individual variation in the extent of raised atherosclerotic lesions in the aorta, the coronary arteries and cerebral arteries[8]. Further, fifty per cent of people who suffer heart attacks cannot be identified with a major risk factor.

These observations taken together indicate that there are undefined mechanisms, including environmental factors, that contribute to the pathogenesis of atherosclerosis and its complications and that defining these mechanisms, as well as those associated with known risk factors, must include understanding why some individuals are more at risk than others.

Because the immune system functions to amplify and diversify the host response to a given stimulus, exposure to substances even in low concentration may have profound effects depending on the capacity of the individual to respond, the nature of the response, e.g. the systems activated, interaction between these systems, the intensity of the challenge, and the capacity of the individual to amplify and to modulate these responses[9]. It is therefore appropriate to study whether immunologic and immunopathologic mechanisms can contribute to the initiation and progression of cardiovascular disease.

HISTORIC PERSPECTIVES BASED ON MORPHOLOGIC OBSERVATIONS

Virchow hypothesized that the development of inflammation in the intima of arteries led to the development of arteriosclerotic plaques[10]. Another hypothesis, raised first by Rokitansky[11] and later by Duguid[12] stated that the formation and organization of thrombi at sites of injury of the vessel wall led to the formation of arteriosclerotic plaques. These two hypotheses were viewed as separate for many years, but the rapidly enlarging body of data demonstrating cooperation between the immune system, pathways leading to generation of inflammatory mediators, and the hemostatic system, unites them.

Empirical support for the concept that immunologic injury could contribute to the pathogenesis of atherosclerosis was obtained nearly 60 years ago. Extending earlier observation of European pathologists, Zeek described the precocious development of arteriosclerosis in patients who had suffered rheumatic heart disease[13,14]. Studies by Karsner and Bayless[15] and Gross, Kugel, and Epstein[16] confirmed and extended these observations. Fahr, 13 years ealier[17], had drawn attention to the resemblance between the arterial lesions of rheumatic fever, poly-arteritis nodosa, and dermatomyositis, an observation supported by similar observations of many of his contemporaries, indicating that at this time there was a large body of evidence supporting the concept of a causal relationship between immunologically mediated arterial injury and the development of arteriosclerosis. Similar arterial lesions involving the intima, media, and adventitia of blood vessels were also described in patients suffering from serum sickness. Seeking a common mechanism, Opie suggested that antigen-antibody complexes precipitating on vascular surfaces initiated a chain of events leading to injury and inflammation of the vessel wall[18]. The authors of these studies also commented on the increased susceptibility of coronary arteries, relative to other arteries, to acute immunologically mediated injury[19,20].

Precocious development of atherosclerosis has been more recently described in association with systemic lupus erythematosus and rheumatoid arteritis, both diseases whose manifestations are mediated at least in part by events resulting from formation of immune complexes[21,22]. Further, patients with S.L.E. have an increased incidence of arterial and venous thrombi suggesting that immune complexes may stimulate thrombus formation[23].

INVESTIGATIONS INTO THE PATHOGENESIS OF IMMUNOLOGICALLY MEDIATED VASCULAR DISEASE

Studies of experimental serum sickness indicated that arteries were targets of injury and that formation of antigen-antibody complexes in moderate antigen excess in the circulation and their deposition in the walls of blood vessels led to the development of arteritis[24]. It was subsequently shown in rabbits that administration of anti-histamine or depletion of platelets inhibited immune complex deposition[25] and that release of histamine from rabbit platelets could be mediated by complement components or by a mechanism involving specific antigen and basophilic leukocytes sensitized with IgE[26]. Later studies revealed that antigen stimulated basophils also released a lipid, initially called platelet activating factor[27] and later structurally characterized as acetyl glyceryl ether phosphorylcholine[28], which caused platelets to aggregate transiently and, in higher doses to secrete[29]. Generation of AGEPC has been observed from rabbit basophils and neutrophils and from human neutrophils, platelets, and mast cells and from rat mononuclear cells. It is an important mediator of the inflammatory response in that it can activate human neutrophils stimulating both chematoxis and secretion, stimulate smooth muscle contraction, and stimulate vascular leakage of macromolecules (reviewed in [30]). It has also been shown that specific antigenic challenge of animals preferentially synthesizing IgE antibodies to that antigen results in activation of the intrinsic pathway of coagulation[31]. It is also known that antigenic challenge of sensitized mast cells results in release of proteolytic activators of prekallikrein[32] and of C3 of the complement system[33].

Thus, antigen triggered IgE mediated release from basophils and/or mast cells results in a highly augmented response generating diverse substances that might alter function of vascular endothelium and perhaps potentiate deposition of immune complexes. Immunologically mediated release by basophiles, mast cells (and other leukocytes) of other mediators of the inflammatory response has been recently and extensively reviewed[30].

Experiments conducted by Minick and colleagues demonstrated that arterial injury induced in rabbits by repeated intravenous injection of foreign serum protein acted synergistically with dietarily induced hyperlipidemia (serum cholesterol levels 200-250 mg/dl), a range comparable to that in the adult population of developed Western countries) to induce atherosclerotic lesions in the aorta and major systemic arteries[34]. The induced lesions strikingly resembled the so called complicated lesions of human atheroarteriosclerosis. Coronary arteries were especially prone to injury in this model and cerebral arteries were virtually entirely spared, drawing attention to important differences in vulnerability and/or response of different segments of the vascular tree and perhaps bearing on the earlier occurrence of heart attacks than of strokes in humans.

In extensions of this experimental model it was observed that sites of intimal thickening that resulted from earlier arterial injury continued to be especially prone to lipid accumulation for at least 80 days after the last injection of foreign serum[35]. These studies raise the possibility that special attention should be paid to dietary lipid intake in patients who have suffered acute arterial injury, e.g. children with Kawasaki's syndrome, and patients with immunologically mediated, systemic diseases.

Unexpectedly severe and rapidly developing atherosclerosis has been found to occur in some human cardiac homografts[36]. Experimentally, heterotopic cardiac homografts in rabbits were shown to develop atherosclerotic change, especially in the presence of dietarily induced hyperlipidemia[37]. Whether injury was induced by humoral or cellular immune mechanisms is not known, but in the light of experiments described below concerning expression of Class I and Class II MHC antigens by vascular endothelial cells, both mechanisms might be operative.

In either the experimental models of serum sickness described above, or in vessels in heterotopically transplanted hearts, platelet aggregates and individual platelets were observed to be adherent to damaged endothelial cells, in gaps between endothelial cells, and in areas of endothelial denudation. It must be pointed out that the injurious stimuli in these models was great, perhaps comparable to that in a patient with fulminant S.L.E. However, other immunologic mechanisms that alter endothelial function without inducing major morphologic changes have been demonstrated and may be relevant to more slowly progressive arterial disease.

The exact mechanisms by which immune complexes deposit in vascular endothelium particularly endothelium of large vessels, whether or not enhanced by IgE mediated release mechanisms, are still subjects of active research. It is conceivable that release of vasoactive amines (histamine or serotonin), or peptides (bradykinin), stimulates endothelial contraction as they appear in post capillary vessels. However, even though contractile proteins are present in arterial endothelial cells, contraction of arterial endothelium in response to these stimuli has not been demonstrated unequivocally. Recently, stimulation by bradykinin of endothelial production of a factor that relaxes vascular smooth muscle has been described[38]. The factor has not been characterized but appears not to be a metabolite of arachidonic acid. It might be hypothesized from these data that relaxation of the arterial wall might result in stretching of the underlying endothelium and opening of gaps.

Modulation of the endothlial surface might also facilitate localization of immune complexes. Camussi and colleagues have recently shown that cationic proteins from platelets were detectable by immunofluorescence microscopy on the walls of glomerular capillaries within 7 to 8 days after intravenous injection of relatively large quantities of bovine serum albumin and preceding or concomittant with the deposition of immune complexes and appearance of proteinuria[39]. Deposition of cationic protein was correlated with loss of anionic sites on the endothelial side, and later, epithelial side of the glomerular basement membrane. The authors suggest that neutralization of polyanionic sites prevented repulsion of immune complexes and plasma proteins. It was not stated in their paper whether cationic proteins derived from either platelets or neutrophiles were deposited on vessels other than glomeruli or peritubular vessels. However, it would be important to know if deposition of cationic proteins from platelets, including platelet factor 4, or leukocytes also enchance the likelihood of immune complex deposition in artery walls rather than physiologic clearance by fixed macrophages.

Similarly, avidity of antigen in immune complexes for tissue structures may also determine whether and where immune complexes deposit in tissue. Gallo and colleagues, in an extension of their earlier studies demonstrated that the more cationic the immunogen the more likely it was to be nephritogenic and to deposit on the glomerular basement membrane, as opposed to the mesangium in experimental serum sickness[40]. It is not known whether immune complexes containing cationic antigen would also be more likely to deposit on arterial endothelium or whether highly cationic antigen might bind directly to arterial or venous endothelium and then react with antibody and complement components. However, a variety of different sites or domains capable of binding cationic molecules have been described on vascular endothelial cells other than renal glomeruli[41].

Vascular endothelium might also bind immune complexes via receptors for Fc fragments of immunoglobulins or for C3b. Endothelial cells cultured from human umbilical veins or pulmonary veins are said not to have Fc and C3b receptors[42]. However, infection of endothelial cells with herpes simplex virus-1 (HSV-1), HSV-2, cytomegalovirus, or varicella virus results in expression of Fc receptors[43,44,45,46]. Infection of endothelial cells with HSV-1 but not HSV-2 results in expression of C3b receptors[47]. Glycoprotein E of HSV-1 has been shown to function as an Fc receptor[48] and glycoprotein C functions as a C3b receptor[49]. These observations suggest the possibility that vascular endothelium expressing these HSV-1 proteins might be more susceptible to immunologically mediated injury induced by immune complexes. In this connection, Marek's disease virus (a herpes virus) has been shown to prevent activation of cytoplasmic cholesteryl esterase in chicken arterial smooth muscle cells leading to accumulation of cholesterol and cholesteryl ester[50]. Infection of smooth muscle cells cultured from human and bovine arteries with HSV-1 also resulted in accumulation of cholesteryl esters in these cells[51]. These observations taken together suggest that infections with certain viruses may contribute to the pathogenesis of arteriosclerosis via several mechanisms, only some of which are immunologic.

The observations cited above concerning the various effects of members of the herpes virus family on infected vascular cells also serve as a paradigm for studying the effects of other viruses on vascular tissues. It is known for example that, many viruses, including strains used for immunization can infect endothelial cells[52] and it has recently been reported that genes responsible for producing IgE binding proteins on murine lymphocytes are members of an endogenous, retrovirus gene family[53].

Although it is not precisely known how circulating immune complexes deposit in or on vessel walls, depletion of complement prevents all but extremely mild changes in artery walls in animals injected with foreign protein[54]. Circulating immune complexes activate the complement cascade and certain components become associated with the complex. Chemotactic factors derived from complement components, especially C5a and C567 complex, attract neutrophils to sites of complement activation[55,56]. Neutrophils are then induced by C5a to produce toxic oxygen radicals which may be injurious to vascular endothelium[57]. Furthermore, when the attracted neutrophils attempt to phagocytize deposited immune complexes, exocytotis occurs along the stimulated portion of the cell membrane, resulting in the release of enzymic consituents, such as elastase and collagenase, destructive to vessel wall constituents[58]. In addition, C3a and C5a, the anaphylatoxic components of complement, can cause discharge of inflamatory mediators from basophils and mast cells also contributing to intensification of the vascular lesion[59,60].

Activation of the alternative pathway of complement which can be achieved by a wide variety of environmental and endogenous substances, including cobra venom, components of microorganisms, and aggregated immunoglobulins, can presumably trigger the same events without the need for antibody[61].

It has also been demonstrated that complement plays a major role in platelet physiology. Thrombin-mediated platelet activation is significantly enhanced by C3-C9[62,63]. At concentrations of 10^{-10}M, C3a (and C3a des-arg) mediate platelet aggregation and release of serotonin. At concentrations below which C3a no longer aggregates platelets directly, it exhibits highly significant synergism with ADP in mediating platelet aggregation and release of serotonin[64]. Assembly of the C5-C9 membrane attack complex of complement on platelets stimulates expression of platelet prothrombinase[65]. These effects may not only be important to normal hemostasis but might also potentiate platelet aggregation and secretion at sites of immunologically mediated vessel injury.

The role of complement may not be limited to immunologically or viral induced atherosclerosis. Severe atherosclerotic changes that characteristically develop in the aortas of rabbits fed cholesterol are very much milder than in rabbits genetically deficient in the sixth component of complement, indicating that activation of the complement cascade and subsequent events described above may play a role in the pathogenesis of diet-induced as well as immunologically mediated atherosclerosis[66].

MODULATION OF VASCULAR ENDOTHELIAL CELL FUNCTION IN IMMUNOLOGIC REACTIONS.

Changes in the expression of surface molecules by vascular endothelial cells can also be stimulated by protein mediators generated as a consequence of exposure to bacterial products such as Gram negative bacterial lipopolysaccharide as well as to proteins produced during the course of the immune response to antigens.

It has been shown in experiments performed for the most part in vitro using endothelial cell monolayers that interleukin-1 and tumor necrosis factor, both products of activated monocytoid cells, can induce a number of changes in the expression of surface molecules by vascular endothelial cells that change the vascular lining from one that is non-supportive of or inhibitory to coagulation to one that favors evolution of both coagulation and the inflammatory response.

Bacterial lipopolysaccharide, interleukin-1 and tumor necrosis factor or cachectin, another product of stimulated monocytes, stimulate expression of tissue factor capable of activating the extrinsic pathway[67], [68,69] and of a number of intercellular adhesion molecules (ICAM's) that cause blood leukocytes including lymphocytes to adhere to endothelial cell monolayers in vitro[70,71], [72,73]. Expression of tissue factor like activity and ICAM's are dependent on protein and RNA synthesis, are maximal 4-6 hours after stimulation, and disappear by 24 hours. It has also been demonstrated recently that heat aggregated human IgG or immune complexes isolated from serum of patients with S.L.E. are also capable of stimulating expression of tissue factor like activity from cultured human endothelial cells. In these experiments expression of tissue factor like activity by endothelial cells was greatly enhanced in the presence of gel filtered platelets[74]. Tumor necrosis factor can also stimulate cultured endothelial cells to express IL-1 activity, thus creating a positive feed back loop for endothelial activation[75].

Two different intercellular adhesion molecules produced by endothelial cells in response to stimulation with IL-1 have been described and monoclonal antibodies have been developed that are reactive with them[76,77,78]. It is likely that many more exist and it is possible that some may be associated with specific vascular beds. In this connection, it has recently been demonstrated that binding of lymphocytes to high endothelium in synovium from humans with rheumatoid arthritis cannot be inhibited with monoclonal antibodies that inhibit binding of lymphocytes to the high endothelium of vessels in Peyer's patches or lymph nodes[79]. These observations and ones yet to be made may bear importantly on the mechanisms by which certain vascular beds and the organs they supply seem to be effected selectively in certain disease states.

It is of considerable interest that both IL-1 and TNF also stimulate endothelial cells to decrease their capacity to activate the anticoagulant,

protein C pathway within the same 4 to 6 hour time period[80].
Interleukin-1 can also modulate endothelial function in the direction
of supporting thrombus formation by decreasing synthesis of tissue plasminogen activator (tPA) and stimulating synthesis of tPA inhibitor[81,82].
These changes peak at 24 hours following stimulation of endothelial cell
monolayers and persist for greater than 48 hours.

Tumor necrosis factor and interferon α stimulate human umbilical
vein endothelial cells to undergo significant rearrangement of active
filaments, to become elongated and to lose their fibronectin matrix.
These changes become most marked by 72-96 hours after stimulation. TNF
and IFNα act synergistically to induce these changes. In higher concentrations these cytokines can induce endothelial shedding[83].

The effects of these various monokines and cytokines are depicted
in the figure below.

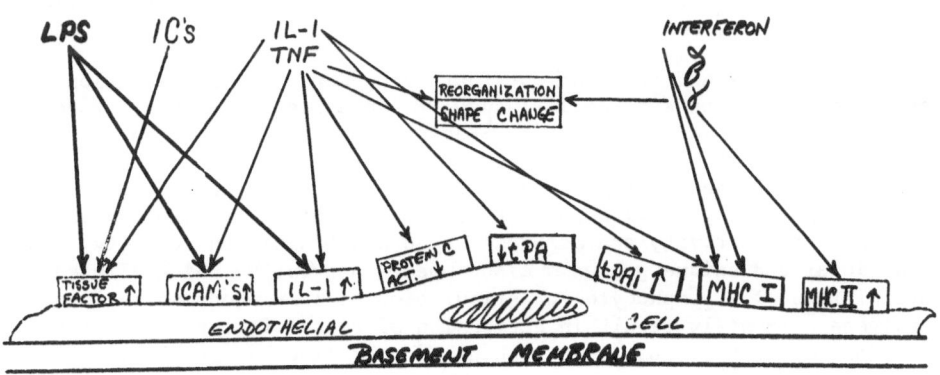

PEAK EXPRESSION OF ACTIVITY IN VITRO

TIME: 6 hrs.   12 hrs.   72 hrs.   96 hrs.

LEGEND

LPS, bacterial lipopolysaccharide; IC's, immune complexes;
IL-1, interleukin-1; ICAM's, intercellular adhesion molecules;
TNF, tumor necrosis factor; protein C act., protein C activating
capacity; tPA, tissue plasminogen activator; tPAi, tissue
plasminogen activator inhibitor, MRC I, Class I major histocompatibility antigens; MCH II, Class II major histocompatibility
antigens.

Although many of the experiments summarized above were performed
in vitro it is likely that they reflect what can occur in vivo since
recombinant TNFα has been shown to induce shock and tissue injury when
infused in rats, thus reproducing many of the effects of injected bacterial endotoxin[84]. The observation that TNFα can cause a reduction in
the capacity of endothelial cells to support activation of protein C is
particularly important in the light of recent experiments demonstrating
that injection of activated protein C into baboons can protect them from
disseminated intravascular coagulation and death when injected intravenously with otherwise lethal doses of Escherichia coli[85]. In other
experiments, injection of baboons with monoclonal antibodies to protein C
rendered them susceptible to otherwise sublethal injections of E. coli[86].

Tumor necrosis factor α, and interferons α and β, products respectively of fibroblasts and leukocytes, have been shown to stimulate
expression of class I major histocompatibility antigens by endothelial
cells. Interferon-γ, a product of lymphocytes, stimulates expression of
class II major histocompatibility antigens by endothelial cells[87]. Thus
altered, the vascular endothelium may become competant to present antigens
to cytotoxic/suppressor T lymphocytes in the context of class I MHC
antigens and to helper T cells in the context of class II MHC antigens[88].
These observations may have important implications for graft rejection,
the interaction of viruses with vascular endothelium and the fate of
infected cells, and for the presentation of antigens derived from
constituents of the vessel wall and the development of autoimmune phenomena
within the walls of vessels.

The series of events described above is depicted in the figure. Viewed from the perspective of a coronary or cerebral artery it is a rather
dismal scenario. Viewed, on the other hand, as a highly integrated system
for defense against infectious organisms it is quite remarkable. Endothelium can be modified to cause adherence of leukocytes early in infection.
Elaboration of tissue factor and down regulation of anticoagulant functions can contribute to isolation of an infected site from the systemic
circulation, and finally, foreign antigens can be presented to the immune system either by modified endothelial cells[88] or monocytic cells adherent to them.

It is important to point out that blood monocytes, in addition to
producing monokines such as IL-1 and TNFα, are also capable of procoagulant
functions. In a series of papers, Edgington and colleagues have demo-
strated that certain T lymphocytes, following stimulation by bacterial
lipopolysaccharide or antigen antibody complexes, are capable of
stimulating monocytes with which they are in contact, to express both
tissue factor activity and membrane bound prothrombinase activity.
Additional and unique pathways also appear to exist by which allogeneic
stimulation of T lymphocytes or stimulation of T lymphocytes by foreign
antigens ultimately result in expression of tissue factor by monocytes.
In addition, other substances such as C5a may also be capable of initiating
expression of procoagulant activity by monocytes. A description of these
pathways and a review of pertinent literature has recently been published
by Edgington and colleagues[89].

Thus it can be seen that environmental stimuli such as bacterial
lipopolysaccharide, foreign antigens and immune complexes can trigger
an almost infinite number of mutually amplifying interactions between
vascular endothelium, monocytes and lymphocytes that can lead to a
thrombotic event. At another level, perhaps with less intense and more
protracted stimulation, these same mechanisms might result in increased
entry of such cells into the arterial wall where local synthesis

of mitogens might contribute to the growth of arteriosclerotic plaques
and where local expression of monokines such as IL-1 and TNF might result
in local and protracted endothelial altered function or dysfunction.
Emigration of lymphocytes into the walls of blood vessels may also have
important immunopathologic consequences. Recently, T lymphocytes of both
helper and cytotoxic/syppressor phenotypes have been identified immuno-
histochemically in arteriosclerotic plaques in human carotid arteries[90].
It has also been demonstrated recently that murine lymphocytes cultured
in vitro with syngeneic vascular smooth muscle cells can mediate vascular
injury in vivo when transferred to syngeneic recipient mice[91]. The
question can be raised as to whether the antigen presenting functions of
monocytes and/or endothelial cells modified as described above would make
such an event more likely in vivo.

In the context of the large number of possible interactions between
components of the walls of blood vessels and fluid and cellular components
of blood involving constituents of both the immune system and the hemostatic system, it is conceivable that prospective approaches to the
identification of potential risk factors for cardiovascular disease can
be constructed. In this construction, potential risk factors could be
identified because of their capacity to stimulate one or more of the
interactions discussed above. Their contributory role in pathogenesis of
cardiovascular disease may then be considered as an accident of their
capacity to pervert highly integrated, adaptive mechanisms. For example,
elevated serum cholesterol levels have long been identified as a major
risk factor for atherosclerosis and its complications. Recent studies
in experimental animal models demonstrate that elevation of plasma
cholesterol levels enhances migration of monocytes into the walls of
arteries[92,93]. Migration and emigration of these cells may be an
important component of blood vessel repair. In the presence of hypercholesterolemia the difference is that such cells may be lipid laden;
if they are also activated by other environmental stimuli to produce
some of the substances mentioned above, then the stage is set for the
synergistic action between hypercholesterolemia and these other activating
stimuli to induce plaque growth and/or thrombus formation.

TOBACCO AND THE IMMUNE SYSTEM

Cigarette smoking, may be a major risk factor for arteriosclerosis
and it complications because constituents of cigarette smoke also prevent
or exaggerate otherwise adaptive defense mechanisms. In the last several
years, our laboratory has investigated this possibility. We have
demonstrated that:
(1) Polyphenol containing glycoprotein antigen(s) isolated from tobacco
    leaves and present in cigarette smoke condensate can activate the
    intrinsic pathway of coagulation in vitro and in vivo[94,95].
(2) This antigen (tobacco glycoprotein or TGP) is by virtue of its poly-
    phenol epitopes mitogenic for vascular smooth muscle cells in vitro
    and for both murine and human B lymphocytes[96,97,98].
(3) TGP can stimulate expression of interleukin-1 activity by human
    peripheral blood adherent leukocytes, e.g. monocytes, as measured by
    thymocyte activation assay[99].
(4) Immunization of mice with TGP or with polyphenol (rutin) epitopes
    coupled to bovine albumin leads to preferential expression of IgE
    antibodies to the carrier molecule[100]. Preferential expression of
    IgE antibodies to TGP has also been demonstrated in humans[101].
    Also, approximately one-third of human volunteers, smokers and
    non-smokers exhibit immediate cutaneous hypersensitivity to TGP[102].
    These observations suggest the possibility that smokers with IgE
    mediated hypersensitivity to antigens present in cigarette smoke
    might repetitively stimulate release of inflammatory mediators from

pulmonary mast cells which could effect the lung but which would also have immediate access to the heart. Further, we have shown that tobacco antigen can trigger cardiac anaphylaxis in appropriately sensitized rabbits and guinea pigs[103]. Because human hearts can also be the target of anaphylactic reactions[104], though the effects of mediators generated in the lung as well as those consequent to IgE mediated release from cardiac mast cells, the question arises as whether some cases of arrhythmia and sudden death are immunologically mediated, and whether the hypersensitive smoker is at greater risk of such an event.

(5) Cigarette smoke also contains a low molecular weight, ca. 97 dalton, substance that is capable of activating the alternative pathway of the complement system, possibly through different mechanisms[105,106]. These effects of cigarette smoke constituents on the alternative pathway of the complement system may be pertinent to cardiovascular disease through multiple effects of activated complement components on platelets as described above as well as those of complement derived anaphylatoxins on vascular tissues including the heart[107].

In view of the known effects of IgE mediated release of effector substances, IL-1, and activation of the complement system, directly or indirectly, on blood vessels and the myocardium, it is reasonable to hypothesize that some of the association of smoking with risk of cardiovascular disease and pulmonary disease may be related to its effects on different limbs of the immune system. Since generation of polyphenols are important to the defense mechanisms of higher plants and substances similar to TGP have been isolated from other commonly ingested or inhaled plant products as coffee, chocolate, or ragweed[108], several questions can be asked. These are: (1) Can similar natural products also contribute to cardiovascular risk when used abusively either by dose or portal of entry?; (2) Can their contribution to cardiovascular risk also occur via perturbation of the adaptive functions of the immune system which, in light of observations, discussed above must now include components of the hemostatic systems and the endothelium of blood vessel?; and (3) Can the same logic be applied to trying to identify the risk factors/mechanisms that may contribute to the 50% of heart attacks that cannot currently be associated with known risk factors? Structural characterization of substances in tobacco that perturb or pervert normally adaptive immune mechanisms and understanding these interactions may permit prediction of as yet unknown environmental substances that contribute to cardiovascular disease through similar interactions.

SUMMARY

A large and rapidly growing quantity of information gained from both clinical and experimental observation strongly indicate that perturbations of the immune system can contribute to the pathogenesis of vessel injury and thrombosis. This is, in part, because the immune system functions to amplify and diversify the host response to a given stimulus often resulting in activation of associated pathways such as the hemostatic system and modulation of endothelial cell function. Studying the pathogenesis of arteriosclerosis and its complications, as well as other vascular disease, from an immunologic or immunopathologic perspective may provide a better understanding of why some some individuals appear to be at greater risk of cardiovascular disease than others, a more precise identification of the mechanisms leading to the expression of increased risk, and because of the structural specificity implicit in immunologic reactions, identification of those environmental factors responsible for inciting such immunologic perturbation. It is conceivable that identification of at least some of the risk factors associated with the 50% of deaths from heart attack that are not associated with known risk factors may be achieved through a consideration of the rôle of immunologic mechanisms in the pathogenesis cardiovascular disease.

140

REFERENCES

1. H. C. McGill, Persistant problems in the pathogenesis of athero-sclerosis, <u>Arteriosclerosis</u> 4:443 (1984).
2. R. G. Gerrity, The role of monocytes in atherogenesis. I. Transition of blood borne monocytes into foam cells in fatty lesions, <u>Am J Path</u> 103:181 (1981).
3. R. Ross, and A. Vogel, The platelet derived growth factor, <u>Cell</u> 14:203 (1978).
4. K. Shimokado, E. W. Raines, D. K. Medtes, T. B. Barrett, and R. Ross, A significant part of macrophage derived growth factor consists of at least two forms of PDGF, <u>Cell</u> 43:277 (1985).
5. L. B. Chen, J. M. Buchanan, Mitogenic activity of blood components. I. Thrombin and prothrombin, <u>Proc Natl Acad Sci</u> (U.S.A.) 72:131 (1975).
6. N. Capurro, and R. Levi, The heart as a target organ in systemic allergic reactions: Comparison of cardiac anaphylaxis <u>in vivo</u> and in vitro, <u>Circ Res</u> 36:520 (1975).
7. T. J. Sullivan, Cardiac disorders in penicillin induced anaphylaxis, <u>JAMA</u> 248:2161 (1982).
8. L.A. Solberg, and J. P. Strong, Risk factors and atherosclerotic lesions. A review of autopsy studies, <u>Arteriosclerosis</u> 3:187 (1983).
9. W. E. Paul, The immune system: An introduction, <u>in</u>: "Fundamental Immunology," W. E. Paul, ed., Raven Press, New York (1984).
10. R. L. K. Virchow, Cellular Pathology as Based Upon Physiological Pathological Histology (1858), translated by F. Chance, Dover, New York (1971).
11. C. Rokitansky, Lehrbuch der Pathologischen Anatomie, Vol 2, ed., W. Bronmueller, Vienna (1856).
12. J. B. Duguid, Pathogenesis of atherosclerosis, <u>Lancet</u> ii:925 (1949).
13. P. Zeek, Studies in Atherosclerosis. I. Conditions in childhood which predispose to the early development of arteriosclerosis, <u>Am J Med Sci</u> 184:350 (1932).
14. P. Zeek, Studies in Atherosclerosis. II. Atheroma and its sequelae in rheumatic heart disease, <u>Am J Med Sci</u> 184:350, (1932).
15. H. T. Karsner, and F. Bayless, Coronary arteries in rheumatic fever, <u>Am Heart J</u> 9:557 (1934).
16. L. Gross, M. A. Kugel, and E. Z. Epstein, Lesions of the coronary arteries and their branches in rheumatic fever, <u>Am J Path</u> 11:253 (1935).
17. T. Fahr, Zür Frage der Polymyositis (Dermatomyositis), <u>Arch Dermatol Syph</u> 130:1 (1921).
18. E. L. Opie, Inflammation and immunity, <u>J Immunol</u> 17:329 (1929).
19. A. R. Rich, Hyersensitivity in disease with especial reference to periarteritis nodosa, rheumatic fever, disseminated lupus erythematosus and rheumatoid arthritis, <u>in</u>: "The Harvey Lecture," Academic Press, New York (1946).
20. A. R. Rich, and J. E. Gregory, Experimental anaphylactic lesions of the coronary arteries of the sclerotic type, commonly associated with rheumatic fever and disseminated lupus erythematosus, <u>Bull Johns Hopkins Hosp</u> 81:313 (1947).
21. V. G. Tsakralides, L. C. Bleiden, and J. E. Edwards, Coronary atherosclerosis and myocardial infarction associated with systemic lupus erythematosus, <u>Am Heart J</u> 87:637, (1974).
22. E. G. L. Bywaters, Peripheral vascular obstruction in rheumatoid arthritis and its relationship to other vascular lesions, <u>Ann Rheum Dis</u> 16:84 (1957).
23. K. S. Kant, V. E. Pollak, A. Dosekun, P. Glas-Greenwalt, M. A. Weiss, and H. I. Glueck, Lupus nephritis with thrombosis and abnornal fibrinolysis, <u>J Lab Clin Med</u> 105:77 (1985).

24. F. J. Dixon, J. J. Vasquez, W. O. Weigle, and C. G. Cochrane, Pathogenesis of serum sickness, Arch Pathol 65:18 (1958).

25. W. T. Kniker, and C. G. Cochrane, The localization of circulating immune complexes in experimental serum sickness, J Exp Med 127:119 (1968).

26. J. Benveniste, P. M. Henson, and C. G. Cochrane, Leukocyte dependent histamine release from rabbit platelets, J Exp Med 136:1356 (1972).

27. J. Benveniste, Platelet activating factor, a new mediator of anaphylaxis and immune complex deposition from rabbit and human basophils, Nature 249:581 (1974).

28. P. O. Clark, D. J. Hanahan, and R. N. Pinckard, Physical and chemical properties of platelet activating factor obtained from human neutrophils and monocytes and rabbit neutrophils and basophils, Biochem Biophys Acta 628:69 (1980).

29. P. M. Henson, Activation of rabbit platelets by platelet activating factor derived from IgE sensitized basophils. Characteristic of the aggregation and its dissociation from secretion, J Clin Invest 60:481 (1977).

30. L. B. Schwartz, and K. F. Austen, Structure and function of the chemical mediators of mast cells, Prog Allergy 34:271 (1984).

31. R. N. Pinckard, C. Tanegawa, and M. Halonen, IgE induced blood coagulation alterations in the rabbit, J Immunol 115:525 (1975).

32. H. L. Meier, A. P. Kaplan, L. M. Lichtenstein, S. D. Revak C. G. Cochrane, and H. H. Newball, Anaphylactic release of a prekallikrein activator from human lung in vitro, J Clin Invest 72:574 (1983).

33. L. B. Schwartz, J. J. Schratz, D. Vik, D. T. Fearon, and K. F. Austen, Generation of C3a anaphylatoxin from human C3 by human mast cell tryptase, J Immunol 130:1891 (1983).

34. C. R. Minick, G. E. Murphy, and W. G. Campbell, Experimental induction of atheroarteriosclerosis by the synergy of allergic injury to arteries and lipid rich diet. I. Effect of repeated injections of horse serum in rabbits fed a dietary cholesterol supplement, J Exp Med 124:635 (1966).

35. N. J. Hardin, C. R. Minick, and G. E. Murphy, Experimental induction of atheroarteriosclerosis by the synergy of allergic injury to arteries and lipid rich diet. III. The role of earlier acquired fibromuscular intimal thickening in the pathogenesis of later developing atherosclerosis, Am J Path 73:301 (1973).

36. A. K. Rider, J. C. Copeland, S. A. Hunt, J. Mason, M. J. Spector R. A. Winkle, C. P. Bieber, M. E. Billingham, E. Doug, R. B. Griepp, J. S. Schroeder, E. B. Stinson, D. C. Harrison, and N. E. Shumway, The status of cardiac transplantation, Circulation 52:531 (1975).

37. D. R. Alonso, P. K. Starek, and C. R. Minick, Studies on the pathogenesis of atheroarteriosclerosis induced in rabbit cardiac allografts by the synergy of graft rejection and hypercholes- terolemia, Am J Path 87:415 (1977).

38. T. M. Cocks, J. A. Angus, J. H. Campbell, and G. R. Campbell, Release and properties of endothelium derived relaxing factor (EDRF) from endothelial cells in culture, J Cell Physiol 123:310 (1985)

39. G. Camussi, C. Tetta, M. Meroni, L. Torri-Tarelli, C. Roffinello, A. Alberton, C. Deregibus, and A. Sessa, Localization of cationic proteins derived from platelets and polymorphonuclear neutrophils and local loss of anionic sites in glomeruli of rabbits with experimentally induced acute serum sickness, Lab Invest 55:56 (1986).

40. G. Gallo, T. Caulin-Glaser, S. N. Emancipator, and M. E. Lamm, Nephritogenicity and differential distribution of glomerular immune complexes related to immunogen charge, Lab Invest 48:353 (1983).

41. N. Simionescu, M. Simionescu, G. E. Palade, Differentiated micro-domains on the luminal surface of the capillary endothelium. I. Preferential distribution of anionic sites, J Cell Biol 90:605 (1981).

42. U. S. Ryan, D. R. Schultz, R. J. Del Vecchio, and J. W. Ryan, Endothelial cells of bovine pulmonary artery lack receptors for C3b and for the Fc portion of immunoglobulin, Science 208:748 (1980).

43. D. Westmoreland, and J. F. Watkins, The IgG receptor induced by herpes simplex virus: Studies using radioiodinated IgG. J Gen Virol 24:167 (1974).

44. R. Keller, R. Peitchel, J. N. Goldman, and M. J. Goldman, An IgG-Fc receptor induced in cytomegalovirus-infected human fibroblasts, J Immunol 116:772 (1976).

45. M. F. Para, L. Goldstein, and P. G. Spear, Similarities and differences in the Fc-binding glycoprotein (gE) of herpes simplex firus types 1 and 2 and tentative mapping of the viral gene for this glycoprotein, J Virol 41:137 (1982).

46. M. Ogata, and S. Shigeta, Appearance of immunoglobulin G Fc receptor in cultured human cells infected with varicella-zoster virus. Infect Immun 26:770 (1979).

47. D. B. Cines, A. P. Lyss, M. Bina, R. Corkey, N. A. Kefalides, and H. M. Friedman, Fc and C3 receptors induced by herpes simplex virus on cultured human endothelial cells, J Clin Invest 69:123 (1982).

48. M. F. Para, R. B. Baucke, and P. G. Spear, Glycoprotein gE of herpes simplex virus type 1: Effects of anti-gE on virion infectivity and on virus-induced Fc binding receptors, J Virol 41:129 (1982).

49. H. M. Friedman, G. H. Cohen, R. J. Eisenberg, C. A. Seidel, and D. B. Cines, Glycoprotein C of herpes simplex virus 1 acts as a receptor for the C3b complement component on infected cells, Nature 309:633 (1984).

50. D. P. Hajjar, Herpesvirus infection prevents activation of cytoplasmic cholesteryl esterase in arterial smooth muscle cells, J Biol Chem 261:7611 (1986).

51. D. P. Hajjar, and A. J. Grant, Herpes simplex virus infection in human arterial cells: Implications in arteriosclerosis, (manuscript in preparation).

52. H. M. Friedman, J. Wolfe, N. A. Kefalides, and E. J. Macarak, Susceptibility of endothelial cells derived from different blood vessels to common viruses, In Vitro Cell and Devel Biology 22:397 (1986).

53. K. W. Moore, P. Jardien, M. L. Mietz, M. L. Trounstine, E. L. Kuff, K. Ishizaka, and C. L. Martens, Rodent IgE-binding factor genes are members of an endogenous, retrovirus like gene family, J Immunol 136:4283 (1986).

54. P. M. Henson, Immune complex diseases. Cellular mediators and the pathogenesis of inflammatory tissue injury produced by immune complexes, in: "Bayer Symposium VI. Experimental Models of Chronic Inflammatory Diseases," L. E. Glynn, and H. O. Schlumberger, ed., Springer Verlag, Berlin-New York (1977).

55. P. M. Henson, and Z. G. Oades, Stimulation of human neutrophils by soluble and insoluble immunoglobulin aggregates, J Clin Invest 56:1053 (1975).

56. J. Fehr, and H. S. Jacob, In vitro granulocyte adherence and in vivo margination: two associated complement-dependent functions, J Exp Med 146:641 (1977).

57. T. Sacks, C. F. Moldow, P. R. Craddock, R. K. Bowers, and H. S. Jacob, Oxygen radicals mediate endothelial cell damage by complement-stimulated granulocytes, J Clin Invest 61:1161 (1978).

58. P. M. Henson, Immune Complex disease. Cellular mediators and the pathogenesis of inflammatory tissue injury produced by immune complexes, in: "Bayer Symposium VI. Experimental M Inflammatory Diseases," L. E. Glynn, and H. O. Schlumberger, ed., Springer Verlag, Berlin-New York (1977).

59. T. E. Hugli, and H. J. Muller-Eberhard, Anaphylatoxins: C3a and C5a, in: "Adv. Immunol. 26," F. J. Dixon, and H. G. Kunkel, ed., Academic Press, New York (1978).

60. E. L. Becker, and P. M. Henson, In vitro studies of immunologically induced secretion of mediators from cells and related phenomena, Adv Immunol 17:193 (1973).

61. M. K. Pangburn, and H. J. Muller-Eberhard, The alternative pathway of complement, Springer Seminars in Immunology 7:163 (1984).

62. M. J. Polley, and R. L. Nachman, Human complement in thrombin mediated platelet function, J Exp Med 150:633 (1979).

63. M. J. Polley, R. L. Nachman, and B. B. Weksler, Human complement in the arachidonic acid transformation pathway in platelets, J Exp Med 153:257 (1981).

64. M. J. Polley, and R. L. Nachman, Human platelets activation by C3a and C3a des-arg, J Exp Med 158:603 (1983).

65. T. Wiedmer, C. T. Esmon, and P. J. Sims, Complement proteins C5b-9 stimulate procoagulant activity through platelet prothrombinase, Blood 68:875 (1986).

66. P. Geertinger, and H. Sorensen, On the reduced atherogenic effect of cholesterol feeding in rabbits with cogenital complement (C6) deficiency, Artery 1:177 (1975).

67. M. P. Bevilacqua, J. S. Pober, G. R. Majeau, R. S. Cotran, and M. A. Gimbrone, Jr., Interleukin 1 (IL-1) induces biosynthesis and cell surface expression of procoagulant activity in human vascular endothelial cells, J Exp Med 160:618 (1984).

68. M. P. Bevilacqua, J. S. Pober, G. R. Majeau, W. Fiers, R. S. Cotran, and M. A. Gimbrone, Jr., Recombinant tumor necrosis factor induces procoagulant activity in cultured human vascular endothelium: Characterization and comparison with the actions of interleukin 1, Proc Natl Acad Sci USA 83:4533 (1986).

69. P. P. Nawroth, and D. M. Stern, Modulation of endothelial cell hemostatic properties by tumor necrosis factor, J Exp Med 163:740 (1986).

70. M. P. Bevilacqua, J. S. Pober, M. E. Wheeler, R. S. Cotran, and M. A. Gimbrone, Jr., Interleukin 1 acts on cultured human vascular endothelium to increase the adhesion of polymorphonuclear leukocytes, monocytes and related leukocyte cell lines, J Clin Invest 76:2003 (1985).

71. J. R. Gamble, J. M. Harlan, S. J. Klebanoff, and M. A. Vadas, Stimulation of the adherence of neutrophils to umbilical vein endothelium by human recombinant tumor necrosis factor, Proc Natl Acad Sci USA 82:8667 (1985).

72. D. E. Cavender, D. O. Haskard, B. Joseph, and M. Ziff, Interleukin 1 increases the binding of human B and T lymphocytes to endothelial cell monolayers, J Immunol 136:203 (1986).

73. R. P. Schleimer, and B. K. Rutledge, Cultured human vascular endothelial cells acquire adhesiveness for neutrophils after stimulation with interleukin 1, endotoxin, and tumor-promoting phorbol diesters, J Immunol 136:649 (1986).

74. S. H. Tannenbaum, R. Finko, D. B. Cines, Antibody and immune complexes induce tissue factor production by human endothelial cells, J Immunol 137:1532 (1986).

75. C. A. Dinarello, J. G. Cannon, S. M. Wolff, H. A. Bernheim,
    B. Beutler, A. Cerami, I. S. Figari, M. A. Palladino, Jr., and
    J. V. O'Connor, Tumor necrosis factor (cachectin) is an endogenous
    pyrogen and induces production of interleukin 1, J Exp Med
    163:1433 (1986).
76. M. L. Dustin, A. K. Rothlein, C. A. Dinarello, and T. A. Springer,
    Induction by IL-1 and interferon-γ, tissue distribution, biochem-
    istry and function of a natural adherence molecule (ICAM-1),
    J Immunol 137:245 (1986).
77. M. P. Bevilacqua, J. S. Pober, M. E. Wheeler, D. Mendrick,
    R. S. Cotran, and M. A. Gimbrone, Jr., Interleukin-1 (IL-1) acts
    on vascular endothelial cells to increase their adhesivity for
    blood leukocytes, Fed Proc 44:1494 (1985).
78. M. P. Bevilacqua, unpublished observations.
79. L. Jalkanen, A. C. Steere, R. I. Fox, and E. C. Butcher, A distinct
    endothelial recognition system that controls lymphocyte traffic
    in inflamed synovium, Science 233:556 (1986).
80. P. P. Nawroth, and D. M. Stern, Modulation of endothelial cell
    hemostatic properties by tumor necrosis factor, J Exp Med 163:740
    (1986).
81. M. P. Bevilacqua, R. R. Schleef, M. A. Gimbrone, Jr., and
    D. J. Loskutoff, Regulation of the fibrinolytic system of
    cultured human vascular endothelium by interleukin-1,
    J Clin Invest 78:587 (1986).
82. R. L. Nachman, K. A. Hajjar, R. L. Silverstein, and C. A. Dinarello,
    Interleukin-1 induces endothelial cell synthesis of plasminogen
    activator inhibitor, J Exp Med 163:1595 (1986).
83. A. H. Stolpen, E. C. Guinan, W. Fiers, and J. S. Pober, Recombinant
    tumor necrosis factor and immune interferon act singly and in
    combination to reorganize human vascular endothelial cell
    monolayers, Am J Path 123:16 (1986).
84. K. J. Tracey, B. Beutler, S. F. Lowry, J. Merryweather, S. Wolpe,
    I. W. Milsark, R. J. Hariri, T. J. Fahey, III, A. Zentella,
    J. D. Albert, G. T. Shires, and A. Cerami, Shock and tissue
    injury induced by recombinant human cachectin, Science 234:470
    (1986).
85. F. B. Taylor, Jr., D. M. Stern, P. P. Nawroth, C. T. Esmon,
    L. B. Hinshaw, and K. E. Blick, Activated protein C prevents
    E. coli induced coagulopathy and shock in the primate
    J Clin Invest (in press).
86. F. B. Taylor, Jr., A. Chang, C. Esmon, A. DiAngelo, S. Vigano,
    D. Stern, P. Nawroth, and L. Hinshaw, Endogenous protein C
    prevents the coagulopathic and lethal effects of E. coli
    infusion in the baboon, J Clin Invest (in press).
87. T. A. Collins, J. Korman, C. T. Wake, J. M. Boss, D. J. Kappes,
    W. Fiers, K. A. Ault, M. A. Gimbrone, Jr., J. L. Strominger,
    and J. S. Pober, Immune interferon activates multiple class II
    major histocompatibility complex genes and the associated
    invariant chain gene in human endothelial cells and dermal
    fibroblasts, Proc Natl Acad Sci USA 81:4917 (1984).
88. T. D. Geppert, and P. E. Lipsky, Antigen presentation by interferon-γ
    treated endothelial cells and fibroblasts: Differential ability
    to function as antigen-presenting cells despite comparable Ia
    expression, J Immunol 135:3750 (1985).
89. T. S. Edgington, H. Helin, S. A. Gregory, G. Levy, D. S. Fair,
    and B. S. Schwartz, Cellular pathways and signals for the induction
    of biosynthesis of initiators of the coagulation protease cascade
    by cells of the monocyte lineage, in: "Mononuclear Phagocytes,:
    R. Van Furth. ed.. Martinus Nvhoff. Boston (1985).

90. L. Joasson, J. Holm, O. Skalli, G. Bondyers, and G. K. Hansson, The human arteriosclerotic plaque: Regional accumulations of T cells, macrophages, and smooth muscle cells, _Arteriosclerosis_ 6:131 (1986).

91. C. F. Moyer, and C. L. Reinisch, The role of smooth muscle cells in experimental autoimmune vasculitis. I. The initiation of delayed type hypersensitivity angiitis, _Am J Path_ 117:380 (1984).

92. I. Joris, T. Zand, J. J. Nunnari, F. J. Krolikowski, and G. Majno, Studies on the pathogenesis of atherosclerosis. I. Adhesion and emigration of mononuclear cells in the aorta of hypercholester-olemic rats, _Am J Path_ 113:341 (1983).

93. A. Fagiotto, R. Ross, and L. Harker, Studies of hypercholesterolemia in the non-human primate. I. Changes that lead to fatty streak formation, _Arteriosclerosis_ 4:323 (1984).

94. C. G. Becker, and T. Dubin, Activation of factor XII by tobacco glycoprotein, _J Exp Med_ 146:457 (1977).

95. L. Dillon, F. Glenn, C. G. Becker, Induction of acalculous chole-cystis and pneumonitis in dogs following inhalation of constituents of cigarette smoke condensate, _Am J Path_ 82:253 (1982).

96. C. G. Becker, D. P. Hajjar, and J. M. Hefton, Tobacco constituents are mitogenic for arterial smooth muscle cells, _Am J Path_ 120:1 (1985).

97. J. W. Choy, C. G. Becker, G. W. Siskind, and T. Francus, Effects of tobacco glycoprotein on the immune system. I. TGP is a T-independent B cell mitogen for murine lymphoid cells, _J Immunol_ 134:3193 (1985).

98. T. Francus, R. F. Klein, L. Staiano-Coico, G. W. Siskind, and C. G. Becker, Effects of tobacco glycoprotein on the immune system. II. TGP stimulates human peripheral blood lymphocytes to proliferate and to differentiate into immunoglobulin secreting cells, (manuscript submitted).

99. T. Francus, L. C. Thompson, B. Y. Rubin, M. K. Crow, G. W. Siskind, and C. G. Becker, Tobacco glycoprotein is a potent inducer of IL-1 production, but does not induce production of IL-2, IL-3, IFN or the expression of IL-2 receptors, (manuscript submitted).

100. T. Francus, G. W. Siskind, and C. G. Becker, The role of antigen structure in the regulation of IgE isotype expression, PNAS 80:3430 (1983).

101. R. F. Klein, and C. G. Becker, Selective expression of IgE reactive with tobacco glycoprotein in human sera, Fed Proc 45:225 (1986).

102. C. G. Becker, T. Dubin, and H. P. Wiedemann, Hypersensitivity to tobacco antigen, _Proc Natl Acad Sci USA_ 73:1712 (1976).

103. R. Levi, A. A. Chenouda, J. P. Trzeciakowski, Guo Zhao-Gui, L. M. Aaronson, R. D. Luskind, C. H. Lee, W. Gay, V. A. Subramanian, J. C. McCabe, and J. C. Alexander, Dysrhythmias caused by histamine release in guinea pig and human hearts, _Klin Wochenschr_ 60:965 (1982).

104. R. Levi, J. Zavecz, J. A. Burke, and C. G. Becker, Cardiac and pulmonary anaphylaxis induced by glycoprotein isolated from tobacco leaves and cigarette smoke condensate, _Am J Path_ 106:318 (1982).

105. A. Firpo, M. J. Polley, and C. G. Becker, The effect of tobacco derived products on the human complement system, _Immunobiology_ 164:318 (1983).

106. A. Firpo, F. Field, D. Wellner, F. Infante, C. G. Becker, and M. J. Polley, On the chemical characterization of a low molecular weight component of cigarette smoke which activates the alternative pathway of complement, in: "Complement: Laboratory and Clinical Research. XIIth International Complement Workshop," J. S. Cooper, and S. Karger, ed., Basel (1985).

107. U. Hachfeld del Balzo, R. Levi, and M. J. Polley, Cardiac dysfunction caused by purified human C3a anaphylatoxin. Proc Natl Acad Sci USA 82:886 (1985).

108. C. G. Becker, N. Van Hamont, and M. Wagner, Tobacco, cocoa, coffee and ragweed: Cross-reacting allergens that activate factor XII dependent pathways, Blood 58:861 (1981).

WHAT'S THE DOSE?

Stanford Wessler

Department of Medicine
New York University School of Medicine
New York, New York

It is doubtful that many in this room would quibble with the statement, in regard to warfarin dosage, that almost every physician appears to behave as if there were no published guidelines for prophylaxis and that he is, so to speak, "therapeutically on his own". What this means in practical terms to individual patients in each of our own communities is that the therapeutic regimen offered depends on which physician is consulted. Moreover, within each category of practitioner, prophylaxis depends on the hospital entered, the service assigned, the specific attending physician responsible for the patient's care, and, at some institutions, the house officer on duty at the time of admission. Private office and clinic outpatient management is no more standardized. In recognition of this absence of consensus it is hoped that several of the presentations to follow may provide some common ground concerning therapeutic regimens that will be of intrinsic value for decision making in cardiac and cerebral vascular disease.

AN HISTORICAL NOTE

The time course of the oral anticoagulant story illustrates the well-known lag phenomenon between discovery of a potential therapeutic agent and the final determination of dose regimens which, in the case of warfarin, is still evolving more than one-half century after the prothrombin time became available. Similar problems exist, of course, for heparin and aspirin both of whose origins date to the 1890's.

Spoiled sweet clover disease was first recognized by the veternarian Schofield in 1922.[1] Paul Link's publications on the synthesis of the coumarin compounds began in 1934,[2] and one year later Quick described the methodology of the prothrombin time.[3] These seminal observations led to the view that coumarin compounds would have antithrombotic efficacy. That thesis was founded, in fact, upon the observations that the oral anticoagulants produced both a bleeding disease in cattle and a few seconds prolongation of a test tube assay designed to recognize hemophilia. Today, hypotheses based on such evidence alone would be unlikely to reach the stage of clinical trial. Yet, clinical trials in 1941-42 [4-6] suggested that the coumarins were effective antithrombotic agents. In short, to quote Peter Medawar: "It doesn't pay to be too clever".[7] This is also one example of how investigators have the ability to imagine what the truth might be, before they establish it.

When, however, the results of a large national trial of the efficacy of Dicumarol in acute myocardial infarction was published more than 30 years ago,[8] disaffection with the original hypothesis gradually developed.

Moreover, skepticism concerning the efficacy of coumarin drugs in coronary artery disease actually increased as further trials were reported, until the value of oral anticoagulants for any type of thromboembolic episode came into serious question.

The credibility of drug efficacy was damaged not so much by any incompetence among the investigators, but rather by the fact that the scientists of that day were prisoners of the state-of-the-art tools of their trade. These limitations, existing in 1941 and unfortunately to some extent, still present today, include: naivete concerning clinical trial technology, incomplete understanding of the pathophysiology of the disease states being treated, rudimentary information of both normal hemostasis and the process of thrombogenesis, meager insight into the pharmacology and toxicity of the coumarin compounds, and last, but in reality what has been most important to clinicians, inadequate knowledge concerning both the standards required for performing the prothrombin time assay as well as identification of those test values that would provide an antithrombotic effect without producing major bleeding. For dosage was regulated by the prothrombin time which predicted bleeding rather than by assays, animal models or clinical trials that determined the minimal amount of drug required for the desired antithrombotic effect.

Accordingly, the so-called therapeutic range was judged to be somewhat below (but ideally just slightly below) the hemorrhagic level--and the same values were recommended not only for all types of antithrombotic prophylaxis, but for the entire course of the thrombotic process (acute and quiescent) in any individual patient. Under these circumstances, the likelihood of hemorrhage became an overriding deterrent to the widespread use of anticoagulants whose efficacy was under challenge in any event. By analogy, if there had been no blood pressure cuff, and shock had been the endpoint by which the value of antihypertensive therapy had been judged, the current reduction in stroke mortality attributable to antihypertensive medications would never have been achieved.

THE PROTHROMBIN TIME

Growing cynicism toward coumarin compounds was abetted by repeated modifications of the Quick assay. Lack of standardization of the test procedure, particularly as to the nature and reproducibility of the thromboplastin reagent as well as the blood collecting system, led to striking discrepancies in prothrombin times. These disparate results were further compounded by the variety of ways in which the data were expressed for clinical use. Such vagaries led not only to confusion, but to different intensities of treatment. Thus, the same coagulation defect accepted as therapeutic at one institution might be considered homeopathic at another or interpreted as a dangerous overdose at a third.

I believe that it may be through the observations made at this symposium that these physician frustrations in regard to the prothrombin time may at last be put to rest.

But after a standardized prothrombin time becomes available to all, the question will still remain: what's the dose?

INTENSITY RANGES OF PROTHROMBIN TIME
RATIOS FOR RABBIT THROMBOPLASTINS EQUIVALENT TO INR'S

COUMARIN INTENSITY	U.S. RANGE	INR RANGE
LOW	1.3 - 1.7	2.0 - 3.5
MEDIUM	1.6 - 1.9	3.0 - 4.2
HIGH	1.8 - 2.1	3.9 - 5.0

THE INTENSITY OF WARFARIN PROPHYLAXIS

It was Geza de Takats, who in 1950, stated his impression that: "It takes much less heparin or Dicumarol to prevent clotting than to treat it" [9]. Not accepted in its day, this view has subsequently prevailed in regard to the quiescent stage of venous thromboembolism: for heparin in the 1970's and for the coumarins in the present decade. And for this latter view we are in large measure indebted to the work of investigators in Great Britain, [10] Hamilton, Ontario [11] and Rochester, NY. [12]

As background for what may be touched on in different ways by some of the subsequent presentations, let me suggest, as shown in the table, that there may be three intensities of coumarin therapy that are prophylactic after different acute thromboembolic episodes have become quiescent, or among patients at risk before such events occur. The data from which these suggested and somewhat overlapping intensities are derived are not as firm as one would desire and are based upon studies of patients with genetic hemostatic defects, well-controlled animal models of thrombosis, a small number of excellent, objective human trials and the clinical impressions of experienced observers. These suggested intensities, moreover, do not have a broad consensus, probably estimate efficacy at 80 per cent for treated patients and will undoubtedly undergo modifications with time.

One result of this symposium may be the recommendation that warfarin intensity be tailored to specific thromboembolic conditions. For this to happen U.S. physicians will have to be weaned from a 40-year old addiction to the view that a single range of prothrombin time ratios will suffice for all clinical circumstances. Initially, the recommended ratios for assays employing rabbit thromboplastins were 1.5 to 3.0, then 1.5-2.5 and more recently 1.5-2.0--reductions decreed by bleeding incidence rather than antithrombotic efficacy. In fact, many physicians, on the basis of their own clinical experience, have kept the prothrombin time ratio as close to 1.5 as possible for all types of thromboembolism. This decision-making has its roots in several phenomena: first, the administration of oral anti-coagulants always confronts clinicians with their failures, be it thromboembolism or hemorrhage, and never with their successes; second, the demonstration in more than one trial, that INR values between 2.0-3.5 (equivalent to rabbit thromboplastin ratios of 1.3 or possibly 1.2-1.7) effectively prevent deep venous rethrombosis with only minor hemorrhage, and third, a hesitancy to accept trial data using more intensive therapy for arterial thromboembolism, for example in the medium intensity range, even if the result is a net gain in the reduction of thromboembolism despite an increased incidence of major hemorrhage.

Physicians instinctively rebel at any decision that will increase bleeding risks particularly among patients such as those with cardiac and cerebrovascular disease in whom life-threatening thromboembolic events are uncommon or in whom the anticipated benefit of anticoagulants is modest.

Accordingly, it becomes essential that anticoagulant administration be associated with a readily acceptable benefit/risk ratio, if warfarin prophylaxis is to be instituted on a much broader scale than is the case today. For it is only under such circumstances that oral anticoagulation can begin to rival the achievements of antibiotic and antihypertensive drugs.

In closing, I believe it is fair to state that physician resistance to the more widespread administration of warfarin, to the use of various intensities of anticoagulation, and to an international nomenclature for expressing the prothrombin time is no minor matter. For the mortality and morbidity from diverse thromboembolic phenomena remain secondary to no other single pathologic process in western society--an issue that is heightened by the increasing documentation that warfarin has a favorable prophylactic effect in preventing or containing many of these episodes.

REFERENCES

1.   F. W. Schofield, A brief account of a disease of cattle simulating hemorrhagic septicaemia due to feeding sweet clover, Can Vet Rec 3:74(1922).

2.   K. P. Link, Anticoagulant from spoiled sweet clover hay, Harvey Lect 39:162(1944).

3.   A. J. Quick, The prothrombin in hemophilia and in obstructive jaundice, J Biol Chem, 109:lxxiii(1935).

4.   J. B. Bingham, O. O. Meyer, and F. J. Pohle, Studies on the hemorrhagic agent 3,3'-methylenebis (4-Hydroxycoumarin). I. Its effect on the prothrombin and coagulation time of the blood of dogs and humans, Am J Med Sci, 202:563(1941).

5.   H. R. Butt, E. V. Allen, and J. L. Bollman, A preparation from spoiled sweet clover [3,3'-methylenebis-(4-hydroxycoumarin)] which prolongs coagulation and prothrombin time of the blood: preliminary report of experimental and clinical studies, Proc Staff Meet Mayo Clin, 16:388(1941).

6.   A. Prandoni, and I. S. Wright, The anticoagulants heparin and the dicumarin -3, 3'-methylenebis-(4-hydroxycoumarin). Bull NY Acad Med, 18:433(1942).

7.   P. B. Medawar, The Limits of Science, Harper and Row, New York (1984).

8.   I. S. Wright, C. D. Marple, and D. F. Beck, Myocardial infarction: its clinical manifestations and treatment with anticoagulants. A study of 1031 cases, Grune and Stratton, New York (1954).

9.   G. deTakats, Anticoagulant therapy in surgery, JAMA, 142:527(1950).

10.   D. A. Taberner, L. Poller, R. W. Burslem, and J. B. Jones, Oral anticoagulants controlled by the British comparative thromboplastin versus low-dose heparin in prophylaxis of deep vein thrombosis. Br Med J 1:272(1978).

11.   R. Hull, J. Hirsh, R. Jay, C. Carter, C. England, R. M. Gent, A. G. Turpie, D. McLoughlin, P. Dodd, M. Thomas, G. Raspob, and P. Ockefford, Different intensities of oral anticoagulant therapy in the treatment of proximal vein thrombosis, N Engl J Med 307:1676(1982).

12.   C. W. Francis, V. J. Marder, C. M. Evarts, and S. Yaukoolbodi, Two-step warfarin therapy: prevention of postoperative venous thrombosis without excessive bleeding. JAMA 249:374(1983).

VENOUS THROMBOEMBOLISM IN MODERATE RISK PATIENTS

Edward Genton

Ochsner Clinic
1514 Jefferson Highway
New Orleans, Louisiana

The incidence and significance of venous thrombosis and pulmonary embolism as a complication in hospitalized patients treated medically or surgically is well established. The incidence of venous thrombosis varies considerably between patient groups based upon numerous factors in addition to the severity of the medical illness or surgical procedure. These other factors include; age of patient, the presence of congestive heart failure, history of prior thromboembolism, etc. The risk of venous thrombosis progressively increases with the number of these risk factors. (Table 1) Therefore, it is possible to categorize patients on the level of their risk for venous thrombosis which is of value not only to identify patients most in need of prophylaxis but also to determine the prophylactic measure because in general the greater the thrombogenic stimulus the more intense the antithrombotic prophylaxis required.

TABLE I

Venous Thromboembolism

R I S K

LOW 10-15%	MODERATE 20-40%	HIGH 50+ %
Abdominal/Thoracic Surgery (< age 50)	Abd/Thoracic Surgery (> age 50)	Abd/Thoracic Surg Malignant Disease
TUR/Vaginal Hysterectomy	Pelvic Surgery	Pelvic Surgery, Extensive
Foot/Ankle Trauma or Surgery	Fx - Long Bones	Hip/Knee Surgery
Cerebral Contusion	Intracranial Surgery	Stroke
MI - Uncomplicated	MI with complications	- - -

Modifying factors: - Agedness   - Heart failure
                    - Immobility - Obesity/Varicosities
                    - Malignancy - Prior thromboembolism

In this presentation, will be considered the effect of oral anticoagulants as prophylaxis for patients at moderate risk for venous thrombosis. We will focus on three issues concerning the oral anticoagulants;
Their effectiveness, 2) Their risks and 3) Comparison with alternative
methods.

Most of the information available on the effect oral anticoagulants
in moderate risk patients in the literature comes from data presented
before currently used objective methods for diagnosis were available and
before the current rigourous guidelines for clinical trials were developed.
Studies for the most part did not use a control group and were either non-
random or used less than optimal methods for randomization and all used
clinical inpoints for the diagnosis of venous thrombosis which are now
known to lack sensitivity and specificity. Most of the trials had small
numbers of patients and those with larger groups were mostly multi-center
trials with the difficulties inherent with that design. Essentially all
the studies reported benefit with treatment. There are several larger
studies that were randomized with a control group in medical or surgical
patients (Table 2). Results in each study demonstrated (1-4) reduction
in incidence of DVT and/or PE with the use of oral anticoagulants. Overall, there was more than a 2/3 reduction in the incidence of clinically
recognized DVT or pulmonary emboli.

Meaningful data on the effect of oral anticoagulants in medical patients is available from the antigoagulant trails in patients with acute
myocardial infarction. In this population venous thrombosis occurs approximately 25% of patients as documented by numerous studies using fibrinogen
leg scans. The risk of the randomized sis varies with clinical parameters
particularly advanced age and compromised hemodynamics. At autopsy pulmonary embolism is found in more than 1/4 of patients dying during the acute phase
of their illness. Examination of the randomized trial reveals a significant reduction in the incidence of thromboembolism during treatment with anticoagulation compared to the control groups. (Table 3) In the three larger trials design was similar in that initial treatment included heparin for several days
followed by oral anticoagulant throughout the hospital stay. The intensity
of anticoagulation in the MRC trial was probably less than the other two.
Results of each study indicated significant decrease in the incidence of
venous thromboembolism by approximately two-thirds. Three smaller trials
documented the effect of oral anticoagulant therapy on the incidence of
venous thrombosis to a similar degree as detected by fibrinogen leg scans.
(8-9-10) The result with oral anticoagulants on venous thrombosis is similar
to that reported using low dose heparin.

TABLE II

DVT PROPHYLAXIS
Random trials with Clinical Endpoints

		#	Control DVT PE		Oral AC DVT PE	
Dick et al 1959	Gen Surg	6500	1.5	1.3	0.1	0.2
Storm* 1958	Thoracotomy	202	9	5	0	1
Anderson & Hill 1950	CHF	297	-	8	-	2
Harvey & Finch 1950	CHF	180	8.0	15	2.5	2.5

* - ℞ begun one week preop

TABLE III

ACUTE MYOCARDIAL INFARCTION
Anticoagulant Effect on Thrombosis

	#	Arterial		Venous (DVT & PE)	
		Control	AC	Control	AC
MRC	1427	3.4	1.3	9.8	3.8
VAH	999	5.6	0.8	3.5	1.4
Drapkin	1136	2.3	1.7	9.2	5.2

Thus, for acute myocardial infarction evidence is persuasive that oral anticoagulants significantly reduce the high incidence of deep venous thrombosis. (DVT)

In surgical patients some of the most interesting and useful data in the literature concerns general and GYN surgical patients. Vroonhoven et al reported a study in 100 patients undergoing general abdominal surgery with DVT diagnosed by leg scan (11). Patients were randomized to receive either low dose heparin or oral anticoagulants begun postoperatively, usually during the first postoperative day. (Table 4) In that study patients given low dose heparin had an incidence of DVT of 2% compared to 18% in those receiving oral anticoagulants. In the nine patients from the oral anticoagulant group developing DVT it is important to note that the positive leg scan developed within the first three postoperative days prior to the time that the desired therapeutic anticoagulation was achieved. Seven of these nine patients had propagation proximally and one developed a pulmonary embolus. From this study it may be concluded that oral anticoagulants begun postoperatively or days after the thrombogenic stimulus do not provide optimal benefit compared to a treatment begun preoperatively that has immediate onset.

The most relevant and revealing study was reported by Taberner et al which evaluated primary prophylaxis in patients over the age of 40 years who were having intraabdominal GYN surgery. (12) 145 patients operated by two surgeons were randomized into treatment with either oral anticoagulants, low dose heparin or saline as a control. The oral anticoagulation patients had treatment begun at least five days preoperatively and received the drug for a total of 14 days. The preoperative PT ratio

TABLE IV

DVT PROPHYLAXIS
General Surgery (abdominal)

	LDH*	Oral AC
n	50	50
DVT% (leg scan)	2	18
Hemorrhage (post-op)	0	0

Random trial (Hosp. number)
Oral AC ℞ started post-op day one
    for 7 days. Thrombotest 5-10% normal
LDH - ℞ 2 hrs preop and 8 days

Lancet 1:376-74 Vroonhoven et al

was established at 2 to 2.5 times control and kept postoperatively between 2 to 4 times. The PTT in these patients was increased by 5 to 15 seconds above control values. The low dose heparin groups received 5,000 units of the drug subcutaneously twice daily beginning two hours preoperatively and continuing for seven days. Thus, both treated groups had "therapeutic" levels at the time of surgery. The saline control patients were treated identically with those receiving heparin. The diagnosis of deep vein thrombosis was made by leg scans performed daily. Bleeding complications were determined by examining wound hematomas at surgery or the hemoglobin values on the second postoperative day. (Table 5) Results in this study confirmed that the oral anticoagulants and low dose heparin significantly reduce the incidence of DVT compared to the control group and equivalently. There was some increase in the incidence of bleeding but this was not statistically significant for the size of the patient groups studied. It was concluded from this study; that surgery was safely performed with a moderately prolonged prothrombin time; that oral anticoagulation of modest levels established preoperatively protected moderate risk patients from developing deep vein thrombosis; and that low dose heparin provides similar protection and is simpler and probably safer.

The risk of oral anticoagulation is hemorrhage. In reported studies an increase in bleeding complications compared to untreated controls was usually observed. The incidence of bleeding varied considerably from 2 to 14% with the majority in the 5 to 6% range. Approximately one half of bleeding complications were of major proportions requiring termination of treatment and/or transfusions. The bleeding usually involves cutaneous hematoma, hematuria or bleeding from the GI track. It is important to note that approximately 25% of patients are considered unsuitable for anticoagulant therapy because of the risk of bleeding.

Alternative approaches to oral anticoagulants for prophylaxis in moderate risk patients of established effectiveness include pneumatic compression stockings, dextran or low dose heparin. Of these low dose heparin has been consistently effective, with low risk of bleeding complications and without the need for dose adjustment or regular monitoring.

TABLE V

DVT PROPHYLAXIS
Gyn Surgery

	Saline	LDH*	Oral AC**	
n	48	49	48	
DVT (%) (leg scan)	23	6	6	.05
Hemorrhage	0	12	7	ns

    * - 5,000 BID begun preop for 7 days

   ** - begun 5 days preop for 14 days

       BCT 2 - 4 times control

BMJ - 1:272-78 Taberner et al

Conclusion

In patients at moderate risk for developing deep vein thrombosis oral anticoagulants offer effective primary prophylaxis. For this purpose the level of anticoagulation required is in the 2 to 2.5 prothrombin ratio range using the British comparative thromboplastin or equivalent INR values with other thromboplastin systems. Results are best if therapy is established prior to the thrombogenic provocation. With this approach bleeding com-

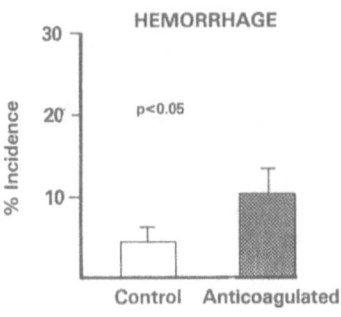

Figure 1

plications are in frequent and approximate 5% of which 1/2 would be considered of major proportion. There are good alternatives to the use of oral anticoagulations in this population and low dose heparin presently represents the most available, least complicated and safest approach. However, in patients already on anticoagulants or where long term treatment is planned warfarin would provide highly effective results.

REFERENCES

1. Dick W Matis, Mayer W Thromb Diath Haemorrh. 3-11-19 1959
   Results of Alternating Prophylaxis in Surgery

2. Storm O - Thromb et Diath Haemorrh 2-484-491 1958. Anticoagulant
   Protection in Surgery.

3. Anderson GM, Hull E - Am Ht J 39-697-701-50. The Effect of
   Dicumarol Upon the Mortality and Incidence of Thromboembolic
   Complications in Congestive Heart Failure.

4. Harvey WP, Finch CA N Engl J Med 242-208-211 1950. Dicumarol
   Prophylaxis of Thromboembolic Disease in Congestive Heart Failure.

5. Members Working Party. Brit Med J. 1-335-342-1969. Assessment
   of Short-term Anticoagulant Therapy in Coronary Thrombosis to the
   Medical Research Council.

6. Anticoagulants in Acute Myocardial Infarction. JAMA 225-724-729
   1973. Results of a Cooperative Clinical Trial.

7. Drapkin A, Merskey C. JAMA 222-541-548 1972. Anticoagulant
   Therapy After Acute Myocardial Infarction.

8. Nicolaides AN, Kakkar V.V., Renney JTG, Ridner PH et al. Brit
   Med J 1-432-434 1971. Myocardial Infarction and Deep Vein Thrombosis.

9. Handley AJ, Emerson PR. Brit Med J 2-436-438 1972. Heparin in
   the Prevention of Deep Vein Thrombosis After Myocardial Infarction.

10. Wray R, Maurer B, Shillingford J. New Engl J. Med 288-815-817
    1973. Prophylactic Anticoagulant Therapy in the Prevention of
    Calf-vein Thrombosis After Myocardial Infarction.

11. Vroonhoven TJ, Zijl J, Muller H. Lancet. 375-377 1974. Low Dose
    Subcutaneous Heparin Versus Oral Anticoagulants in the Prevention
    of Postoperative Deep Venous Thrombosis.

12. Taberner DA Poller L, Burslem RW, Jones JB. Brit Med J 1-272-274
    1978. Oral Anticoagulants Controlled by the British Comparitive
    Thromboplastin Versus Low Dose Heparin in Prophylaxis of Deep Vein
    Thrombosis.

TWO-STEP WARFARIN THERAPY FOR THE PROPHYLAXIS OF

VENOUS THROMBOSIS AFTER ELECTIVE SURGERY

Victor J. Mader and Charles W. Francis

Hematology Unit, Department of Medicine
University of Rochester School of Medicine
Rochester, N.Y.

A recurrent theme in the management of patients subjected to major surgical procedures has been the need for safe but effective anti-thrombotic treatment. This is an especially difficult dilemma for extensive bone or joint repair or replacement surgery, during which the prothrombotic tendencies would appear to require the use of more intensive anticoagulant therapy. Thus, Sevitt and Gallagher[1] demonstrated a clearcut decrease in clinical deep vein thrombosis and pulmonary embolism and in autopsy-proven thrombotic disease with coumarin therapy before repair of hip fracture, but this was achieved at an increased risk of bleeding complication (Table 1).

Table 1. COUMARIN VS NO COUMARIN IN ASSOCIATION
WITH REPAIR OF FRACTURED HIP
(Sevitt & Gallagher, Lancet 2:981, 1959).

	CONTROL (150)	PHENINDIONE (150)
DVT	29%	3%
PE	18%	0%
Fatal PE	10%	0%
Thrombosis at autopsy	83% of 35	14% of 21
Bleeding		
Minor	8%	20%
Major	2 cases	5 cases

Because of the increase in clinically-apparent bleeding, there has not been a general acceptance of this treatment regimen, even though the more serious complication of fatal pulmonary embolism was essentially avoided. The confusion regarding "therapeutic" prothrombin time results obtained with human brain thromboplastin, as utilized by Sevitt and Gallagher[1], or with the less sensitive rabbit brain thromboplastin may have contributed to such continued problems with hemostasis at surgery. Still, information available in the literature suggested that surgery could be safely performed during continued coumarin therapy (Table 2).

Table 2. EARLY STUDIES REPORTING SURGERY
ON ANTICOAGULATED PATIENTS

	SURGERY	PROTHROMBIN TIME	SAFETY	THROMBOSIS
Vanderveer et al (1952) (USA)	Appendectomy	Corrected	Yes	-
Mullertz & Storm (1954) (Denmark)	"Major surgery"	p < 30%	Yes	None (clinical)
Littman & Brodman (1955) (USA)	Vascular	Therapeutic	Yes	-
Sevitt & Gallagher (1959) (UK)	Hip fracture	15-30%	More bleeding	Decreased (clinical)
Rustad & Myhre (1963) (Norway)	Cholecystectomy Gastrectomy	15-25%	Yes	-

In 1952, Vanderveer and colleagues[2] performed an appendectomy on a single patient who was on coumarin therapy, although the risk was no doubt lessened by partial correction of the prothrombin time by vitamin K administration preoperatively. Mullertz and Storm[3] reported on a series of 11 patients who underwent "major surgery" some 2-4 days after starting Dicoumrol therapy, usually with the "prothombin/proconvertin" assay indicating less than 30% of initial activity during and after the procedure. While only clinical endpoints of thrombosis were monitored, the results were impressive, with neither thromboembolic nor hemorrhagic events occurring. Littman and Brodman[4] reported a retrospective analysis of 11 patients who had safe vascular surgery while on therapeutic levels of coumarin. Following the Sevitt and Gallagher report[1] showing an increased incidence of minor bleeding (20% vs 8%) in patients receiving phenindione, Rustad and Myhre[5] compared operative and post-operative blood loss in a blinded study of patients undergoing cholecystectomy or gastrectomy who were untreated or receiving anticoagulant therapy. Safety was clearly documented by virtue of their having been no difference between the two groups of patients.

The situation for bone surgery thus appeared to be a particularly difficult management problem, and our rationale for the development of a safe yet effective treatment regimen evolved from guidelines based on the following principles. First, surgery could be performed safely after significant reductions in vitamin K dependent coagulation factor activity, but greater safety against hemorrhage could perhaps be assured at lesser degrees of anticoagulation. Second, the precise degree of anticoagulation required for preventing thrombosis was not certain, but if this could be achieved at a minimum level, then safety also would be guaranteed. Satisfying both aspects would require that surgery be performed when the prothrombin time is clearly in a hemostatically-safe range, and that a minimal "therapeutic" level for thrombus prophylaxis be achieved rapidly after surgery.

The "two-step warfarin" plan[6] begins therapy about 10-14 days prior to surgery, slowly decreasing all of the vitamin K-dependent factors to approximately 60% of initial, with a resultant slight increase in prothrombin time ratio to about 1.2 (1.5-3.0 seconds prolonged using rabbit brain thromboplastin), corresponding to an International Normalized Ratio (INR) of about 1.5[7,8]. This "priming" of anticoagulant therapy was initiated slowly, to avoid an exaggerated effect of rapid factor VII decrease on the prothrombin time, yet to allow for a subsequent additional effect within 24 hours after surgery to antithrombotic therapeutic levels (prothrombin time ratio 1.5, INR 2.5) (Fig. 1).

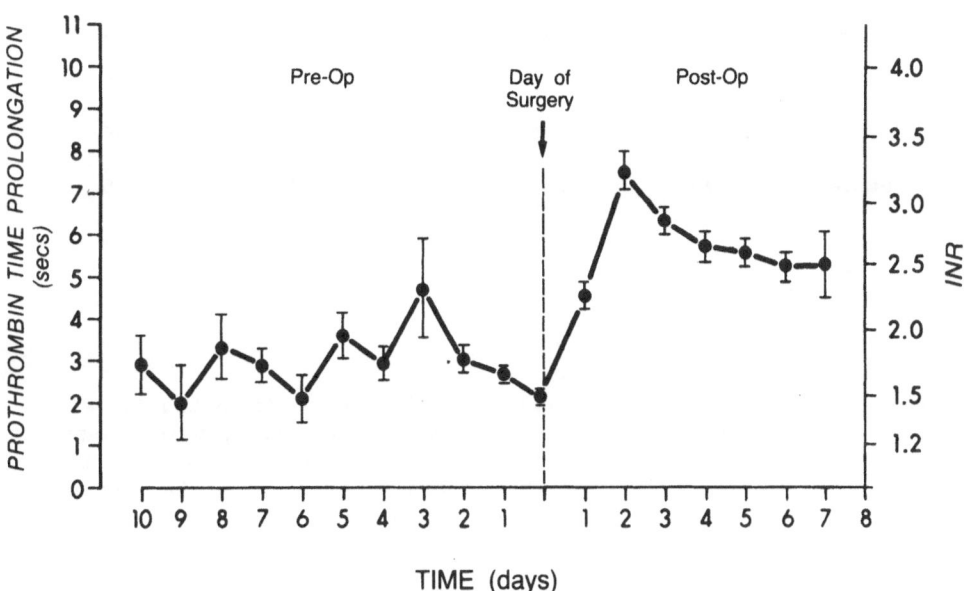

TIME (days)

The latter value would still fall within the lower therapeutic range of coumarin therapy and minimize post-operative bleeding complications. This approach paralleled the independent studies of Gitel and Wessler[9], showing an antithrombotic effect of a 50% reduction in vitamin K-dependent factors, associated with an increase in factor X inhibitory activity to 125%, using a rabbit jugular vein thrombosis model.

In practical terms, the mean daily dose of warfarin administered in the study by Francis et al[6] was 3.0 mg/day preoperatively (0.5-10 mg range), with about twice the maintenance dose administered following surgery to achieve "therapeutic" levels. This objective was achieved in 20 of 57 patients on the first post-operative day and in 43 of 57 patients on the second post-operative day. Of the 53 patients so managed, two instances of bleeding occurred, on post-operative days 2-3 and 5-7, each of which was associated with an excessively prolonged prothrombin time (ratio greater than 2.0). Both instances of bleeding were minor (wound hematoma and bleeding from an operative drain) and both were managed easily by withholding warfarin and administering plasma, then continuing therapy without untoward sequelae.

Therapeutic benefit relative to intravenous dextran, administered as a continuous infusion beginning one hour before surgery and continuing for 4.5 days post-operatively, was demonstrated by follow-up venography at post-operative day 5-7. The overall incidence of deep vein thrombosis in hip and knee prosthetic surgery was 21% versus 51% for dextran therapy and proximal deep vein thrombosis was present in only 2% of cases, versus 16% for dextran (Table 3).

Table 3. INCIDENCE OF VENOGRAPHICALLY DEMONSTRATED VENOUS THROMBOSIS AFTER PROSTHETIC HIP OR KNEE REPLACEMENT SURGERY (Francis et al, JAMA 249:374, 1983).

VENOUS THROMBI	DEXTRAN (37)	WARFARIN (53)	p
Minor veins only	19%	0%	<.005
Deep veins of calf	16%	19%	NS
Femoral-popliteal	16%	2%	<.05
TOTAL	51%	21%	<.005

Using a radiolabeled fibrinogen uptake assay in patients with gynecologic surgery, Taberner et al[10] also showed therapeutic benefit, with thrombosis noted in 3 of 48 patients treated with coumarin to a 2-2.5 prothrombin time ratio (human brain thromboplastin reagent) versus 11 of 48 positive assays in the untreated group. A similar approach in prophylaxis of recurrent deep vein thrombosis after heparin therapy for acute disease has been reported by Hull and colleagues[11], in which "less intense" therapy to produce a prothrombin time of 15 seconds (using rabbit brain thromboplastin) was equally effective as "more intense" therapy in which the prothrombin time was 19.4 seconds, but without the bleeding complications associated with the latter regimen.

In summary, several independent studies support the use of lower dosages of coumarins than have been used heretofore. "Two-step" therapy is both safe and effective after hip or knee prosthetic replacement. Still to be determined is the lowest effective dose that will prevent thrombosis and the shortest "priming" time required prior to the surgical procedure. Since bleeding complications are usually associated with deviation from the low dose guidelines, simpler regimens that are less likely to produce exceptionally long clotting time results will likely find the widest acceptance.

REFERENCES

1. S. Sevitt and N.G. Gallagher, Prevention of venous thrombosis and pumonary embolism in injured patients. Lancet 2:981 (1959).

2. J.B. Vanderveer, A.P. Parker, and F.R. Boyer, Emergency appendectomy in a patient receiving anticoagulants for myocardial infarction. JAMA 149:1307 (1952).

3. S. Mullertz and O. Storm, Anticoagulant therapy with dicumarol maintained during major surgery. Circulation 10:213 (1954).

4. J.K. Littman and H.R. Brodman, Surgery in the presence of the therapeutic effect of dicumarol. Surg Gyne Obstet 101:709 (1955).

5. H. Rustad and E. Myhre, Surgery during anticoagulant treatment. THe risk of increased bleeding in patients on oral anticoagulant treatment. Acta Med Scand 173:115 (1963).

6. C.W. Francis, V.J. Marder, C. McCollister Evarts, and S. Yaukoolbodi, Two-step warfarin therapy. Prevention of postoperative venous thrombosis without excessive bleeding. JAMA 249:374 (1983).

7. E.A. Loeliger, The optimal therapeutic range in oral anticoagulation. History and proposal. Thrombos Haemost 42:1141 (1979).

8. E.A. Loeliger, A.M.H.P. van den Besselaar, and S.M. Lewis, Reliability and clinical impact of the normalization of the prothrombin times in oral anticoagulant control. Thrombos Haemost 53:148 (1985).

9. S.N. Gitel and S. Wessler, Dose-dependent antithrombotic effect of warfarin in rabbits. Blood 61:435 (1983).

10. D.A. Taberner, L. Poller, R.W. Burslem, and J.B. Jones, Oral anticoagulants controlled by the British comparative thromboplastin versus low-dose heparin in prophylaxis of deep vein thrombosis. Br Med J 1:272 (1978).

11. R. Hull, J. Hirsh, R. Jay, C. Carter, C. England, M. Gent, A.G.G. Turpie, D. McLoughlin, P. Dodd, M. Thomas, G. Raskob, and P. Ockelford, Different intensities of oral anticoagulant therapy in the treatment of proximal-vein thrombosis. New Engl J Med 307:1676 (1982).

PREVENTION OF VENOUS THROMBOEMBOLISM IN HIGH-RISK PATIENTS

BY PROPHYLACTIC ADMINISTRATION OF ORAL ANTICOAGULANTS

Edwin W. Salzman

Harvard Medical School, Beth Israel Hospital

330 Brookline Avenue   Boston, MA   02215

In recent years the development of sensitive and specific noninvasive methods for diagnosis of venous thrombosis, with confirmation by phlebography, and improvements in the diagnostic methods available for detection of pulmonary embolism have made it possible to identify a number of major risk factors for venous thromboembolism. These features of a patient's illness may be employed as criteria for selection of the patient as a candidate for prophylactic administration of antithrombotic agents. The more important risk factors that predispose to venous thromboembolism are shown in Table 1.

In Table 2 the impact of such risk factors on the prevalence of thromboembolic complications is illustrated[1]. The combination of several risk factors may put a surgical patient in a high risk group in which the frequency of postoperative venous thrombosis may exceed 50% unless anti-thrombotic agents are administered prophylactically. For example, the operation of total hip replacement may be followed by venous thrombosis in over 50% of cases and by fatal pulmonary embolism in over 3%. An extensive surgical dissection with tissue trauma and blood loss is compounded by local injury to the femoral vein from the torsion that occurs with disloca-tion of the hip at operation and the heat of polymerization of the acrylic, and the procedure is followed by convalescence in bed. Age is an additional risk factor in many cases. All these factors contribute to the high risk of thromboembolism. Widely performed (estimated at over 100,000 per year

Table 1. Risk Factors in Post-Operative Thromboembolism

Age
History of previous thromboembolism
Obesity
Operations in the lower extremities or pelvis
Malignant tumors
Tissue trauma
Immobility
Increased blood viscosity (dehydration, polycythemia)
Oral contraceptives
Congestive heart failure
Varicose veins
Inherited factors (family history)

Table 2. Classification of Disease or Risk (Based upon Published Data).

NATURE OF THROMBOEMBOLIC EVENT	LOW RISK (Uncomplicated surgery in patients under 40 years of age with no other risk factor)	MODERATELY HIGH RISK* (Surgery in patients over the age of 40 years lasting 30 minutes or myocardial infarction or heart failure)	VERY HIGH RISK (Surgery in patients over the age of 40 years plus previous DVT or PE or extensive malignant disease or major orthopedic surgery or stroke)
Calf-vein thrombosis (%)	2	10-40	40-80
Proximal vein thrombosis (%)	0.4	2-8	10-20
Clinical pulmonary embolism (%)	0.2	1-8	5-10
Fatal pulmonary embolism (%)	0.002	0.1-0.4	1-5

* Risk increased by obesity, age, malignancy, varicose veins, or prolonged bedrest.

in the United States), the operation presents a particularly valuable
opportunity to study the use of prophylactic agents to prevent thromboembolism and has contributed important data to the understanding of antithrombotic prophylaxis. The patient undergoing hip replacement is the
prototypical high risk case, and extension of lessons about the efficacy
of prophylactic methods learned after total hip replacement to other high
risk situations not specifically studied in this context is reasonable,
albeit tentative. Much the same can be said for patients with fractures
of the hip.

An important consideration in regard to high risk patients, first
clearly demonstrated in patients undergoing hip operations, is that
popular prophylactic regimens such as the use of subcutaneous "mini-heparin"
(5000 units subcutaneously twice or three times daily) are inadequate to
the task of preventing thromboembolism in such patients[2,3]. More aggressive
methods must be used to protect the high-risk patient. Modifications in the
use of heparin such as the administration of titrated doses[4] or a combination of heparin with dihydroergotamine[5] have their advocates. Alternatively, it is in such patients that prophylactic administration of oral anticoagulants has the most to offer the clinician. The choice of warfarin or
other oral anticoagulants as the prophylactic agent in high-risk patients
has several advantages over other forms of preventive therapy.

1. Widely used and established historically, oral anticoagulants are
familiar to most clinicians and the control of dosage is straightforward
and relatively simple in practice. Drug interactions that affect the
response of the clotting system to oral anticoagulants are well understood
and have been extensively reviewed.

2. Oral anticoagulants administered prophylactically are prescribed
in the same dose that would be given for treatment of patients with
established venous thromboembolism, a distinct advantage in surgical
practice. It is not unusual for the surgeon to be referred a patient who
has already languished for several days at bed rest on the medical service
or at home, often with unrecognized venous thrombosis. Thus administration
of the drug may actually be therapeutic rather than prophylactic. This
advantage of oral anticoagulants is not shared by any other form of antithrombotic prophylaxis.

3. Oral anticoagulants are economical. Warfarin sufficient for one
week's treatment costs less than $1.00[6]. Its administration prophylactical-
ly to high-risk patients is cost effective, even considering the cost of
laboratory control. This point will be discussed in more detail later.

4. Although oral anticoagulants have not been universally adopted
by practitioners in the past because of fear of hemorrhagic complications,
recent evidence that the proper dose of warfarin may be lower than that
conventionally prescribed offers promise of reducing the bleeding side
effects. Sevitt and Innes[7] first showed that the degree of prolongation
of the prothrombin time is closely linked to the frequency of bleeding
complications in patients receiving oral anticoagulants. Hull and
associates[8] found the frequency of bleeding reduced by a factor of 5 when
they lowered their prescribed therapeutic intensity to a prothrombin time
of 15 sec.

The first prospective controlled clinical trial of an antithrombotic
agent in the prophylaxis of venous thromboembolism was conducted in high-
risk patients with fractures of the hip and reported in 1959 by Sevitt and
Gallagher[9]. This study included 319 patients over age 55 with subcapital,
intertrochanteric, or subtrochanteric fractures of the hip. Patients ad-

mitted on even numbered days of the month received prophylactic phenindione, a synthetic Vitamin K antagonist; those admitted on odd numbered days served as controls. Patients were followed for as long as 4 months. Those in the phenindione group received the drug until they were ambulatory, ranging from 2 to 12 weeks (mean 5 weeks). Twenty-three patients were excluded for various reasons, and the group was then supplemented by additional cases until the study groups were each made up of 150 patients. Dosage was based on the prothrombin time, aiming for a prolongation to 2½ to 3 times the control value.

Diagnosis of DVT in surviving patients was made according to clinical criteria and strongly favored the phenindione group (4 vs. 43 cases). Of more importance is consideration of patients who died; this included 42 controls and 25 anticoagulated patients. Autopsies were carried out in 35 controls (83%) and 21 anticoagulated patients (84%), and the principal conclusions of the study were based on anatomic evidence. Major pulmonary embolism was found in 15 (43%) of the autopsied controls and in two (10%) of the phenindione cases, both of the latter having occurred after the drug had been discontinued. Extensive thrombi were found in the lower extremities of 29 controls (83%) and 3 phenindione patients (14%). Of the excess mortality in the control group (17 deaths), 13 cases were accounted for by the difference in the incidence of PE in the two groups. Two controls (1.3%) and five phenindione patients (3.3%) had major bleeding complications, none of which were fatal. The authors conclude that "phenindione effectively prevents thrombosis in veins and eliminates the risk of pulmonary embolism in patients under its influence provided that the drug is given early, for sufficient time, and under laboratory control." This classic paper invites rereading. Its conclusions would be hard to improve on today.

In 1985, Gruber[10] published a comparison of the results of Sevitt's study with a contemporary trial of heparin/dihydroergotamine vs. dextran in patients with hip fractures, including as an endpoint fatal pulmonary embolism verified at autopsy. The well-known defects in studies based on retrospective comparisons are evident in this analysis, but the data probably justify the author's conclusion, which is that all three forms of prophylaxis are highly effective in preventing death from PE (2.0% with phenindione, 2.3% with heparin/dihydroergotamine, and 3.8% with dextran, vs. 10% in controls). Differences in the several trials prevent one from drawing more sweeping conclusions.

The landmark publication of Sevitt and Gallagher was followed by more than thirty reports, largely confirmatory, many of which considered other types of patients. The earlier examples of this genre have been reviewed in detail[11]. Although their experimental design was in many instances inferior to that employed by Sevitt and Gallagher, these papers in the aggregate provide strong support for the use of oral anticoagulants in a variety of high risk patients, fear of hemorrhagic side effects not withstanding. The reports that meet modern standards for prospective randomized trials are listed in Table 3, which considers only diagnoses established by objective techniques, such as labelled fibrinogen scanning or phlebography.

In general they confirm the results of Sevitt and Gallagher in other patient groups at high risk. The exceptions are worth noting. The papers of Pinto[15] and van Vroonhafen[17] are noteworthy, as neither investigator found a reduction in venous thrombosis in patients given oral anticoagulants after hip reconstruction or general surgical operations, respectively. Diagnosis in both studies was by labelled fibrinogen scanning, which provided clear and objective evidence of a high incidence of venous thrombosis within the first 72 hours after operation. However, in both studies

Table 3. Oral Anticoagulant Prophylaxis Against Venous Thromboembolism.

Authors	Surgery	End Point	Patients					
			Untreated			Treated		
			No.	DVT(%)	"Fatal" PE(%)	No.	DVT(%)	"Fatal" PE(%)
Sevitt and Gallagher, 1959[9]	Fractured hip	Autopsy	150	83	10	150	14	1.3
Eskeland et al., 1966[12]	Fractured hip	Autopsy	100		7.0	100		1.0
Borgstrom et al., 1965[13]	Fractured hip	Venography	29	56.5		29	9.5	
Hamilton et al., 1970[14]	Fractured hip	Venography	38	49		38	26	
Pinto, 1970[15]	Fractured hip	Leg scan	25	32	0	25	36	0
Hume et al., 1973[16]	Elective hip	Leg scan	19	42		17	59	
Van Vroonhoven et al., 1974[17]	General	Leg scan	50	2 (Heparin)	0	50	18	0
Morris and Mitchell, 1976[18]	Fractured hip	Autopsy	74	68	8	75	31	0
Taberner, 1978[19]	Gynecologic	Leg scan	48	23		48	6	
Francis et al., 1983[20]	Elective hip or knee	Venography	37 (Dextran)	51		53	21	
Harris et al., 1986[24]	Hip replacement	Venography	66	17 (EPC)	0	72	17	0

169

the administration of warfarin was commenced at the time of operation or even later. This was unfortunately too late for warfarin to have had any possible effect in the early postoperative period, and provides an obvious explanation for the failure of the drug to reduce the frequency of early postoperative thrombi. Nonetheless, despite the high rate of venous thrombi detected by labelled fibrinogen scanning in the first three days after operation, pulmonary embolism was observed in only one patient, and this was not a fatal embolus. Thus the therapeutic properties of oral anticoagulants intervened to prevent progression of the thrombi that had developed during the initiation of therapy while the warfarin effect was gaining momentum. This was of course entirely predictable from the pharmacology of the drug and represents a flaw in design of the trials, but the experience serves to highlight an important feature of warfarin's effect.

Coventry et al.[22] reported a 3.4% mortality following total hip replacement among 58 patients who received no prophylactic agents, a startling figure after an elective operation. Practice subsequently changed at his institution, the Mayo Clinic; prophylactic anticoagulation was adopted, and he then reported a mortality of 0.05% from fatal pulmonary embolism in 1950 patients in whom warfarin administration was begun on the fifth postoperative day and continued for three weeks, aiming for a prothrombin time $1\frac{1}{2}$ to 2 times the control value. Many of these patients were also given aspirin in the early postoperative period. There was no simultaneous comparison group and the study was not randomized, but the large numbers involved and the striking difference in mortality provides circumstantial supportive evidence for the efficacy of oral anticoagulants. Eighty-three patients (4.1%) in the Mayo Clinic series had bleeding complications, of which 1% were major. No patient died of hemorrhage.

Crawford[23] in 1968 reported the experience in Charnley's clinic, where the use of phenindione in 450 patients reduced the mortality from fatal PE after hip replacement from 1.8% to 0.8%. Unfortunately, the occurrence of three deaths from bleeding complications offset the benefits of preventing fatal PE. The prescribed range of Thrombotest values in these patients was 10 to 25%.

Several recent studies are of particular interest. Francis and associates[20] studied patients with elective surgery of the hip or knee, beginning prophylactic warfarin in small doses 10 to 14 days preoperatively with the aim of keeping the prothrombin time at $1\frac{1}{2}$ to 3 seconds longer than the control. Immediately after operation the dose was increased to produce a prothrombin time of 1.5 times the control, which was maintained until the patient was ambulatory. Fifty-three patients received warfarin and the results were compared with those in 37 similar patients given dextran. DVT was diagnosed by phlebography. The condition was found in 51% of the dextran patients, compared with 21% in the warfarin group, and the incidence of thrombi in proximal veins (popliteal or femoral) was 16% and 2%, respectively. Bleeding complications were infrequent and occurred with the same frequency in the two groups.

Harris and associates[21] reported a comparison of warfarin with external pneumatic compression of the lower extremities after total hip replacement in patients who had a history of prior thromboembolism, an exceedingly high risk group with multiple risk factors. All patients were studied by phlebography both before and after operation. External pneumatic compression was equivalent in efficacy to warfarin in patients whose preoperative phlebogram was normal, showing no evidence of residual venous damage from the presumed previous episode of venous thrombosis. In patients whose preoperative venogram was abnormal, however, revealing residual structural changes in the veins of the lower limbs, warfarin was substantially superior: 55% vs. 25%.

170

More recently Harris et al.[24] studied patients undergoing total hip replacement treated with warfarin in small doses (prothrombin time 1.3 times the control: approximately 15 sec.). The frequency of venous thrombosis among patients receiving low dose warfarin was 17%, the same rate as that in a comparison group receiving external pneumatic compression of the legs and thighs, vs. 35 to 50% in comparable patients studied earlier and given no prophylaxis. Harris also reported his total experience with low dose warfarin, administered to 195 patients. DVT developed in 14.4% of patients, and in 7.2% of cases the thrombus was in a proximal vein. Bleeding into the wound was a major complication in 1.5% of cases. No patient died.

The cost of prophylactic administration of warfarin was modest. Harris et al.[25] compared the cost effectiveness of five strategies for prevention of DVT and PE, including a control group given no prophylaxis, a group subjected to routine phlebography 10 to 14 days postop as the sole prophylactic measure (based on the view that early treatment of asymptomatic DVT can prevent PE), groups given warfarin for 10 days, with or without phlebography, and a group given warfarin for three months. All of the latter four strategies saved lives by preventing PE, but the cost was very great in the approaches that included phlebography. The most economical practice, and the one advocated by Harris et al., was the routine administration of warfarin for three months, which was calculated to have a marginal cost of only $70 for each death averted, after taking into account the costs of the prophylactic program and the costs of the complications that were prevented.

Guyer and associates[26] undertook to study the ability of warfarin in low doses to prevent PE after total hip replacement. Eighty-eight patients received warfarin in a dose intended to prolong the prothrombin time to 1.2 to 1.4 times the control, begun on the first postop night and continued until discharge. A comparison group of 96 patients received aspirin. Nineteen of the aspirin patients developed a "high probability" perfusion lung scan, eight of which were accompanied by symptoms, and in one patient who received aspirin, the PE led to his death. In contrast, a high probability lung scan was found in only 6 of the warfarin patients, 5 of whom were symptomatic. Seven of the patients given warfarin developed a wound hematoma, compared with 10 given aspirin. Because the aspirin and warfarin groups were not concurrent and because of uncertainty about the accuracy of diagnosis based on clinical criteria or a perfusion lung scan without a ventilation scan or corroborative angiography, these data cannot be regarded as conclusive, but they are at least consistent with the rest of the evidence.

The required duration of prophylaxis is under dispute and clearly varies from patient to patient. It is certain that the danger of thromboembolic complications persists in many high-risk patients after hospitalization: in patients with fractures of the hip, for example, at least until the patient is capable of vigorous ambulation[27]. Thus, prophylactic administration of oral anticoagulants should be continued in many patients after they are discharged from the hospital and until full ambulation is achieved, often several months later. Fortunately, this is less of a problem than might be feared since bleeding complications of oral anticoagulation most frequently develop in the early weeks of therapy when unsuspected underlying lesions that predispose to bleeding are provoked to manifest themselves (for example, carcinoma fo the cecum or peptic ulcer). Zweifler[28] showed that bleeding in patients receiving warfarin may be a clue to the existence of an underlying silent lesion. In his study, if a hemorrhagic complication occurred while the prothrombin time was excessively prolonged, investigation for the presence of an underlying lesion was usually unproductive, whereas in patients who bled at a time when they were not clearly overdosed, investigation often revealed a separate explanation for the bleeding.

The conduct of surgery in patients receiving oral anticoagulants is worth mention. It is usually safer to maintain an anticoagulated patient on his oral anticoagulant during and following an operation, accepting a finite hazard of bleeding complications, than it is to discontinue the drug during the perioperative period and expose the patient to the thrombotic complication for which the drug was initially prescribed[29,30]. Experience has shown that general surgical operations can be safely conducted while the prothrombin time is prolonged, as long as it does not exceed twice the control. With the current enthusiasm for lower doses of warfarin, the prescribed range is generally substantially below this level, so the rate of bleeding complications of surgery in patients receiving oral anticoagulants can be expected to decline, provided that increasing experience confirms the efficacy of a low dose program.

Sevitt and Innes[7] showed almost 25 years ago that the rate of complications in patients receiving oral anticoagulants is a function of the prothrombin time, increasing in parallel with the antithrombotic effectiveness of the drug. If any aphorism concerning anticoagulant therapy is immutable, that is it, although the data available in support of this thesis have some shortcomings, by modern standards[31]. One hopes that the demonstration of the prophylactic efficacy of modest doses of warfarin in high risk patients will be accompanied by a substantial reduction in hemorrhagic side effects, and that the preliminary reports that have brought us to our present position will be rapidly and consistently confirmed.

REFERENCES

1. J. Hirsh and E.W. Salzman, Prevention of venous thromboembolism, in: "Hemostasis and Thrombosis, " R.W. Colman, J. Hirsh, V.J. Marder, E.W. Salzman, eds., J.B. Lippincott Company, Philadelphia (1982).
2. C.M. Evarts and R.J. Alfidi, Thromboembolism after total hip reconstruction: Failure of low doses of heparin in prevention, J Am Med Assn. 225:515 (1973).
3. W.G.J. Hampson, F.C. Harris, H.K. Lucas, P.H. Roberts, I.W. McCall, P.C. Jackson, N.L. Powell, and G.E. Staddon, Failure of low-dose heparin to prevent deep-vein thrombosis after hip replacement arthroplasty, Lancet 2:795 (1974).
4. P.F. Leyvraz, J. Richard, F. Bachmann, G. Van Melle, J.M. Treyvaud, J.J. Livio, and G. Candardjis, Adjusted versus fixed-dose subcutaneous heparin in the prevention of deep-vein thrombosis after total hip replacement, N Engl J Med 309:954 (1983).
5. V.V. Kakkar, P.J. Fok, W.J.G. Murray, T. Paes, D. Mereustein, R. Dodds, R. Farrell, R.Q. Crellin, E.M. Thomas, T.R. Morley, A.J. Price, Heparin and dihydroergotamine prophylaxis against thromboembolism after hip arthroplasty, J Bone Joint Surg. (Br) 67:538 (1985).
6. E.W. Salzman and G.C. Davies, Prophylaxis of venous thromboembolism, Ann Surg. 191:207 (1980).
7. S. Sevitt and D. Innes, Prothrombin time and thrombotest in injured patients on prophylactic anticoagulant therapy, Lancet 1:124 (1964).
8. R. Hull, J. Hirsh, R. Jay, D. Carter, C. England, M. Gent, A.G.G. Turpie, D. McLoughlin, P. Dodd, M. Thomas, G. Raskob, and P. Okelford, Different intensities of oral anticoagulant therapy in the treatment of proximal vein thrombosis, N Engl J Med. 207:1676 (1982).
9. S. Sevitt and N.G. Gallagher, Prevention of venous thrombosis and pulmonary embolism in injured patients, Lancet 2:981 (1959).

10. U.F. Gruber, Prevention of fatal pulmonary embolism in patients with fractures of the neck of the femur, Surg Gynecol Obstet. 161:37 (1985).
11. G.P. Clagett and E.W. Salzman, Prevention of venous thromboembolism, in: "Pulmonary Embolism," A.A. Sasahara, E.H. Sonnenblick, M. Lesch, eds., Grune & Stratton, New York (1974, 1975).
12. G. Eskeland, K. Solheim, and F. Skjorten, Anticoagulant prophylaxis, thromboembolism, and mortality in elderly patients with hip fractures: Controlled clinical trial, Acta Chir Scand. 131:16 (1966).
13. S. Borgstrom, T. Greitz, W. Van der Linden, J. Molin, I. Rudics, Anticoagulant prophylaxis of venous thrombosis in patients with fractured neck of the femur: A controlled clinical trial using venous phlebography, Acta Chir Scand. 129:500 (1965).
14. H.W. Hamilton, J.S. Crawford, J.H. Garginer, and A.M. Wiley, Venous thrombosis in patients with fracture of the upper end of the femur, J Bone Joint Surg. (Br) 52:268 (1970).
15. D.J. Pinto, Controlled trial of an anticoagulant (warfarin sodium) in the prevention of venous thrombosis following hip surgery, Brit J Surg. 57:349 (1970).
16. M. Hume, X. Kuriakose, L. Zuch, and R.H. Turner, ^{125}I fibrinogen and the prevention of venous thrombosis, Arch Surg. 107:803 (1973).
17. T.J.M.V. van Vroonhoven, J. van Zijl, and H. Muller, Low-dose subcutaneous heparin versus oral anticoagulants in the prevention of postoperative deep-venous thrombosis, Lancet 1:375 (1974).
18. G.K. Morris and J.R.A. Mitchell, Warfarin sodium in prevention of deep venous thrombosis and pulmonary embolism in patients with fractured neck of femur, Lancet 2:869 (1976).
19. D.A. Taberner, L. Poller, R.W. Burslem, and J.B. Jones, Oral anticoagulants controlled by the British comparative thromboplastin versus low-dose heparin in prophylaxis of deep vein thrombosis. Br Med J. 1:272 (1978).
20. C.W. Francis, V.J. Marder, C.M. Evarts, and S. Yaukoolbodi, Two-step warfarin therapy: Prevention of postoperative venous thrombosis without excessive bleeding, JAMA 249:374 (1983).
21. W.H. Harris, J.K. Raines, C. Athanasoulis, A.C. Waltman, and E.W. Salzman, External pneumatic compression versus warfarin in reducing thrombosis in high-risk hip patients, in: "Venous Thrombosis: Prevention and Treatment," J.L. Madden and M. Hume, eds., Appleton-Century, NY (1976).
22. M.B. Coventry, D.R. Nolan, and R.D. Beckenbaugh, "Delayed" prophylactic anticoagulation: A study of results and complications in 2,012 total hip arthroplasties, J Bone Joint Surg. 55A:1487 (1973).
23. W.J. Crawford, F. Hillman, and J. Charnley, A clinical trial of prophylactic anticoagulant therapy in elective hip surgery, Wrightington Internal Publications No. 14 (1968), cited in R. Johnson, J.R. Green, and J. Charnley, Pulmonary embolism and its prophylaxis following the Charnley total hip replacement, Clinical Orthopaedics and Related Research 127:123 (1977).
24. G. Paiement, S.J. Wessinger, A.C. Waltman, and W.H. Harris, Low-dose warfarin versus external pneumatic compression for prophylaxis against venous thromboembolism following total hip replacement, Submitted for publication.
25. G. Paiement, S.J. Wessinger, and W.H. Harris, Cost effectiveness of prevention and early detection of venous thromboembolism in total hip replacement patients, Submitted for publication.
26. R.D. Guyer, R.E. Booth, and R.H. Rothman, The detection and prevention of pulmonary embolism in total hip replacement, J Bone Joint Surg. 64A:1040 (1982).
27. E.W. Salzman, W.H. Harris, and R.W. DeSanctis, Anticoagulation for prevention of thromboembolism following fractures of the hip, N Engl J Med. 275:122 (1966).
28. A.J. Zweifler, Relation of prothrombin concentration to bleeding during oral anticoagulant therapy: Its importance in detection of latent

organic lesions, <u>N Engl J Med</u>. 267:283 (1962).

29. O. Storm, Anticoagulant protection in surgery. <u>Thromb Diath Haemorrh</u>. 2:484 (1958).

30. H. Rustad and E. Myhre, Surgery during anticoagulant treatment: the risk of increased bleeding in patients on oral anticoagulant treatment, <u>Acta Med Scand</u>. 173:115 (1963).

31. M.N. Levine, G. Raskob, and J. Hirsh, Hemorrhagic complications of long-term anticoagulant therapy, <u>Chest</u> 89:16S (1986).

GENETIC COAGULATION DEFECTS

Ewa Marciniak

Department of Medicine
University of Kentucky College of Medicine
Lexington, Ky.

Normal hemostasis in response to blood vessel injury results from sequential activation of coagulation enzymes and culminates in formation of a stabilized fibrin clot. Complex natural mechanisms are known to exist for deterring this process. The principal components that suppress intravascular clotting thereby ensuring unobstructed blood flow are the coagulation inhibitors and the fibrinolytic system. When defects of these components occur the disrupted balanced between procoagulant and anticoagulant activities in blood may lead to thrombosis.

The purpose of this presentation is to review and summarize current knowledge regarding hereditary defects in coagulation inhibitors and evaluate the extent to which these disorders contribute to the risk of thromboembolism in man.

HEREDITARY DEFICIENCY OF ANTITHROMBIN III

Antithrombin III, a 58-kd plasma glycoprotein produced by hepatocytes represents the primary inhibitor of serine proteinases that participate in the intrinsic and common pathways of blood coagulation[1]. It is estimated that about 85 percent of thrombin potentially generated in plasma and most of the available factor Xa are neutralized by antithrombin III[2]. Catalytically active thrombin, and possibly other enzymes, cleave a specific $arginine_{385}-serine_{386}$ bond in the C-terminal portion of the antithrombin III molecule, which leads to formation of a stable inactive equimolar complex between the inhibitor and the active serine center of the protease[3]. With time active thrombin may slowly dissociate from the complex releasing the antithrombin III moiety which no longer has an inhibitory activity[4,5]. Both the inhibition of enzymes[1] and the formation of an inactive antithrombin III derivative[6] are markedly enhanced by heparin.

As early as 1914 Howell[7] suspected that thrombosis might be prevented by a natural plasma protein. More than half a century later, Egeberg[8] described a familial disorder characterized by low levels of antithrombin III in blood and a high incidence of venous thromboembolism. Subsequently, a number of families with similar characteristics have been reported[9-13]. The disorder is inherited as an autosomal dominant trait[14] but appears to be heterogeneous. In most cases antithrombin III

is qualitatively normal but is present in plasma at about 50 percent of
the normal concentration. It's catabolic rate as well as its distribution
between plasma and noncirculatory compartments remain unchanged; the
defect lies in the synthesis of the protein which occurs at half the
normal rate[15]. Studies of families with this so-called "classical"
form of deficiency provided evidence for the linkage between the
antithrombin III locus and the locus of the Duffy blood group in the
heterochromatic region of the long arm of chromosome 1 [16,17].
The location of the structural antithrombin III gene in human chromosome 1
was recently confirmed by genetic mapping[18]. With the use of
recombinant-DNA techniques a common DNA polymorphism within the gene was
identified[19]. While in some families the deficiency is associated
with structural gene deletion, in other families both parental
antithrombin III genes are detectable in the affected members[19,20].
The disorder has a relatively low frequency of occurrence and is estimated
to appear in approximately 1 in 5,000 persons[21]. Males and females
are equally affected. According to Vikydal et al[22], inherited
antithrombin III deficiency occurs in less than 2 percent of all patients
presenting with venous thromboembolism. Clinically, the deficiency is
characterized by recurrent thromboembolism with onset at a relative early
age often in the absence of other predisposing factors. Exceptional
subjects may have arterial thrombosis. We have investigated 43 deficient
members of six unrelated families. Cumulative risk of thrombosis in this
group exceed 90 percent (Fig 1). This flagrant thrombotic tendency
emphasizes the importance of procoagulant-anticoagulant balance,
particularly in areas of prolonged venous stasis. Total homozygous
deficiency in man is unknown and is most likely incompatible with survival
beyond fetal life.

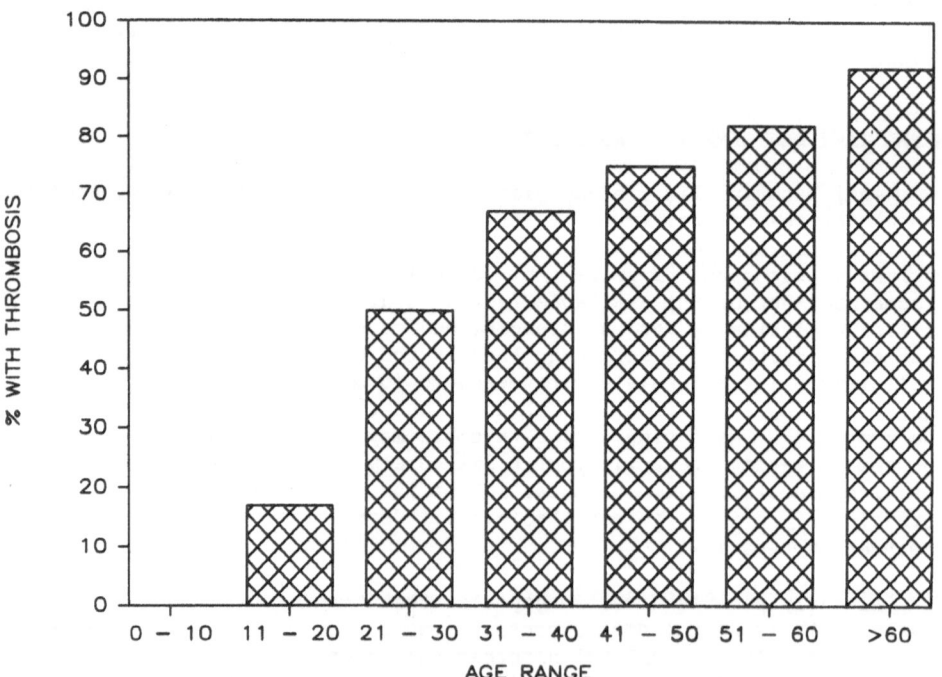

Fig. 1. Cumulative incidence of thromboembolism related to age,
as estimated in a population of 43 subjects with "classical"
type of hereditary antithrombin III deficiency.

Infrequently, a heritable defect is associated with the presence of an abnormal antithrombin III protein. Heterozygotes for this type of disorder have normal quantities of immunoreactive antithrombin III in blood with markedly impaired functional properties. Some of these dysfunctional proteins were shown to derive from one-step mutations resulting in single amino acid substitutions[23,24]. The first rare genetic variant incapable of binding both thrombin and heparin was described by Sas et al[25] in a family with extensive history of venous thromboembolism. Subsequently, variants with selective defects in heparin binding but normal reactivity with enzymes were reported in four families[26-29]. Among the numerous heterozygotes of these four families only one case of recurrent thromboembolism was documented[27] and another subject presented with superficial phlebitis[28]; most severly affected was a third patient who proved to be homozygous for the trait inherited from both asymptomatic parents[29]. Clinical manifestations associated with the presence of the mutant protein which binds thrombin but can not interact with heparin, assume unique significance in that they seem to confirm an increasing body of evidence that endogenous heparin or a similar substance expressed in a receptor form on vascular endothelium, plays an important role in fending off thrombosis when acting in conjunction with antithrombin III[30,31]. The third group of dysfunctional disorders is characterized by mutant antithrombin subtypes which bind heparin with normal or even increased affinity, but do not react with thrombin[32-39]. The incidence of thrombosis among heterozygotes for this trait is high and most likely equals that observed in the "classical" type of deficiency.

Although there are no controlled clinical trials to provide evidence for the efficacy of therapy in the high-risk group of antithrombin III deficient patients, existing data are sufficient to warrant recommendations for long-term warfarin prophylaxis[2]. Oral anticoagulants impair synthesis of clotting factors thereby lowering potential need for neutralization of coagulation enzymes and for utilization of the inhibitor. The anticoagulant effect of therapy with warfarin may be further potentiated by an increase in plasma antithrombin III levels, although, there is a lack of general agreement between investigators on this issue. Results obtained in six of our patients in whom antithrombin III was recently evaluated before and during anticoagulation with warfarin are shown in Fig. 2. Five of these subjects had an apparent increase in both functional and antigenic antithrombin III concentration, but only differences in functional inhibitor levels proved to be statistically significant ($P<0.05$). These data are in agreement with the observation made by Wessler et al[40] that warfarin therapy increases the rate at which plasma inhibits clotting proteases. Warfarin-induced increase in the circulating antithrombin protein is less certain although it might be in line with decreased requirement for the inhibitor in the anticoagulated patient and would suggest a cause-effect relationship.

A long-term therapy with heparin alone may not prevent recurrent thrombosis. In a number of patients with hereditary antithrombin III deficiency, death due to extensive intravascular clotting occurred during heparin administration[10,14,37]. This therapy accelerates the breakdown of the inhibitor further lowering the content of circulating antithrombin III[41,42]. Within two to three days of treatment, antithrombin III in a deficient subject may decrease below 20 percent of the normal level. A distinct reduction is also noted during therapy with low dose heparin[43]. The pathway by which exogenous heparin exerts its effect on antithrombin III catabolism is not clear. Recent data suggest that binding to a heparin-like endothelial receptor site not only mediates the inhibition of enzymes by antithrombin III but may accelerate the breakdown of the inhibitory protein during passage through endothelial cell cytoplasm[44]. A possibility exists that exogenous heparin potentiates this natural mechanism thereby lowering circulating antithrombin III levels. In vitro heparin affects adversely the inhibitory capacity of antithrombin III enhancing its limited proteolysis by thrombin[6,45]. For all these reasons, intravenous heparin therapy should not be given to an antithrombin III deficient patient unless normal plasma or antithrombin III concentrates are administered concurrently. In Europe, antithrombin III concentrates have been successfully used for protection of deficient subjects during surgical

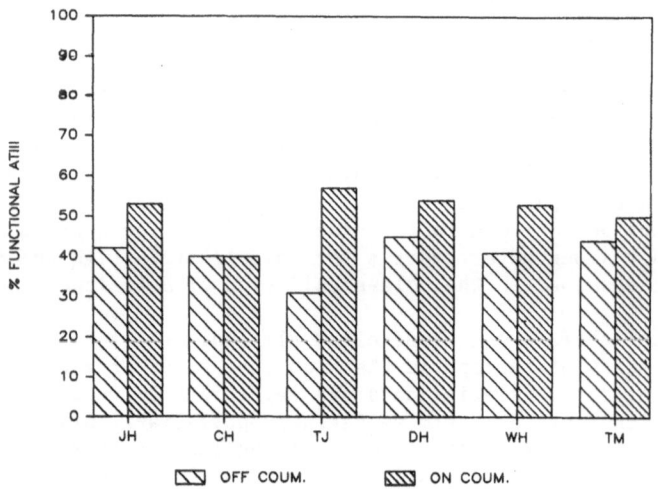

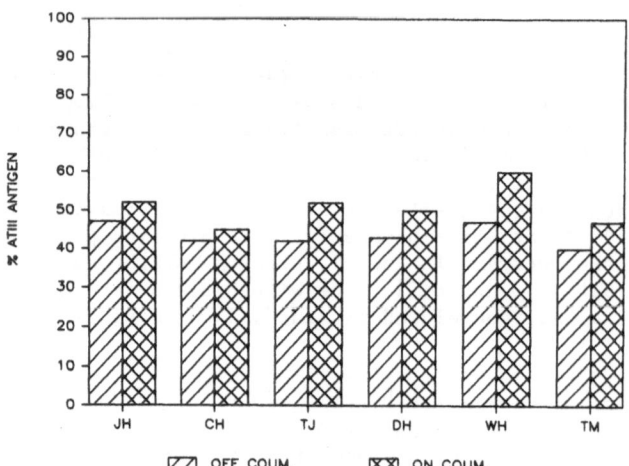

Fig. 2. The effect of warfarin therapy on functional activity and antigenic concentrationof antithrombin III in plasma of six subjects with hereditary antithrombin III deficiency (the "classical" form). Functional activity was measured as antifactor Xa-heparin cofactor; antigen was determined by rocket immunoelectrophoresis.

procedures, pregnancy complications and obstetrical delivery.
Antithrombin III prepared for clinical usage has an effective half-life of
about 60 hrs in which it resembles the native plasma protein[46]. No
differences were found in the catabolism and distribution of the
concentrate between normal and antithrombin III deficient subjects. The
therapy appears to be safe and protective without causing adverse
reactions[47].

HEREDITARY DEFICIENCY OF PROTEIN C AND PROTEIN S

Protein C, a vitamin-K dependent glycoprotein, is regarded as a
second major component of the inhibitory mechanism regulating coagulation
pathways[48]. Produced in the liver, protein C circulates as a 62-kd
zymogen[48,49]. When cleaved by thrombin, the zymogen is
converted to a potent anticoagulant enzyme[49,50]. Since
activation of protein C in purified systems proceeds slowly and only trace
quantities of active enzyme appear during spontaneous blood clotting,
there were initially some doubts about the physiologic importance of this
inhibitor. A major step forward was made when Esmon and Owen[51] showed
that thrombin bound to thrombomodulin, an endothelial cell cofactor,
activates protein C at a much accelerated rate. The key regulatory role
of activated protein C in blood coagulation is the prevention of thrombin
formation through degradation of the heavy chain of factor Va located on
the outer surface of platelets where it serves as the receptor site for
factor Xa[52,53]. Events accompanying the activation of factor V
by thrombin and its cleavage by activated protein C, such as the ability
of factor Xa to protect factor Va from proteolysis, and the ability of
factor Va to protect factor Xa from inactivation by antithrombin III, have
been documented in model systems employing isolated platelets and purified
proteins[54,55]. Thus, by destroying factor Va, activated protein
C not only limits a further generation of thrombin but also makes factor
Xa more accessible to inhibition by antithrombin III. This in turn may
faciliate factor Va proteolysis. From these considerations it appears
that the platelet membrane and the phospholipid vesicle might be the
central stage for critical events in which both major inhibitors,
antithrombin III and activated protein C, participate and work in concert
to limit intravascular clotting. Activated protein C also inactivates

Table 1.   Incidence of Thromboembolism in Protein C
            Deficient Families without Known Homozygosity

REFERENCE	NO OF STUDIED FAMILIES	HETEROZYGOTES TOTAL	HETEROZYGOTES WITH THROMBOEMBOLISM
Griffin et al.[58]	1	3	3
Wintzen et al.[66]	20	53	42
Pabinger-Fashings et al.[66]	2	9	5
Herellou et al.[67]	9	22	16
McGehee et al.[69]	1	5	1
Total	33	92	67 (73%)

Table 2.   Incidence of Thromboembolism in Protein C
Deficient Families with Known Homozygosity

REFERENCE	NO OF STUDIED FAMILIES	HETEROZYGOTES TOTAL	HETEROZYGOTES WITH THROMBOEMBOLISM
Branson et al.[59]	1	3	0
Marciniak et al.[60]	2	27	0
Seligsohn et al.[61]	1	12	0
Sills et al.[62]	1	4	1
Estelles et al.[63]	1	7	0
Yuen et al.[64]	1	3	0
Subcommittee ICTH*[68]	3	11	0
Total	10	67	1 (1%)

*) cases published separately are not included

factor VIIIa[56] and supports fibrinolysis[57] most likely by
stimulating release or preventing inhibition of tissue plasminogen
activator. The biologic significance of these effects is not yet well
defined.

The importance of protein C for control of the coagulation cascade is
confirmed by clinical manifestations in persons who have a selective,
hereditary deficiency of protein C. Numerous families with this disorder
have been investigated[58-69]. Decreased protein C levels ranging
from 30 to 60 percent of the normal concentration are inherited through
autosomal transmission in a dominant fashion. In most cases, the disorder
is detected in association with a positive family history for thrombosis
in a symptomatic heterozgous patient and is characterized by high
incidence of recurrent thromboembolism often with onset in the third
decade of life[58,65-67,69].   Occasionally, however,recognition of the
familial abnormality occurs by the existence of a homozygous offspring who
developes lethal manifestations of purpura fulminans or extensive organ
thrombosis in the neonatal period while numerous heterozygous relatives
remain free of major thrombotic complications through life[59-64,68].

The incidence of thrombosis among families without and with known
homozygosity is presented in Tables 1 and 2. The difference in the
numbers of clinically affected persons in these two groups of families
raises tantalizing questions. Is the clinical expression of the
deficiency based on some genetically transmitted properties of protein C
not presently accounted for in laboratory observations or do other
heritable properties influence the prevalence of thrombosis in a given
family? Since venous thromboembolism is a final expression for multiple
pathogenic pathways and adverse events, further thorough and unbiased
clinical and laboratory studies of deficient families may resolve this
critical issue.

Some cases of functional protein C deficiency with normal antigen
levels have been detected [70,71]. The defect appears to be
associated with an increased risk of thrombosis.

Generalized thrombotic manifestations which appear in infants
homozygous for protein C deficiency shortly after birth are invariably
fatal unless protein C is administered by infusion of plasma or
concentrates of factor IX rich in protein C. Purpuric and thrombotic

lesions are successfully averted as long as protein C in plasma is supported at measurable levels. Heparin therapy in these infants is ineffectual; their antithrombin III plasma levels are generally normal even during extensive thrombotic activity. Anticoagulation with warfarin is an alternative to the replacement therapy. Homozygous children treated with warfarin alone remain free of thrombosis for several weeks or months. The therapy which induces a decrease of biological activities of procoagulants appears to eliminate the necessity for anticoagulation by protein C.

Long-term warfarin prophylaxis may also prevent the recurrence of thrombosis in symptomatic heterozygotes despite further depression of their functional protein C levels. One possible complication of this therapy is warfarin-induced skin necrosis[69,72]. This rare syndrome characterized by capillary thrombosis and necrosis of surrounding tissues may develop during initial stages of the therapy. After administration of warfarin, functional protein C in blood decreases more rapidly than do the procoagulants with a slower catabolic rate. In subjects with pre-existing protein C deficiency this may lead to thrombotic activity localized to the skin which resembles the purpuric lesions that characterize the homozygous protein C deficiency. So far there has been no direct measurements of protein C activity in warfarin treated patients. Since factor Va is selectively degraded by activated protein C and some of this enzyme generates during clotting, we utilized the rate at which factor V activity disappears from clotted plasma to assess the presence of functional protein C[73]. Using this method, we were able to show that functional protein C decreases in parallel with the degree of anticoagulation by warfarin. When prothrombin time exceeds 30 seconds little if any of functional protein C could be accounted for in plasma[74]. This observation supports the concept that impairment of hemostasis induced by therapy with oral anticoagulants is invariably associated with an equal impairment of natural suppression of clotting by the protein C system. Therefore, this therapy eliminates the damage caused by protein C deficiency once a suffcent anticoagulation is achieved.

The function of activated protein C depends to a notable extent on the presence in plasma of protein S, an additional vitamin K-dependent glycoprotein[75]. Protein S serves as a cofactor enhancing proteolysis of factor Va by activated protein C. Partial deficiency of protein S has been detected in several patients with recurrent thrombosis and some data obtained in family studies suggest that it might be inherited as an autosomal dominant trait[76-79]. But protein S exists in plasma in two forms, free protein S and protein S bound to C4b-binding protein, a component linked to the complement system[80]. Comp and Esmon[77] demonstrated that protein S is active only in the free form which varies quantitatively in individual subjects and may decrease considerably in some clinical disorders such as sytemic lupus erythematsus[81]. Although decreased protein S levels are likely to precipitate thrombosis, the diagnosis of a heritable deficiency of protein S in a patient with thrombosis must be based on a thorough evaluation of immunologic and functional properties of this protein in several family members as well as in the patient.

In summary, laboratory and clinical investigations of patients with hereditary deficiencies of coagulation inhibitors have provided a new insight into the physiology of hemostasis as well as the pathogensis of thrombosis and may have important bearing on the management of thromboembolic disease. The invariable association of homozygous protein C deficiency with onset of disseminated thrombotic activity immediately after birth or even in utero, is strong evidence for continuous

181

elaboration of thrombin within the vascular tree. This evidence
highlights the importance of physiological defense mechanisms which must
continuously counteract thrombosis. The outcome of anticoagulant therapy
in a patient with the genetic defect in whom the procoagulant tendencies
distinctly prevail provides important data in support of the potency and
the efficacy of this therapy not otherwise obtainable in clinical trials.

REFERENCES

1. P. C. Harpel, and R. D. Rosenberg, Alpha-2 macroglobulin and
   antithrombin-heparin cofactor: Modulators of hemostatic and
   inflammatory reactions, Prog.Hemostsis Thromb., 3:145 (1976).
2. S. Wessler, and S. N. Gitel, Warfarin from bedside to bench,
   N.Engl.J.Med., 311:645 (1984).
3. I. Bjork, C. M. Jackson, H. Jornvall, K. K. Lavine, K. Nordling and
   W. S. Salsgiver, The active site of antithrombin, J.Biol.Chem.,
   257:2406 (1982).
4. J. Jesty, The kinetics of formation and dissociation of the bovine
   thrombin-antithrombin III complex, J. Biol.Chem., 254:10044
   (1979).
5. W. W. Fish, K. Orre, and I. Bjork, The production of an inactive form
   of antithrombin through limited proteolysis by thrombin, FEBS
   Letters, 98:103 (1979).
6. E. Marciniak, Thrombin-induced proteolysis of human antithrombin III:
   an outstanding contribution of heparin, Brit.J.Haematol., 48:325
   (1981).
7. W. H. Howell, The Condition of the blood in hemophilia, thrombosis
   and purpura, Arch.Intern.Med., 13:76 (1914).
8. O. Egeberg, Inherited antithrombin deficiency causing thrombophilia,
   Thromb.Diath.Haemorrh., 13:516 (1965).
9. E. Marciniak, C. H. Farley, and P. A. DeSimone, Familial thrombosis
   due to antithrombin III deficiency, Blood, 43:219 (1974).
10. D. J. Filip, J. D. Eckstein, and J. J. Veltkamp, Hereditary
    antithrombin III deficiency and thromboembolic disease,
    Am.J.Hematol., 2:343 (1976).
11. J. van der Meer, E. A. Stoepman-van Dalen, and J. M. S. Jansen,
    Antithrombin-III deficiency in a Dutch family, J.Clin.Pathol.,
    6:532 (1973).
12. M. Mackie, B. Bennett, D. Ogston, and A. S. Douglas, Familial
    thrombosis: Inherited deficiency of antithrombin III, Br.Med.J.,
    1:136 (1978).
13. W. R. Pitney, A. Manoharan, and S. Dean, Antithrombin III deficiency
    in an Australian family, Br.J.Haematol., 46:147 (1980).
14. T. M. Cosgriff, D. T. Bishop, E. J. Hershgold, M. H. Skolnick, B. A.
    Martin, B. J. Baty, and K. S. Carlson, Familial antithrombin III
    deficiency: Its natural history, genetics, diagnosis and
    treatment, Medicine, 62:209 (1983).
15. D. R. Ambruso, B. D. Leonard, R. D. Bies, L. Jacobson, W. E.
    Hathaway, and E. B. Reeve, Antithrombin III deficiency: Decreased
    synthesis of a biochemically normal molecule, Blood, 60:78
    (1982).
16. E. W. Lovrien, R. E. Magenis, M. L. Rivas, S. Goodnight, R. Moreland,
    and S. Rowe, Linkage study of antithrombin III,
    Cytogenet.Cell.Genet., 22:319 (1978).
17. J. Winter, B. Bennett, J. Watt, T. Brown, C. San Roman, A. Schinzel,
    J. King, and P. Cook, Confirmation of linkage between antithrombin
    III and Duffy blood group and assignment of AT 3 to 1q22-q25,
    Ann.Hum.Genet., 46:29 (1982).
18. F. T. Kao, H. G. Morse, M. L. Law, A. Lidsky, T. Chandra, and S. L.

C. Wood, Genetic mapping of the of the structural gene for antithrombin III to human chromosone 1, Hum.Genet. 67:34 (1984).

19. E. V. Prochownik, S. Antonarakis, K. A. Bauer, R. D. Rosenberg, E. R. Fearon, and S. H. Orkin, Molecular heterogeneity of inherited antithrombin III deficiency, N.Eng.J.Med., 308:1549 (1983).

20. S. C. Bock, J. F. Harris, C. E. Schwartz, J. H. Ward, E. J. Hershgold, and M. H. Skolnick, Hereditary thrombosis in a Utah kindred is caused by a dysfunctional antithrombin III gene, Am.J.Genet., 37:32 (1985).

21. O. R. Odegard, M. K. Fagerhol, and M. Lie, Heparin cofactor activity and antithrombin III concentration in plasma related to age and sex, Scand.J.Haematol., 17:258 (1976).

22. R. Vikydal, C. Korninger, P. A. Kyrle, H. Niessner, I. Pabinger, E. Thaler, and K. Lechner, The prevalence of hereditary antithrombin III deficiency in patients with history of venous thromboembolism, Thrombos,Haemostas., 54:744 (1985).

23.J. Y. Chang, and T. H. Tran, Antithrombin III Basel: identification of a pro-leu substitution in a hereditary abnormal antithrombin with impaired heparin cofactor activity, J.Biol.Chem., 261:1174 (1986).

24. T. Koide, S. Odani, K. Takahasi, T. Ono, and H. Sakuragawa, Antithrombin III Toyama: replacement of arginine-47 by cysteine in hereditary abnormal antithrombin III that lacks heparin-binding ability, Proc.Natl.Acad.Sci.USA, 81:289 (1984).

25. G. Sas, D. Blasko, D. Banhegyi, J. Jako, and L. A. Palos, Abnormal antithrombin III (antithrombin III "Budapest") as a cause of a familial thrombophilia, Thromb.Diath.Haemorrh., 32:105 (1974).

26. J. A. Penner, H. Hassouna, M. J. Hunter, and M. Chockley, A clinically silent antithrombin III defect in an Ann Arbor family, Thromb.Haemostasis, 42:186 (1979).

27. M. Wolf, C. Boyer, J. M. Lavergne, and M. J. Larrieu, A new familial variant of antithrombin III: antithrombin III Paris, Br.J.Haematol., 51:285 (1982).

28. T. H. Tran, H. Bounameaux, C. Bondeli, T. H. Tran, H. Bounameaux, C. Bondeli, H. Honkanen, G. A. Marbet, and F. Duckert, Purification and partial characterization of a hereditary abnormal antithrombin III fraction of a patient with recurrent thrombophlebitis, Thrombos.Haemostas., 44:87 (1980).

29. N. Sakuragawa, K. Takahashi, S. Kondo, and T. Koide, Antithrombin III Toyama: a hereditary abnormal antithrombin III of a patient with recurrent thrombophlebitis, Thromb.Res., 31:305 (1983).

30. P. Lollar, and W. G. Owen, Clearance of thrombin from circulation in rabbits by high-affinity binding sites on endothelium, J.Clin.Invest., 66:1222 (1980).

31. R. D. Rosenberg, and J. S. Rosenberg, Natural anticoagulant mechanism, J.Clin.Invest., 74:1 (1984).

32. A. Girolami, F. Fabris, G. Cappellato, L. Sainati, and G. Boeri, Antithrombin III (AT III) Padua$_2$: a new congenital abnormality with defective heparin-co-factor activities but no thrombotic disease, Blut, 46:1 (1983).

33. T. Barbui, G. Finazzi, F. Rodeghiero, and E. Dini, Immunoelectrophoretic evidence of a thrombin induced abnormality in a new variant of hereditary dysfunctional antithrombin III (At III Vicenza), Br.J.Haemat., 54:116 (1983).

34. P. J. Sorensen, G. Sas, I. Peto, Gy Blasko, T. Kremmer, A. Samu, Distinction of two pathologic antithrombin III molecules: Antithrombin III "Aalborg" and antithrombin III "Budapest", Thromb.Res., 26:211 (1982).

35. M. L. Jorgensen, C. Petersen, and S. Thorsen, Purification and characterization of hereditary abnormal antithrombin III with impaired thrombin binding, J.Lab.Clin.Med., 104:245 (1984).

36. A. Girolami, F. Marafioti, M. Rubertelli, M. A. Vicarioto, G. Cappellato, and M. Mazzuccato, Antithrombin III Trento. A "new" cogenital AT-III abnormality with a peculiar crossed immunoelectrophoretic pattern in the absence of heparin, Acta.Haematol., 72:73 (1984).

37. K. A. Bauer, J. B. Ashenhurst, J. Chediak, and R. D. Rosenberg, Antithrombin "Chicago": a functionally abnormal molecule with increased heparin affinity causing familial thrombophilia, Blood, 62:1242 (1983).

38. M. Wolf, C. Boyer, A. Tripodi, D. Meyer, M. J. Larieu, and P. Mannucci, Antithrombin Milano: a new variant with monomeric and dimeric inactive antithrombin III, Blood, 65:496 (1985).

39. J. E. Sambrano, L. J. Jacobson, E. B. Reeve, M. J. Manco-Johnson, and W. E. Hathaway, Abnormal antithrombin III with defective serine protease binding (antithrombin III Denver), J.Clin.Invest., 77:887 (1986).

40. S. Wessler, S. N. Gitel, H. Bank, U. Martinowitz, and R. C. Stephenson, An assay of the antithrombotic action of warfarin: its correlation with the inhibition of stasis thrombosis in rabbits, Thromb.Haemost., 40:486 (1976).

41. D. Collen, J. Schetz, De Cock F., E. Holmer, M. Verstraete, Metabolism of antithrombin III (heparin cofactor) in man: effects of venous thrombosis and heparin administration, Eur.J.Clin.Invest., 7:27 (1977).

42. E. Marciniak, and J. P. Gockerman, Heparin-induced decrease in circulating antithrombin III, Lancet, 2:581 (1977).

43. M. Hellgren, L. Tengborn, and U. Abildgaard, Pegnancy in women with cogenital antithrombin III deficiency: experience of treatment with heparin and antithrombin, Gynecol.Obstet,Invest., 14:127 (1982).

44. T. H. Carlson, A. C. Atencio, and T. L. Simon, In vivo behavior of radioiodinated rabbit antithrombin III. Demonstration of a noncirculating vascular compartment, J.Clin.Invest., 74:191 (1984).

45. E. Marciniak, Differential role of fractionated heparin in antithrombin III proteolysis, Blood, 59:576 (1982).

46. E. Marciniak, and E. H. Romond, Catabolism and distribution of functionally heterogenous human antithrombin III, J.Lab.Clin.Med., (in press).

47. N. Miller, M. B. Hultin, M. Gounder, and M. H. Zarrabi, Hereditary antithrombin III deficiency: case report and review of recent therapeutic advances, Am.J.Hematol., 21:215 (1986).

48. J. Stenflo, A new vitamin K-dependent protein: purification from bovine plasma and preliminary characterization, J.Biol.Chem., 251:355 (1976).

49. W. Kisiel, Human plasma protein C: isolation, characterization, and mechanism of activation by α-thrombin, J.Clin.Invest., 64:761 (1979).

50. E. Marciniak, G. Murano, and W. H. Seegers, Inhibitor of blood clotting derived from prothrombin, Thromb.Diath.Haemorrh., 18:161 (1967).

51. C. T. Esmon, and W. G. Owen, Identification of an endothelial cell cofactor for thrombin-catalyzed activation of protein C, Proc.Natl.Acad.Sci.USA, 78:2249 (1981).

52. F. J. Walker, P. W. Sexton, and C. T. Esmon, The inhibition of blood coagulation by activated protein C through the selective inactivation of activated factor V, Biochim.Biophys.Acta., 571:333 (1979).

53. B. Dahlback, and J. Stenflo, Inhibitory effect of activated protein C on activation of prothrombin by platelet-bound factor X, Eur.J.Biochem., 107:331 (1980).

54. J. P. Miletich, C. M. Jackson, and P. W. Majerus, Properties of the factor X, binding site on human platelets, J.Biol.Chem., 253:6908 (1977).

55. P. B. Tracy, M. E. Nesheim, and K. G. Mann, Proteolytic alterations o f factor Va bound to platelets, J.Biol.Chem., 258:662 (1983).

56. C. A. Fulcher, J. E. Gardiner, J. H. Griffin, and T. S. Zimmerman, Proteolytic inactivation of human factor VIII procoagulant protein by activated human protein C and its analogy with factor V, Blood, 63:486 (1984).

57. P. C. Comp, and C. T. Esmon, Generation of fibrinolytic activity by infusion of activated protein C into dogs, J.Clin.Invest., 68:1221 (1981).

58. J. H. Griffin, B. Evatt, T. S. Zimmerman, A. J. Kleiss, and C. Widerman, Deficiency of protein C in cogenital thrombotic disease, J.Clin.Invest., 68:1370 (1981).

59. H. E. Branson, J. Katz, R. Marble, and J. H. Griffin, Inherited protein C deficiency and coumarin-responsive chronic relapsing purpura fulminans in a newborn infant, Lancet 2:1165 (1983).

60. E. Marciniak, H. D. Wilson, and R. A. Marlar, Neonatal purpura fulminans: a genetic disorder related to the absence of protein C in blood, Blood 65:15 (1985).

61. U. Seligsohn, A. Berger, M. Abend, L. Rubin, D. Attias, A. Zivelin, and S. I. Rapaport, Homozygous protein C deficiency manifested by massive venous thrombosis in the newborn, N.Engl.J.Med., 310:559 (1984).

62. R. H. Sills, R. A. Marlar, R. R. Montgomery, G. N. Deshpande, and J. R. Humbert, Severe homozygous protein C deficiency, J.Pediatr., 105:409 (1984).

63. A. Estelles, I. Garcia-Plaza, A. Dasi, J. Aznar, M. Duart, G. Sanz, J. L. Perez-Requejo, F. Espana, C. Jimenez, and G. Abeledo, Severe inherited "homozygous" protein C deficiency in a newborn infant, Thromb.Haemostas., 52:53 (1984).

64. P. Yuen, A. Cheung, H. Ju Lin, F. Ho, J. Mimuro, N. Yoshida, and N. Aoki, Purpura fulminans in a Chinese boy with congenital protein C deficiency, Pediatrics, 77:670 (1986).

65. A. R. Wintzen, A. W. Broekmans, R. M. Bertina, E. Briet, P. E. Briet, A. Zecha, G. J. Vielvoye, and G. Th. Bots, Cerebral haemorrhagic infarction in young patients with hereditary proteinc C deficiency: evidence for "spontaneous" venous thrombosis, Br.Med.J., 290:350 (1985).

66. I. Pabinger-Faschings, R. M. Bertina, K. Lechner, H. Niessner, and Ch. Korninger, Protein C deficiency in two Austrian families, Thromb.Haemostas., 50:810 (1983).

67. M. H. Horellou, J. Conard, R. M. Berina, and M. Samama, Congenital protein C deficiency and thrombotic disease in nine French families, Br.Med.J., 289:1285 (1984).

68. Report of the Subcommittee on Protein C, Xth International Congress on Thrombosis and Haemostasis, 1985.

69. W. G. McGehee, T. A. Klotz, D. J. Epstein, S. I. Rapaport, Coumarin necrosis associated with hereditary protein C deficiency, Ann.Intern.Med., 101:59 (1984).

70. P. C. Comp, R. R. Nixon, and C. T. Esmon, Determination of functional levels of protein C, an antithrombotic protein, using thrombin-thrombomodulin complex, Blood, 63:15 (1984).

71. T. Barbui, G. Finazzi, L. Mussoni, M. Riganti, M. B. Donati, M. Colucci, and D. Collen, Hereditary dysfunctional protein C (protein C Bergamo) and thrombosis, Lancet, 2:819 (1984).

72. A. W. Broekmans, R. M. Bertina, E. A. Loelinger, V. Hofmann, and H. G. Klingemann, Protein C and the development of skin necrosis during anticoagulant therapy, Thromb.Haemost., 49:251 (1983).

73. E. Marciniak, Inactivation of factor V in clotted plasma as a

function of protein C content and activation, <u>Thromb.Haemostas.</u>, 54:84 (1985).

74. E. Marciniak, and M. C. Hermansen, Factor V utilization during clotting observations made in a case of homozygous protein C deficiency and in warfarin treated patients, (manuscript in preparation).

75. F. J. Walker, Regulation of activated protein C by a new protein: a possible function for bovine protein S, <u>J.Biol.Chem.</u>, 255:5521 (1980).

76. H. P. Schwarz, M. Fischer, P. Hopmeier, M. A. Batard, and J. H. Griffin Plasma protein S deficiency in familial thrombotic disease, <u>Blood,</u> 64:1297 (1984).

77. P. C. Comp, and C. T. Esmon, Recurrent venous thromboembolism in patients with a partial deficiency of protein S, <u>N.Engl.J.Med.</u>, 311:1525 (1984).

78. P. C. Comp, R. R. Nixon, M. R. Cooper, and C. T. Esmon, Familial protein S deficiency is associated with recurrent thrombosis, <u>J.Clin.Invest.</u>, 74:2082 (1984).

79. A. W. Broekmans, R. M. Bertina, J. Reinalda-Poot, L. Engesser, H. P. Muller, J. A. Leeuw, J. J. Michiels, E. J. P. Brommer, and E. Briet, Hereditary protein S deficiency and venous thromboembolism. A study in three Dutch families, <u>Thromb.Haemostas.</u>, 52:273 (1985).

80. B. Dahlback, and J. Stenflo, High molecular weight complex in human plasma between vitamin K-dependent protein S and complement component C4b-binding protein, <u>Proc.Natl.Acad.Sci.USA</u>, 78:2512 (1981).

81. P. C. Comp, J. P. Miletich, and R. A. Marlar, The protein C pathway and thrombosis, Hematology 1985. Educational Program American Society of Hematology, New Orleans (1985).

TREATMENT OF FIRST EPISODE OF VENOUS THROMBOSIS

J. Hirsh, M. Levine, and R. Hull

Department of Medicine
McMaster University
Hamilton, Ontario, L8N 3Z5

Patients with venous thrombosis are usually treated with heparin and then with oral anticoagulants. The pattern of practice related to the continued use of oral anticoagulants after the patient with venous thromboembolism is discharged from hospital varies considerably from centre to centre. Some clinicians use no anticoagulants after the patient is discharged, while others treat the patient for up to a year.

In this chapter we propose to discuss a number of practical issues related to the use of oral anticoagulants in the treatment of venous thromboembolism. These are: 1) the evidence supporting the use of oral anticoagulants after an initial course of heparin in the treatment of venous thromboembolism; 2) the optimal therapeutic range for the control of oral anticoagulant therapy; 3) the optimal duration of treatment with oral anticoagulants; and 4) the need to treat calf vein thrombosis with oral anticoagulants.

1. Evidence Supporting the Use of Oral Anticoagulant Therapy Following an Initial Course of Heparin

The clinical practice of using anticoagulant therapy (heparin plus oral anticoagulants) for the treatment a venous thromboembolism is supported by the results of one randomized trial performed by Barrett and Jordan in 35 patients with clinically suspected pulmonary embolism (1). In this study, the use of heparin (administered for 36 hours by intermittent intravenous injection) plus oral anticoagulant therapy for 14 days was found to be much more effective than the results in an untreated control group. Five of 19 patients died of pulmonary embolism compared to none in the treated group (P = 0.036). Since heparin was used in combination with oral anticoagulants, this study does not provide definitive evidence that oral anticoagulants are necessary for the treatment of patients with venous thromboembolism.

The first study which examined the need for oral anticoagulants following initial heparin therapy in patients with deep vein thrombosis or pulmonary embolism was reported by Coon and Willis (2). They carried out a retrospective survey and reported that the frequency of clinically diagnosed recurrent venous thrombosis was lower in patients who were treated with oral anticoagulants after discharge from hospital then in a group that did not receive long term anticoagulant therapy. This study, which formed the basis for continuing anticoagulant therapy after hospital discharge was retrospective, lacked a clear inception cohort of patients, and used clinical features only, for both the initial diagnosis and for the diagnosis of recurrent thromboembolism.

In 1979, Hull and associates (3) performed a randomized trial to evaluate the need for long term treatment in patients with acute venous thrombosis. Patients with venographically confirmed proximal deep vein thrombosis were treated with an initial course of heparin and were then randomized to receive either sodium warfarin controlled by a prothrombin time using a relatively insensitive rabbit brain thromboplastin at a targetted therapeutic range of 1 1/2 to twice control (International Normalized Ratio (INR) of 2.6-4.4) or fixed low dose subcutaneous heparin (5000 units every 12 hours); both treatments were for three months. All patients were assessed for evidence of recurrence using reliable objective tests. Low dose subcutaneous heparin proved to be ineffective since the rate of recurrent venous thromboembolism was 47% in the 19 patients in this group compared to 0% in the 17 patients treated with warfarin sodium. This study therefore provided definitive evidence that patients with proximal vein thrombosis who are treated with an initial course of heparin therapy have a very high rate of recurrence unless effective anticoagulant therapy is continued for weeks or months after their discharge from hospital.

In a recent Scandinavian trial (4), patients with symptomatic venographically confirmed calf vein thrombosis were randomized either to heparin for five days followed by warfarin for three months (23 patients) or only heparin for five days (28 patients). In the patients who were treated with warfarin, there were no recurrences compared to eight venographically documented recurrences (29%) in the control group. The results of this study provide further support for the use of oral anticoagulants after heparin treatment in patients with venous thrombosis and indicate that there is a high rate of recurrence or extension of calf vein thrombosis unless anticoagulants are continued for up to six weeks.

2.   The Optimal Therapeutic Range for the Control of Oral Anticoagulant Therapy

The study by Hull and associates (3) was the first of three randomized clinical trials which were designed both to evaluate the need for long term treatment in patients with acute venous thrombosis and to determine the optimal therapeutic range for monitoring oral anticoagulants in patients with proximal vein thrombosis. Although the more

intense oral anticoagulant regimen was found to be much more
effective than subcutaneous heparin in preventing recurrent
venous thromboembolic events, it was associated with a 21%
rate of clinically overt bleeding (3). A second trial was
therefore performed in which sodium warfarin (adjusted to
maintain the prothrombin time using a commercial rabbit
brain thromboplastin at a prothrombin ratio in the range of
1 1/2 to twice control (INR 2.6-4.4)) was compared with an
adjusted dose of subcutaneous heparin with the hope that
adjusted dose heparin might be associated with a low risk of
hemorrhage without loss of effectiveness (5). The dose of
subcutaneous heparin was adjusted to maintain the
mid-interval activated partial thromboplastin time
(determined six hours after injection) at 1 1/2 times the
control value. The dose was then fixed after the initial
three days and no further anticoagulant monitoring was
performed throughout the three months of long term therapy.

Both forms of therapy proved to be effective in
preventing recurrent venous thromboembolism but the adjusted
dose subcutaneous regimen was associated with a
significantly lower incidence of bleeding than sodium
warfarin, 2% versus 17% respectively. The results of the
second study raised the possibility that a less intense
anticoagulant regimen using sodium warfarin might be as
effective in preventing recurrent venous thromboembolism but
have a lower risk of bleeding than the accepted conventional
dosage regimen. A third randomized trial was therefore
performed to determine whether a less intense regimen using
sodium warfarin would be effective in preventing recurrent
venous thrombosis but would be associated with a lower risk
of bleeding (6). The same therapeutic range and
thromboplastin (1 1/2 to twice control, INR 2.6-4.4) was
used in the standard more intensely treated group to provide
continuity with the previous two randomized trials and this
was compared to a less intense regimen monitored by human
brain thromboplastin (Manchester Comparative Reagent) at an
INR of 2. This intensity in anticoagulant effect is
equivalent to a PT ratio of 1.25 using the commercial rabbit
brain thromboplastin. This third study demonstrated that
sodium warfarin administered to provide a less intense
anticoagulant effect retained its effectiveness against
recurrent venous thromboembolism (incidence of recurrence
was less than 2%) with a greatly reduced frequency of
bleeding (less than 5%) compared to an incidence of bleeding
of 20% in the conventional warfarin sodium group (Table I).
On the basis of these studies we recommend that patients
with a first episode of deep vein thrombosis or pulmonary
embolism should be treated with initial course of heparin
followed by oral anticoagulant therapy with a targetted
therapeutic range equivalent to an INR of 2.0 - 3.0 (less
responsive rabbit brain thromboplastin of 1.2 - 1.5).

THE OPTIMAL DURATION OF ORAL ANTICOAGULANT THERAPY

The pattern of practice across North America and Europe
related to the duration of oral anticoagulant therapy in
patients with venous thrombosis varies markedly, with some
authorities recommending one month, others three to six
months, and some even twelve months of treatment.

Until recently, only two studies were reported which addressed this issue. In the study by Coon and Willis which was a retrospective review of 1500 patients with deep vein thrombosis or pulmonary embolism the risk of recurrent venous thromboembolism was observed to be highest in the first nine weeks after hospital discharge and then plateaued after four months. On this basis, they recommended that patients with an initial episode of deep vein thrombosis should be treated for four months (2). In 1972, O'Sullivan reported on a trial in which patients with a clinical diagnosis of deep vein thrombosis or pulmonary embolism were randomized following 10 days of heparin therapy to either six weeks (94 patients) or six months (92 patients) of oral anticoagulant therapy (7). There were six (6.4%) recurrent thromboembolic episodes in the former group and nine (9.8%) in the latter group; a difference which is not statistically significant and which does not favour the longer duration of therapy.

Both of these studies suffered from a number of methodologic problems which limit the validity of their findings. In the first study, neither the initial diagnosis of thrombosis nor the outcomes of recurrent venous thromboembolism were confirmed objectively, and the different durations of anticoagulant therapy were not predetermined nor allocated randomly among patients. In addition, there was no clear inception cohort of patients. In the second study, objective outcome criteria were not used, nor was the period of follow-up specified.

Recently Holmgren er al performed a randomized trial to evaluate the optimal duration of oral anticoagulant therapy in patients with proximal vein thrombosis using objective outcomes (8). In this study, 135 patients were randomized to receive oral anticoagulant therapy for either one or six months. In each treatment group, the rate of recurrent thrombosis was approximately 5% during the period of anticoagulant therapy, and approximately 17% in the first year after initiating anticoagulant therapy. The post-therapy recurrences (12%) were distributed over an 11 month period following completion of anticoagulant therapy in the first group and over a six month period in the second group suggesting that the addition of five months of oral anticoagulant therapy merely delayed recurrences and that one month of oral anticoagulant therapy is as effective (or ineffective) as six months.

Our approach has been to treat all patients having a first episode of proximal venous thrombosis with an initial course of heparin, and then to continue oral anticoagulants for three months providing there is no continuing risk factor such as antithrombin III or protein C deficiency.

In the three randomized trials in patients with proximal deep vein thrombosis performed by Hull et al, at least one treatment group received standard intensity warfarin for three months (3,5,6) (Table 1). The average rates of recurrence during warfarin therapy for the 166 patients were 1.8% during anticoagulant therapy, 4.2% during the subsequent nine months, and 6.0% in the year following initiation of anticoagulant therapy.

It is clear, therefore, that there is a substantial
risk of recurrence when oral anticoagulants are
discontinued, and that the optimal duration of anticoagulant
therapy following initial heparin remains unresolved. At
present, the decision to stop oral anticoagulants is based
on regional preferences and is purely arbitrary. It is
likely that recurrence would be reduced if anticoagulant
therapy was continued indefinitely in all patients, but with
this approach the majority of patients would be exposed to
the unnecessary inconvenience, risk, and expense of
anticoagulant therapy. Alternatively, treatment could be
stopped after one to three months which would result in an
expected recurrence rate of between 4 to 12% (based on the
data from Holmgren et al (8), and Hull et al (3,5,6)) over
the next year.

It is unlikely that the question of the optimal
duration of anticoagulant therapy will be resolved by simply
performing further studies in which patients are randomized
to treatments of varying duration, since none of the
previous studies has provided definitive answers. It is
possible however, that the decision to stop or continue
warfarin therapy in patients with proximal vein thrombosis
could be based on the continuing presence or absence of risk
factors such as stasis which can now be assessed by objective
methods such as the IPG (9). But this approach needs to be
evaluated formally before it can be recommended.

4.   The Need to Treat Calf Vein Thrombosis

While there is general agreement that patients with
proximal vein thrombosis should be treated with either
anticoagulants or thrombolytic agents, the treatment of calf
vein thrombosis remains controversial (10). Untreated,
between 20% and 30% of calf vein thrombi extend into the
proximal venous segment (11,12). The proponents of
non-treatment of calf vein thrombosis recommend that
patients with clinically suspected venous thrombosis should
be investigated by non-invasive tests such as impedance
plethysmography or Doppler ultrasound which are sensitive to
proximal (popliteal, femoral or iliac) vein thrombosis but
insensitive to calf vein thrombosis (12,13). The safety of
this approach has been demonstrated in four large studies of
patients with clinically suspected venous thrombosis who
were followed by serial impedance plethysmography (12-15).
The results of these studies indicate that calf vein thrombi
are rarely associated with clinically significant pulmonary
embolism, provided that they remain confined to the calf and
provided that proximal extension is detected by serial
impedance plethysmography and treated promptly. On the
other hand, there is now good evidence that some patients
with calf vein thrombosis should be treated with
anticoagulants.

In a study reported by Hull and associates 32 patients
with calf vein thrombosis were randomized to receive either
six weeks of conventional sodium warfarin therapy or
low-dose subcutaneous heparin therapy (5,000 units every 12
hours) (3). There were no recurrences in either group
suggesting that patients with calf vein thrombosis require
less intense anticoagulant treatment than those with
proximal vein thrombosis.

In a more recent randomized study which has been
discussed earlier in this chapter (4), patients with calf
vein thrombosis had a substantial frequency of recurrence or
extension when they were treated for only five days with
intermittent intravenous heparin; this recurrence rate was
markedly reduced in the group who received concurrent oral
anticoagulant therapy which was continued for six weeks.

A review of the seven studies which have addressed the
issue of management of calf vein thrombosis reveals a
consistent message (3,4,11-15). Untreated, calf vein
thrombosis has a substantial (20-30%) risk of extension
(11,12) which can be readily and safely detected by serial
impedance plethysmography (12-15). Symptomatic calf vein
thrombi that extend usually do so in the first five days of
presentation, and extension or recurrence of untreated calf
vein thrombosis is rare after the first week of presentation
(12,14). Treatment with intermittent intravenous heparin
for 5 days does not eliminate extension but appears to delay
this complication until after anticoagulant therapy has been
discontinued (4). Treatment of calf vein thrombosis with
anticoagulants for at least six weeks virtually eliminates
extension (3,4,16).

In institutions with proper facilities to monitor for
extension, the potential benefits of treating patients with
calf vein thrombosis that may extend should be weighed
against the risks and cost of anticoagulant therapy in the
much larger group of patients whose thrombi will not
extend. For example, if the IPG is used as the method of
choice for the diagnosis of venous thrombosis, then of 1000
symptomatic patients with clinically suspected venous
thrombosis approximately 300 will have a positive IPG (and
most will have proximal vein thrombosis) and 700 will have a
negative IPG. Of these 700, 100 will have calf vein
thrombosis and 20 will extend and develop a positive IPG.
Of the remaining 680 patients whose IPG remains negative on
serial testing only one patient will develop recurrent
symptomatic disease. Our approach, therefore, is to
disregard (not treat) clinically suspected calf vein thrombi
in symptomatic patients (i.e.: those with a negative IPG on
presentation) provided that they can undergo serial testing
with impedance plethysmography (15). On the other hand, if
facilities are not available for serial IPG testing then
patients with calf vein thrombosis confirmed by venography
should be treated with anticoagulants for six weeks to
prevent recurrence in 20 to 30% of patients.

From a practical point of view the approach to the
management of calf vein thrombosis depends upon the clinical
circumstances and the availability of non-invasive
diagnostic tests. If calf vein thrombosis is diagnosed by
venography in either a symptomatic or asymptomatic patient
then it would be reasonable to treat with heparin followed
by oral anticoagulants or subcutaneous heparin for six
weeks. If there is a contraindication to anticoagulant
therapy and facilities are available to monitor for
extension with impedance plethysmography then this approach
would be a reasonable alternative. If, as in our practice,
patients with clinically suspected venous thrombosis are
investigated by impedance plethysmography, most patients

with calf vein thrombosis will remain undetected because the IPG will be negative in these patients and the small number of calf vein thrombi that extend can be detected by serial IPG.

REFERENCES

1. Barritt DW, Jordan SC: Anticoagulant drugs in the treatment of pulmonary embolism. Lancet 1960; 2:1309-1312.
2. Coon WW, Willis PW: Recurrence of venous thromboembolism. Surgery 1973; 73:823-827
3. Hull R, Delmore T, Genton E, et al: Warfarin sodium versus low-dose heparin in the long-term treatment of venous thrombosis. N Engl J Med 1979; 301:855-858
4. Lagerstedt CI, Olsson CT, Fagher BO, Oqvist BW, Albrechtsson U: Need for long-term anticoagulant treatment in symptomatic calf vein thrombosis. Lancet 1985; 2:515-518
5. Hull R, Delmore T, Carter C, et al: Adjusted subcutaneous heparin versus warfarin sodium in the long-term treatment of venous thrombosis. N Engl J Med 1982; 306:189-194
6. Hull R, Hirsh J, Jay R, et al: Different intensities of oral anticoagulant therapy in the treatment of proximal-vein thrombosis. N Engl J Med 1982; 307:1676-1681
7. O'Sullivan EF: Dura;tion of anticoagulant therapy in venous thromboembolism. Med J Aust 1972; 2:1104-1107
8. Holmgren K, Andersson G, Fagrell B, et al: One month versus six month therapy with oral anticoagulants after symptomatic deep vein thrombosis. Acta Med Scand 1985; 218:279-284
9. Jay R, Hull R, Carter C, et al: Outcome of abnormal impedance plethysmography results in patients with proximal vein thrombosis: frequency of return to normal. Thromb Res 36:259-263, 1984
10. Adar R, Salzman EW: Treatment of thrombosis of veins of the lower extremities. N Engl J Med 1975; 292:348
11. Kakkar Vv, Flanc C, Howe CT, et al: Natural history of post-operative deep vein thrombosis. Lancet 1969; 2:230
12. Hull RD, Hirsh J, Carter CJ, et al: A randomized trial of non-invasive testing for clinically suspected deep vein thrombosis: the diagnostic efficacy of impedance plethysmography. Ann Intern Med 1985; 102:21-28
13. Wheeler HB, Anderson FA, Jr.: Can noninvasive tests be used as the basis for treatment of deep vein thrombosis? In: Noninvasive Diagnostic Techniques in Vascular Disease, Chapter 58, 1982; pp. 545
14. Huisman MV, Buller HR, ten Cate JW, et al: Evaluation of serial impedance plethysmography in the diagnosis of symptomatic deep vein thrombosis (DVT). Thromb Haemostas 1985; 54:157 (Abstract)
15. Jonker JJC, de Boer AC, den Ottolander GJH: Impedance plethysmography (IPv) in the management of patients with deep vein thrombosis (DVT) at home. Thromb Haemostas 1985; 54:99 (Abstract)
16. Bentley PG, Kakkar VV, Scully MF, et al: An objective study of alternative methods of heparin administration. Thromb Res 1980; 18:177

MANAGEMENT OF RECURRENT

VENOUS THROMBOEMBOLISM

Kenneth M. Moser

Professor of Medicine
University of California, San Diego
   School of Medicine
San Diego, CA

INTRODUCTION

Despite gains in our abilities to identify patients at
high risk of venous thromboembolism and provide them with
rather safe and effective forms of primary prophylaxis (1-5),
venous thromboembolism (V T-E) continues to occur at a
substantial rate. Part of the problem is a failure to
recognize the high risk patient; part, limited application of
the available prophylactic options. Clearly, educative and
logistic initiatives are still needed in many health care
facilities, the key ingredient being a physician catalyst who
can carry forward a primary prophylaxis program.

However, the current reality is that acute venous
thromboembolism continues to be a common event. Even in
facilities which neglect primary prophylaxis, the occurrence of
acute V T-E attracts substantial attention. A positive venogram
or positive angiogram in a patient with signs and symptoms of
acute embolism (Fig. One) generate major interest. Much
discussion usually surrounds initial management decisions. Some
controversies regarding initial treatment of V T-E still exist
(6), and ongoing studies of newer thrombolytic agents will fuel
others. Nonetheless, the acute therapeutic approach is now
reasonably uniform and successful. Quite different, however, is
the situation with respect to the long-term management of V T-E;
that is, therapy designed to prevent recurrent V T-E.

One key difference between the acute and chronic management
of V T-E is that substantially less physician interest and
concern attach to therapy once the initial diagnostic-management
decisions have been made. My observations suggest that, beyond
the acute event, the decision-making process becomes anti-
climactic and, unfortunately, substantially less careful and
uniform. Furthermore, in these days of heavy emphasis on cost
containment and reducing hospital stays, there is a tendency to
rush toward discharge. Considerations regarding prevention of
recurrence often are neglected in this harried environment.

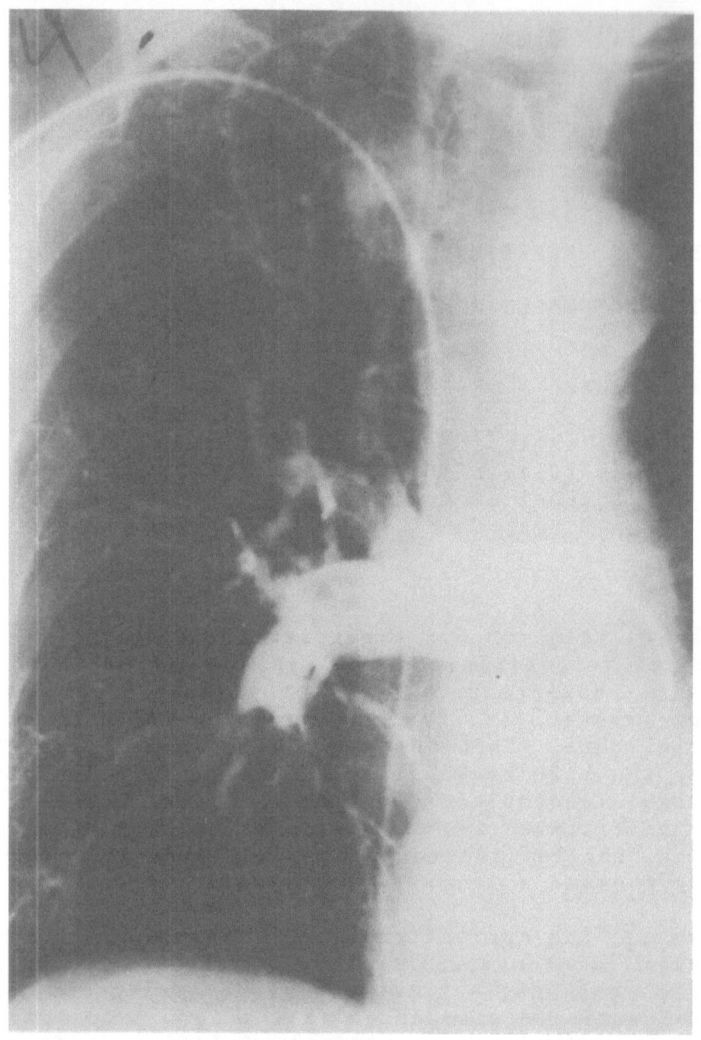

Figure One. Angiogram in patient with acute
embolism who was admitted to the intensive
care unit in shock. Extensive occlusion is
present.

     The effects of these practical considerations are compounded
by the relative dearth of hard information upon which long-term
prophylactic decisions can be made. There are several reasons
that we lack such data. These studies are logistically complex.
They require long-term follow-up of a significant number of
patients, a mandate which, at least in the current U.S. health
care system, is difficult to follow. Furthermore, such studies
may lack the allure (and funding) of more fundamental
investigations regarding thrombogenesis and its consequences.

     These considerations have led to a paradox in the logic
applied to the management of V T-E. The primary goal of _initial_
therapy, including some aspects of thrombolytic therapy, is to

prevent thromboembolic recurrence and extension. This is, of course, the _identical_ goal of long-term therapy. Yet, in pre-discharge planning and post-discharge management, this identity of goals is often poorly recognized. The goal of long-term prevention is, therefore, neglected. We have done several informal surveys of attending physicians and house officers at our institution and others in recent years. These have disclosed significant uncertainty about the pre- and post-discharge management of V T-E. Specifically, there are uncertainties about _transition options_ from acute to chronic therapy, about _who merits_ longer-term protection -- and _with what_; and about _how long_ is long enough. This uncertainity also is reflected by our growing experience with an unusual, but particularly instructive, group of patients; namely, those with massive, chronic thromboembolic obstruction of the major pulmonary arteries (7,8). We have now seen some 90 such patients and have performed thromboendarterectomy in 60 of them for relief of pulmonary hypertension. The histories of these patients, who are drawn from all parts of the North American continent, disclose that there is great non-uniformity in the long-term management of V T-E. The nature and duration of anticoagulant protection they have received beyond an acute venous thrombotic or pulmonary embolic event has been highly variable (8). Indeed, in these patients, the persistence of chronic venous obstruction, often severe and coupled with evidence of chronic pulmonary embolic obstruction, usually has _not_ led to their receiving prolonged anticoagulant protection.

SELECTION OF PATIENTS FOR LONG-TERM PROTECTION

Based on the considerations reviewed above, and the modest available data, we have developed a plan for long-term management. This plan is clearly subject to revision as new data appear; but it represents our own best thoughts at this juncture.

The first element of the plan is to decide who merits long-term protection; or, put another way, "Does _every_ patient with proven acute V T-E warrant such protection?" The answer to that question drives acute to chronic therapy transition policies as well as post-discharge decisions. [It should be noted that, at present, we do not acutely treat calf-limited thrombosis (9-11), so those patients are not included in this discussion].

The data elements we consider in selecting patients for long-term protection are as follows:

(1) The results of impedance plethysmography (IPG) (or contrast venography).
(2) The results of the perfusion lung scan.
(3) The presence of persistent clinical risk factors for recurrent DVT.
(4) The individual patient's hemorrhagic risk, should long-term prophylaxis be instituted.

Unfortunately, there are reasonable, though incomplete, statistical data regarding only the first criterion. Data with respect to the other criteria are quite soft.

Implicit in applying these criteria are two management

concepts: (1) all patients with pulmonary embolism should have
a lung scan and IPG done not only initially but also pre-
discharge; and (2) similarly, all patients with DVT should
have an initial and pre-discharge lung scan and IPG.

With respect to the first concept, it is not routine now to
obtain a impedance plethysmography (IPG) in all patients with
proven embolism. We submit that it should be. In our experience
(8) and that of others (12), a positive IPG is present in 75-80%
of patients with acute or chronic pulmonary embolism. Not only
is this a useful initial diagnostic finding, but also it may
condition initial management. For example, a positive IPG is an
indication for anticoagulant therapy whether or not the diagnosis
of embolism is confirmed. Less well established is the routine,
pre-discharge repetition of the lung scan and IPG. Both, we
feel, are essential to proper decisions regarding long-term
management.

More controversial is the proposal that all patients with
deep venous thrombosis have a lung scan. The proposal is based
on the fact that emboli, even of some size, may be asymptomatic
or promote so few symptoms that they are overlooked (13,14).
Therefore, if vague symptoms (or more provocative ones such as
pleuritic chest pain) appear during initial treatment of DVT, and
no baseline lung scan was obtained, the finding of defect(s) may
suggest recurrence -- even though, had a lung scan be obtained at
the outset, the defect(s) may have been present at that time.
The pre-discharge repetition of the scan serves a similar purpose
in clarifying post-discharge management. It documents the
presence (or absence) of embolic events during initial therapy of
DVT; and it serves as an invaluable baseline should post-
discharge symptoms lead to another lung scan.

Impedance Plethysmography

With respect to impedance plethysmography, we do not yet
have precise data regarding the frequency with which a positive
IPG reverts to negative during acute therapy with heparin. Nor
do we have good evidence as to the basis for such reversion when
it occurs; that is, whether reversion is due to thrombus
clearance or collateral vein formation around a persistent,
obstructing thrombus. However, some data do exist which bear on
this point. We recently have reviewed some 40 patients with
initially positive IPG results and found that, after 7-10 days of
heparin therapy, over 70% remained positive. In the very few
reported studies in which serial venograms have been done in
patients with DVT, total resolution during heparin therapy has
been uncommon, ranging from 0 - 15% (15-17). Lesser degrees
of lysis occurred in up to 38% (17), but it is not known how such
resolution would have influenced IPG results. It should be noted
that, with thrombolytic therapy, complete resolution also was
uncommon, while lesser degrees of lysis were observed in 53 - 88%
(17). Again, how such data may translate into IPG results is
unknown.

There have been several studies in which patients with a
positive IPG have been treated with anticoagulants and followed
for three months or more. In some studies, the test was done
because of a initial episode of clinically-suspected DVT (10.11)
and in one report because recurrent DVT was suspected (18). No

definitive data are available from these studies which document the incidence of IPG reversion to normal after given intervals of therapy. However, it is clear that patients with a positive IPG in either group (clinically-suspected initial or recurrent DVT) have a significant frequency of subsequent recurrence of V T-E, ranging from 3 - 20%, including fatal pulmonary embolism (18). The duration of anticoagulant protection beyond the positive IPG was variable in these series, and it appears that the majority of recurrences developed after such protection was discontinued (11,18).

Finally, in our patients with chronic thromboembolic pulmonary hypertension -- who often have gone months to years without clinical evidence of acute V T-E -- over 50% have a positive IPG at entry to our Center (8).

While these data are imperfect, they certainly indicate that a positive IPG is an indication not only for acute treatment but also for long-term prophylaxis. Therefore, our current policy is to repeat the IPG at 5-7 days after initiation of therapy for DVT and/or P.E. and take a persistent positive as an indication for long-term therapy.

Lung Scan

We use the perfusion lung scan as our second criterion for considering long-term therapy. If the lung scan repeated on the fifth to seventh day of treatment shows persistent, or new, perfusion defects which are segmental or larger in size, we institute long-term therapy. This criterion has not been validated. Our rationale for employing it is two-fold. First, we feel that an embolic event of this size establishes the diagnosis of antecedent venous thrombosis in the larger, above-knee veins (or another source), even if the initial and/or follow-up IPG is negative. Second, we have concern that an unresolved embolus of this size may serve as a site from which proximal or distal thrombotic extension may occur in the absence of anticoagulant protection. Also, as already noted, the follow-up scan is useful in assessing embolic recurrence in the post-discharge period. Finally, such follow-up will assist in earlier detection of that small number of patients with extensive embolization who, despite clinical improvement, fail to resolve their emboli and may maintain chronic pulmonary hypertension (7).

Clinical Risk Factors

The role of clinical risk factors as a determinant of recurrence and, therefore, as an indication for long-term therapy, has not been studied. However, as already noted, it is well-established that clinical risk factors relate closely to the incidence of acute initial episodes of V T-E. Therefore, as in the case of assessing patients for primary prophylaxis, we feel it is rational to accept the continued presence of these factors as an indication for post-discharge therapy. Such factors include the many medical, post-traumatic and post-surgical conditions associated with persistent immobility or venous stasis; and patients with thrombogenic coagulopathies (e.g., Protein C, Protein S, anti:thrombin III deficiencies; lupus anticoagulant). In our view, these factors place the patient at special risk of recurrence and warrant application of long-term therapy.

Hemorrhagic Risk

The fourth consideration -- hemorrhagic risk -- is one of the most difficult to assess. In some instances, the risk is clear; for example, individuals with a known bleeding diathesis or a recent, significant episode of gastrointestinal hemorrhage. [Of course, such patients may not be candidates for initial therapy]. Patients with a more remote history (weeks, months) of a bleeding site are more difficult to assess, and no hard and fast rules can be applied. Individual risk/benefit ratios must be determined. Our experience has indicated that patients with other significant illnesses that are associated with tissue injury (e.g., cancer, connective tissue diseases, chronic infections) also pose special bleeding risk during initial therapy (19). We assume these same factors place such patients at special risk during long-term therapy, though no data bearing on this point are available. But the most difficult element to assess with regard to hemorrhagic risk is the intellectual and/or psychological status of the patient, particularly when an inadequate support system exists outside the hospital. Concern about hemorrhagic risk on this basis is, in fact, the most frequent reason we withhold long-term therapy in our patient population. Included among such patients are those with compromised cerebral function, a limited ability for any reason to follow instructions, and an established history of ethanol or other substance abuse.

As we analyze these four criteria, a decision about the risk/benefit of long-term protection is made. We do not provide long-term protection to all patients beyond acute therapy for V T-E. If a patient has a negative pre-discharge IPG and lung scan and has no persistent clinical risk factors, [or poses special hemorrhagic risks], post-discharge anticoagulant therapy is not provided. We do provide it to all others -- approximately 80% of our patients with acute V T-E.

A recently-published retrospective study by Petitti et al takes issue with this approach, concluding that long-term hemorrhagic risks outweigh the benefits of reduced recurrence rates (20). However, neither the methods used to identify recurrence nor the details of anticoagulant management are stipulated in that report; nor is the nature of the patient population clear. Our own experience, and that of others reported here, has led us to adopt the criteria we have described according to which a majority of, but not all, patients with acute V T-E merit long-term protection.

Other Options

What options exist for the patient in whom clear indications for long-term protection do exist, but the use of anticoagulant drugs is contraindicated or considered unwise? This is a difficult problem with no answer applicable to all patients. However, our very positive experience with the Greenfield filter (21, 22) over the last 5 years has made this our primary option in such patients. We now routinely place these inferior vena caval filters pre-operatively in patients undergoing pulmonary thromboendarterectomy. More than 20 such patients now have been followed for at least two years. In addition, more than 30 other patients with V T-E have received this device. In none of these patients, to this time, has there been embolism, bleeding, migration or filter occlusion.

WITH WHAT AND FOR HOW LONG?

Having decided to protect patients against recurrence with long-term use of anticoagulant drugs, the next questions to be answered are "with what?" and "for how long?"

We regard warfarin and subcutaneous heparin as equally attractive options in term of risk/benefit ratios (23,24). We often offer patients these options, after discussing the practical pros and cons of each. Some patients prefer subcutaneous heparin because regular monitoring of blood tests is not required or difficulties may exist in obtaining such tests. Further, should bleeding occur, cessation of effect is quickly achieved. Others find repetitive injections cumbersome or unacceptable.

If subcutaneous heparin is used, we either adjust the dose to keep the activated partial thromboplastin time at 1.5 times control values at 6 hours after injection; or simply prescribe 10,000 units every twelve hours. We do not monitor the APTT in these patients after discharge. If warfarin is chosen, we attempt to maintain patients in the range of 1.5 - 1.8 times control.

Transition Options

To keep the total hospital stay as short as possible, three acceptable scenarios can be followed for instituting long-term prophylaxis. First, if a decision for long-term warfarin is made early, the drug can be initiated after several days of intravenous heparin therapy and an overlap of at least 3 or 4 days can be assured. If, later in the hospital stay, long-term warfarin is deemed unnecessary, warfarin is discontinued.

Alternatively, the patient can be simply changed from therapeutic intravenous to prophylactic subcutaneous doses of heparin after the first week. A third option we often employ is to discharge the patient on subcutaneous heparin and make the transition to warfarin as an outpatient.

The last question -- "how long is long enough" -- is still poorly answered. We need better data, using objective criteria for defining the frequency of bleeding and recurrence, to determine the optimal duration of anticoagulant protection following an acute episode of V T-E. Our own current policy with respect to duration is based on essentially the same criteria as our decision to initiate long-term protection. We routinely continue protection for six months. If, at the end of that period, the IPG is negative, the scan no longer shows segmental defects and clinical risk factors have abated, we discontinue therapy. However, if only the IPG remains positive, we also discontinue therapy, but advise patients to receive prophylaxis in any future risk situation. When therapy is maintained beyond six months, we periodically review with the patient the risks and benefits of continued anticoagulant protection. The decision to maintain or discontinue therapy is an interactive one. Until studies become available regarding recurrence rates at specific intervals after the initial episode of V T-E, we will continue this policy. At the moment, patients cannot be offered hard data regarding recurrence versus bleeding risk over the very long term.

SUMMARY

We have described our current criteria for selecting those patients with acute V T-E who merit long-term protection, for accomplishing the acute to long-term transition efficiently and for deciding when such protection can be interrupted. Naturally, in individual patients, special circumstances may exist which alter these decisions. Also, it is evident that additional studies are needed so that this sequence of decision-making can be improved. Our current approach contains a number of rather arbitrary components. Furthermore, if effective thrombolytic therapy does become available, we will need to reevaluate current criteria for long-term protection from recurrence.

References

1.   Crandon, A.J., Peel, K.R., Anderson, J.A., Thompson, V., McNicol, G.P. Post-operative deep vein thrombosis: identifying high risk patients. Brit. Med. J., 281:343-44, 1980.

2.   Sue-Ling, H.M., McMahon, M.J., Johnston, D., Philips, P.R., Davies, J.A. Pre-operative identification of patients at high risk of deep venous thrombosis after major abdominal surgery. The Lancet, 1:1173-1176, 1986.

3.   Consensus Conference: Prevention of Venous Thrombosis and Pulmonary Embolism. JAMA, 256:744-749, 1986.

4.   Havig, O. Deep vein thrombosis and pulmonary embolism. Chir. Scand., 478, 1-93, 1978.

5.   The Epidemiology of Venous Thrombosis. The Milbank Memorial Fund Quarterly, 50:1-283, 1972.

6.   Moser, K.M. and Fedullo, P.F., Venous thromboembolism: three simple decisions, 83:117-121, 256-260, 1983.

7.   Moser, K.M., Spragg, R.G., Utley, J., Daily,, P.O. Chronic thrombotic obstruction of major pulmonary arteries. Ann. Int. Med., 99:299-305, 1983.

8.   Moser, K.M., Daily, P.O. and Peterson, K.L. Management of chronic unresolved large vessel thromboembolism in the Pulmonary Circulation in Health and Disease (Ed: J.A. Will) Academic Press. (In press)

9.   Moser, K.M., LeMoine, J.R. Is embolic risk conditioned by location of deep venous thrombosis? Ann. Int. Med, 94:439-434, 1981.

10. Hull, R.D., Hirsh, J., Carter, C.J, et al. Diagnostic efficacy of impedance plethysmography for clinically suspected deep vein thrombosis. Ann. Int. Med., 102:21-28, 1985.

11. Huisman, M.V., Buller, H.R., Ten Cate, J.W, Vreeken, J. Serial impedance plethysmography for suspected deep venous thrombosis in outpatients. New Engl. J. Med., 314:823-828, 1986.

12. Hull, R.D., Hirsh, J., Carter, C.J. et al. Pulmonary angiography, ventilation lung scanning and venography for clinically suspected pulmonary embolism with abnormal perfusion lung scan. Ann. Int. Med., 98:891-899, 1983.

13. Moser, K.M. Asymptomatic pulmonary embolism. JAMA, 247:1049, 1982.

14. Brach, B.B., Moser, K.M., Cedar, L., et al. Venous thrombosis in acute spinal cord paralysis. J. Trauma, 17:289-292, 1977.

15. Marder, V.J., Souler, R.L., Aticharthkarn, V., et al. Quantitative venographic assessment of deep vein thrombosis in the evaluation of streptokinase and heparin therapy. J. Lab. Clin. Med., 89:1018-24, 1977.

16. Robertson, B.R., Nilsson, I.M., and Nylander, G. Thrombolytic effect of streptokinase as evaluated by phlebography of deep venous thrombi of the leg. Act. Chir. Scand., 136:173-178, 1970.

17. Goldhaber, S.Z., Buring, J.E., Lipnick, R.L., Hennekens, C.H. Pooled analysis of randomized trials of streptokinase and heparin in phlebographically documented acute deep venous thrombosis. Am. J. Med., 76:393-397, 1984.

18. Hull, R., Carter, C., Jay, R.M., et al. The diagnosis of acute, recurrent deep vein thrombosis: A diagnostic challenge. Circ., 67:901-906, 1983.

19. Nelson, P.H., Moser, K.M., Stover, C., Moser, K.S. Risk of complications during intravenous heparin therapy. West J. Med., 136:189-197, 1982.

20. Pettiti, D.R., Strom, B.L., Melmon, K.L. Duration of warfarin anticoagulant therapy and the probabilities of recurrent thromboembolism and hemorrhage. Am. J. Med., 81:255-259, 1986.

21. Greenfield, L.J. A new intracaval filter permitting continued flow and resolution of emboli. Surg., 73:599-605, 1973.

22. Greenfield, L.J. Greenfield vena caval filter experience. Arch. Surg., 116:1451-55, 1981.

23. Hull, R., Delmore, T., Carter, C., et al. Adjusted subcutaneous heparin vs warfarin sodium in the long-term treatment of venous thrombosis. New Engl. J. Med., 306:189-194, 1982.

24. Hull, R., Hirsh, J., Jay, R., et al. Different intersities of oral anticoagulant therapy in the treatment of proximal-vein thrombosis. New Engl. J. Med., 307:1676-1681, 1982.

WARFARIN METABOLISM AND DRUG-DRUG INTERACTIONS

Robert A. O'Reilly

Departments of Medicine
Santa Clara Valley Medical Center
Stanford University School of Medicine
University of California, San Francisco
San Jose, California

I. INTRODUCTION

Drug interactions with warfarin vary from useful to disastrous. The
pharmacologic combination of warfarin and a platelet inhibitor can be
clinically efficacious. Contrarily, the increasing number of drugs that
interact with warfarin can potentiate its anticoagulant effect and cause
life-threatening hemorrhagic events. To avoid the futility of memorizing
long lists of these drugs, guidelines will be presented for the prescribing
physician. These concepts are understood best after the metabolism of
warfarin in man is reviewed.

II. CLINICAL PHARMACOLOGY OF RACEMIC WARFARIN

Warfarin is a racemic mixture composed of two optical isomers, R- and
S-warfarin. Racemic warfarin is usually administered to patients as the
highly water-soluble sodium salt. This aqueous solubility, the drug's
favorable pKa, and the hydrophobic nature of the coumarin-ring structure
assure the 100% bioavailability of racemic warfarin, even with severe bowel
disease and the virtual absence surgically of the small intestine.[1] The
biologic half-life of racemic warfarin in man is 36 hours. The high degree
of binding of racemic warfarin to plasma albumin, over 99% at therapeutic
concentrations, can explain its clinical pharmacology: the prolonged half-
life and biologic effect, the absence of warfarin in red blood cells or
cerebrospinal fluid, and the lack of excretion of unchanged warfarin into
the urine or stool.[2] Thus, warfarin is administered therapeutically at time
intervals of 24 hours, which is shorter than its half-life of 36 hours.
This practice permits a patient to reach a "steady state" with respect to

warfarin dose and prothrumbin time. Bodily accumulation of drug is safest when long-term therapy is initiated without any "loading" dose, but can be dangerous when <u>any other drug</u> is added to a chronic anticoagulant regimen.[3]

III. STEREOCHEMISTRY OF RACEMIC WARFARIN

R- and S-warfarin have substrate stereospecificity during their metabolic transformation. R-warfarin is metabolized primarily by reduction of the acetonyl sidechain into secondary warfarin alcohols that are excreted mainly by the kidneys into the urine. S-warfarin is metabolized primarily by oxidation of the coumarin ring to 7-hydroxy-S-warfarin, which is excreted mainly by the liver into the bile and stool.[4] Several drug-drug interactions with racemic warfarin are stereoselective, because only the oxidative metabolism of S-warfarin is altered (Table 1). This stereoselective interaction is important heuristically and dangerous clinically because S-warfarin has five times more anticoagulant activity than R-warfarin.

Table 1. Pharmacokinetic and Pharmacodynamic Drug
Interactions with Warfarin

Increased Prothrombin Time

<u>Pharmacokinetic</u>	<u>Pharmacodynamic</u>
Cimetidine	Aspirin
Disulfiram	Cephalosporins, 3rd generation
Metronidazole*	<u>Heparin</u>
Phenylbutazone*	<u>Hepatic disease</u>
Sulfinpyrazone*	
Trimethoprim-Sulfamethoxazole*	

Decreased Prothrombin Time

Barbiturates	Diuretics
<u>Cholestyramine</u>	Heredity resistance
Rifampin	Vitamin K

---

*Stereoselectively inhibits the oxidative metabolism of the S-warfarin enantiomorph of racemic warfarin.

———— indicate a clinically important drug combination and interaction.

IV. DRUG INTERACTIONS WITH RACEMIC WARFARIN: GENERAL ASPECTS

Drug interactions with oral anticoagulants may be all too obvious because excessive effect can be readily detectable as bleeding.[5] Furthermore, bleeding is often forewarned by marked prolongation of the one-stage prothrombin time, the test used to monitor therapy in all patients. The ease of measuring warfarin in the plasma facilitates the study of its drug interactions.

Drug interactions with warfarin have two mechanisms: pharmacokinetic, or drug-drug, and pharmacodynamic (Table 1). For pharmacokinetic mechanisms, the interacting drug alters the amount of warfarin delivered to its receptor site. For pharmacodynamic mechanisms, the interacting drug alters the effect of warfarin at its receptor site. With pharmacokinetic interactions, the alterations of the warfarin concentration in plasma and of the prothrombin time are correlated. With pharmacodynamic interactions, the warfarin concentration in blood is unaltered and the prothrombin-time response varies widely.

V. PHARMOCOKINETIC OR DRUG-DRUG INTERACTIONS WITH WARFARIN

A. Absorption

Cholestyramine. The interaction of cholestyramine with warfarin has become clinically important because of recently demonstrated efficacy of cholestyramine in the secondary prophylaxis of coronary artery disease.[6] Thus, patients may be treated simultaneously with both drugs. Cholestyramine lessens the hypoprothrombinemic effect of warfarin by decreasing its bioavailability. The cholestyramine resin binds warfarin in the intestinal tract, which interrupts its enterohepatic circulation and increases the excretion of unchanged warfarin into the stool.[7] The interaction is reduced when cholestyramine is omitted for a few hours after the daily warfarin dose.[8]

B. Decreased Metabolic Clearance

Several drugs reduce the metabolic clearance of racemic warfarin and increase its hypoprothrombinemic effect: phenylbutazone, sulfinpyrazone, disulfiram (Antabuse), metronidazole (Flagyl), and trimethoprim-sulfamethoxazole (Bactrim, Septra).[2] All these drugs have a similar mechanism of interaction with racemic warfarin. They decrease the clearance of S-warfarin, but have no effect on the clearance of R-warfarin or its hypoprothrombinemic effect. These stereoselective effects have more pharmacologic than clinical interest because these drugs at this time are seldom used concurrently with warfarin. Even sulfinpyrazone, when it failed to receive FDA approval for use in the secondary prophylaxis of coronary artery disease, has showed a marked decrease in concurrent use with warfarin. The anti-arrhythmic drug amiodarone is being used more frequently in patients taking warfarin. Amiodarone decreases the clearance of both R- and S-warfarin and markedly increased the hypoprothrombinemia of racemic warfarin (O'Reilly, 1986; unpublished observations).

C. Increased Metabolic Clearance

Barbiturates and rifampin. Barbiturates and rifampin induce the activity of hepatic mixed-function oxidases.[9] Both drugs reduce the hypoprothrombinemia of racemic warfarin, which correlates with lower blood concentrations of the anticoagulant as a result of its more rapid clearance.[10] These interactions are not stereoselective; the clearance of both enantiomorphs of racemic warfarin is increased.

Ethanol. Ethanol reportedly alters the anticoagulant effect of warfarin: ethanol taken acutely increasing the effect by inhibited metabolic clearance of warfarin and ethanol taken chronically decreasing the effect by induction of hepatic microsomal enzymes.[2] However, prospective studies showed that large quantities of ethanol in wine both with meals and in the fasting state had no significant effect during chronic anticoagulant therapy.[11,12]

D. Excretion

Diuretics. Diuretics reportedly reduce the response to oral anticoagulants by increasing the renal excretion of unchanged anticoagulant drug. In a prospective study the chronic administration of the diuretic chlorthalidone (Hygroton) caused no significant changes in the plasma concentrations of racemic warfarin and no renal excretion of unchanged drug.[13] The diuretic caused a highly significant loss of plasma water associated with increased clotting-factor activity. It was concluded that diuretics lessen anticoagulant activity by concentrating clotting factors. Another prospective study with the diuretic spironolactone (Aldactone) showed the same results.[14]

VI. PHARMACODYNAMIC INTERACTIONS WITH WARFARIN

A. Vitamin K

Sulfonamides and antibiotic drugs. Sulfonamides and antibiotic drugs reportedly potentiate the anticoagulant effect of warfarin by eliminating the intestinal bacterial flora and thereby producing vitamin-K deficiency. Most studies show that oral antibiotics caused no significant effect on long-term anticoagulant therapy except in patients on a vitamin-K deficient diet.[15] Third-generation cephalosporin antibiotics markedly augment the anticoagulant effect of warfarin by directly inhibiting the vitamin-K dependent carboxylase.[16] Dietary sources rich in vitamin K can lead to "acquired resistance" to warfarin: liquid nutritional supplements and excessive broccoli ingestion.[17,18] Acquired resistance to warfarin can also result from administration of vitamin K subcutaneously, which apparently acts as a slow-release repository.[1]

B. Aspirin

The use of aspirin in patients on warfarin is dangerous. In a prospective study, six tablets of aspirin daily to subjects on long-term therapy with warfarin caused significant prolongation of the bleeding time without any change in the prothrombin time.[13] Thus, the dual impairment of hemostasis by the effect of aspirin on platelet activity and by the effect of warfarin on fibrin formation causes increased susceptibility to hemorrhagic episodes.

C. Production of Clotting Factors

Hepatic disease. Hepatic disease in patients administered warfarin results in an exaggerated anticoagulant response. The interaction is pharmocodynamic; there is no change in the blood concentrations of warfarin.[2]

Clofibrate. The hypolipidemic drug clofibrate (Atromid-S) augments the anticoagulant effect of warfarin. In a prospective study with racemic warfarin in man, the co-administration of clofibrate reduced platelet adhesiveness and aggregation, increased the one-stage prothrombin time and turnover rate of clotting factors II and X, but had no effect on the blood concentrations of the anticoagulant.[19] It was concluded that the hemorrhagic complications of simultaneous therapy with clofibrate and warfarin may result from the combined hemostatic defect of reduced platelet function and increased turnover of clotting factors dependent on the activity of lipid-soluble vitamin K.

VII. PREVENTION OF HEMORRHAGIC DRUG INTERACTIONS WITH WARFARIN

A. General

The hemorrhagic consequences of warfarin, particularly from the interaction of another drug, are all too familiar. Bleeding is usually associated with extension of the anticoagulant effect of warfarin. Therefore, the physician and patient must avoid all possible factors that can augment its hypoprothrombinemic effect.[20] It was generally believed that warfarin would be an effective antithrombotic drug only if doses producing a coagulation defect so intense that the risk of bleeding was just being avoided.[21] However, recent studies have shown that smaller doses of warfarin may be effective not only in preventing thrombosis but also in reducing the risk of bleeding.[22] The critical factors for safe anticoagulant therapy are a carefully selected patient, an experienced physician and a reliable laboratory.

B. The Patient

Patients or their surrogates must take responsibility for their anticoagulant therapy. They must be intelligent enough to understand the serious nature of the therapy and the need for close supervision. They must have literacy in a language mutual to the patient and physician and enough visual acuity to read instructions. The patient must be compliant and show consistency in keeping appointments.

C. The Physician

Physicians should perform a thorough history and examination of the patient to detect any bleeding or potentially hemorrhagic lesions. They should identify the relative and absolute contraindications to anticoagulant therapy, and assess the risk for intracranial hemorrhage in hypertensive patients. All patients should be screened for potential sources of gastrointestinal, urologic, and gynecologic bleeding.

Physicians experienced with anticoagulant therapy provide their patients with detailed verbal and written instructions.[20] They describe the danger signs of bleeding and the symptoms of thromboembolic disease, the times to contact the physician, the danger of relying on memory and the utility of a calendar to record doses of anticoagulant taken and appointment dates and prothrombin-time results, a wallet card or Med-alert bracelet to identify the patient as an anticoagulant user, and a supply of vitamin-K tablets for emergency use.

D. Laboratory Control

For laboratory control of therapy with the one-stage prothrombin time, the most important factor is the brand of tissue thromboplastin used.[20] Physicians must know the values in their laboratory for the therapeutic range of the prothrombin time, and those beyond which the potential for hemorrhage exists. The results of the prothrombin time can be expressed in seconds, or the ratio of patient and control times in seconds, or in percent of normal activity. Recent redefinitions of the therapeutic range as a coagulation defect of lessened intensity should lower the risks of bleeding in patients.[22]

E. Bleeding

Bleeding episodes occur most often during the first two months or beyond three years of therapy. For outpatient therapy physicians initially should examine their patients at weekly intervals for evidence of bleeding, patient comprehension, and result of the prothrombin time. There are many risk factors for hemorrhagic complications: the existence of medical contraindications, poor patient supervision, poor laboratory control, large loading doses of drug, therapy too intense for the patient, intercurrent disease particularly in the elderly, and drug interactions especially with over-the-counter preparations containing aspirin.

VIII. CONCLUSION

In conclusion, all drug interactions with warfarin are potentially dangerous.[20] Beware of adding any drug or "food" to the regimen of a patient on warfarin. Choose your patients for warfarin therapy carefully. Continuously re-educate yourself and your patients about this therapy. Finally, drug interactions with warfarin will end only when it's no longer used.

IX. REFERENCES

1. P. J. Kearns, and R. A. O'Reilly, Bioavailability of warfarin in a patient with short bowel syndrome, J. Paren. Ent. Nutr. 10:100 (1986).
2. R. A. O'Reilly, Drug-induced vitamin K deficiency, resistance and drug interactions, in: "Prothrombin and Other Vitamin K Proteins," Vol. II. W. H. Seegers and D. A. Walz, ed., CRC Press, Boca Raton (1986).

3. R. A. O'Reilly and P. A. Aggeler, Determinants of the response to oral anticoagulant drugs in man, Pharmacol. Rev. 22:35 (1970).

4. R. J. Lewis, W. F. Trager, K. K. Chan, A. Breckenridge, M. Orme, M. Roland, and W. Schary, Warfarin: stereochemical aspects of its metabolism and the interaction with phenylbutazone, J. Clin. Invest. 53:1607 (1974).

5. R. A. O'Reilly, Anticoagulant, antithrombotic, and thrombolytic drugs, in: "Goodman and Gilman's The Pharmacological Basis of Therapeutics," A. G. Gilman, L. S. Goodman, T. W. Rall, and F. Murad, eds., Chap. 58, Macmillan, New York (1985).

6. B. M. Rifkind, Lipid Research Clinics Program, J.A.M.A. 252:2547 (1984).

7. R. A. O'Reilly, Drug interactions involving oral anticoagulants, Cardiovasc. Cl. 6:23 (1974).

8. D. B. Hunninghake and D. M. Hibbard, Influence of time intervals for cholestyramine dosing on the absorption of hydrochloro-thiazide, Clin. Pharmacol Ther. 39:329 (1986).

9. J. M. Van den Broek, H. C. Ten Wolde-Kraamwinkel, C. H. Klein-bloesem and D. D. Breimer, Effect of rifampicin treatment on in vitro drug-metabolizing activities in the pig, Biochem. Pharmacol. 33:325 (1984).

10. R. A. O'Reilly, Interaction of chronic, daily warfarin therapy and rifampin, Ann. Int. Med. 83:506 (1975).

11. R. A. O'Reilly, Lack of effect of mealtime wine on the hypoprothrombinemia or oral anticoagulants, Am. J. Med. Sci. 277:189 (1979).

12. R. A. O'Reilly, Lack of effect of fortified wine ingested during fasting and anticoagulant therapy, Arch. Int. Med. 141:458 (1981).

13. R. A. O'Reilly, M. A. Sahud, and P. M. Aggeler, Impact of aspirin and chlorthalidone on the pharmacodynamics of oral anticoagulant drugs in man, Ann N. Y. Acad. Sci. 179:173 (1971).

14. R. A. O'Reilly, Interaction of spironolactone and racemic warfarin in man, Clin. Pharmacol. Ther. 27:198 (1980).

15. P. G. Frick, G. Riedler, and H. Brögli, Dose response and minimal daily requirement for vitamin K in man, J. Appl. Physiol. 23:387 (1967).

16. L. Uotila, J. W. Suttie, Inhibition of vitamin K-dependent carboxylase in vitro by cefamandole and its structured analogs, J. Infect. Dis. 148:571 (1983).

17. R. A. O'Reilly and D. A. Rytand, "Resistance" to warfarin due to unrecognized vitamin K supplementation, N. Engl. J. Med. 303:160 (1980).

18. S. J. Kempin, Warfarin resistance caused by broccoli, N. Engl. J. Med. 308:1229 (1983).

19. R. A. O'Reilly, M. A. Sahud, and A. J. Robinson, Studies on the interaction of warfarin and clofibrate in man, Throm. Diath. Haemorrh. 27:309 (1972).

20. R. A. O'Reilly, Editorial: complications of anticoagulant therapy, West. J. Med. 132:453 (1980).

21. T. W. Meade, Safety of oral anticoagulation, Lancet 1:1387 (1986).

22. R. Hull, J. Hirsh, R. Jay, C. Carter, C. England, M. Gent, A. G. G. Turpie, D. McLoughlin, P. Dodd, M. Thomas, G. Raskob, and P. Ockelford, Different intensities of oral anticoagulant therapy in the treatment of proximal-vein thrombosis, N. Engl. J. Med. 307:1676 (1982).

IMPROVING THE BENEFIT/RISK RATIO

Stanford Wessler

Department of Medicine
New York University School of Medicine
New York, New York

Using the smallest effective dose of warfarin, clearly will diminish hemorrhage. But there are more than a dozen factors other than dose that can either favorably effect the benefit/risk ratio or tell the physician that he should or should not consider using warfarin in specific patient groups. Three of these factors, the prothrombin time, warfarin resistance, and drug-drug interactions, have already been commented upon at this symposium and so I shall discuss several other factors.

HEMOSTATIC COMPETENCE

Since the primary hazard in anticoagulant prophylaxis is bleeding, the hemostatic competence of the patient must be established before or, in emergencies, as soon as possible after institution of therapy. It is through the history, including current drug use, the physical examination, and several readily available laboratory tests, that hemostatic competence is defined. Such competence can be determined with minimum effort, time, and cost by ascertaining that the patient does not have a tendency to bleed easily, has never hemorrhaged excessively when cut, bruised, or subjected to dental procedures or surgery; that bleeding is not occurring from any site at the time of examination; and that the hematocrit, platelet count, partial thromboplastin time, prothrombin time, and bleeding time as well as urinanalysis and stool examination for gross or occult hemorrhage are normal.[1]

INTERVAL SURGERY

For minor surgery such as tooth extraction, interruption of warfarin therapy is rarely necessary. In contrast, guidelines have been less clearly defined for patients facing major elective general surgery who are already on a maintainance dose of warfarin. One choice is to discontinue the drug for four days before operation and for one to two days postoperatively before resuming oral anticoagulation. A second alternative is to discontinue warfarin four days before operation, substituting a low-dose heparin regimen in the perioperative period (as outlined for primary prophylaxis among surgical patients) and then reinstituting warfarin prophylaxis. Finally, there is the option of limiting the prothrombin time ratio to or slightly below 1.5 prior to surgery and maintaining this intensity in the perioperative and immediate postoperative period. Published trial data do not identify the extent of the hemorrhagic risk, if any, with this third alternative. Whether the risk is as low as starting warfarin on the day before or the day of operation has not been established. Nevertheless, some knowledgeable investigators believe that it is safe to continue the preoperative warfarin regimen through the surgical procedure, provided the prothrombin time is not excessively prolonged.[2]

DIET

There are no food restrictions per se for patients on warfarin. The public, however, receives advice about pharmaceuticals in lay publications. There are statements in this literature to the effect that patients maintained on oral anticoagulants should avoid excessive consumption of foods rich in vitamin K because the compound promotes clotting. Listed among such foods are leafy greens, asparagus, bacon, broccoli, brussels sprouts, and beef liver. Physicians should advise patients that these foods are entirely safe in and of themselves, and should not be restricted because of warfarin administration. The point, rather, is that any **major change** in diet, as with the addition or deletion of other drugs, should be reported to the patient's physician so that drug dosage can be adjusted based on more frequent determinations of the prothrombin time. The recommendation to delete from the diet leafy vegetables, moreover, stands in conflict with the suggestion that these vegetables may form part of an anticancer diet.

DIABETIC RETINOPATHY

Among diabetic patients requiring long-term warfarin therapy, the question often arises whether anticoagulation represents a risk of vitreous or retinal hemorrhage, particularly among patients with advanced retinopathy. Not only are there no data to support such concerns, but trials of anticoagulants initiated to treat retinal venous occlusion complicated by retinal hemorrhage have not been associated with any enhancement of existing bleeding.

TERATOGENICITY

Fertile women receiving warfarin must be warned of the risks of teratogenicity if they become pregnant. When pregnancy is an immediate possibility, consideration should be given to substituting heparin for the oral anticoagulant. Specific warfarin-induced embroyopathies occur in the sixth to the 12th week of pregnancy, and central nervous system and ocular fetal anomolies may occur at any time during pregnancy.[3] If the patient has been alerted to notify her physician that her menstrual period is late by only a few days, there is a human, β-chorionic gonadotropin radioimmunoassay specific for detecting pregnancy from the 14th postconception day. Even when menses are delayed by one to two weeks, there is still time to discontinue warfarin therapy and markedly diminish, if not avoid, the likelihood of a teratogenic outcome. If pregnancy is recognized too late, abortion should be considered. Sonography provides no assistance in making this decision.

BREAST FEEDING

During metabolism warfarin is hydroxylated to an inactive compound. The drug appears in the urine almost entirely as its metabolite. Although warfarin does pass the placental barrier, it appears in the milk of nursing mothers in an inactive form. Direct testing has shown no unchanged drug in maternal milk.[4] Accordingly, and contrary to prevailing opinion, warfarin given postpartum to nursing mothers poses no hazard to the full-term infant.[5]

This is of particular importance for women such as those with prosthetic heart valves who become pregnant and whose anticoagulant is changed from warfarin to heparin for the 9 months of their pregnancy. These women, postpartum, can again take warfarin, even if they nurse, thus diminishing their long exposure to heparin with its attendant risk of osteoporosis.

CONJOINT USE OF ANTIPLATELET AGENTS

Stated simply: on the basis of currently available data, aspirin and anticoagulant therapy should not be administered concurrently because of the increased risk of bleeding. This observation confronts physicians with a special dilemma because aspirin, aside from its several non-vascular indications, has been approved by the FDA for transient ischemic attacks, unstable angina, and secondary myocardial infarction. A review of the available evidence suggests that in patients with transient ischemic attacks, aspirin should take precedence over warfarin for the first six months following the onset of TIA. If there has been a prior stroke, atrial fibrillation or a failure of aspirin to prevent further TIA's, then warfarin should be considered in place of aspirin. In patients with unstable angina, aspirin should also take precedence over warfarin for the first six months unless an acute myocardial infarction supervenes in which case anticoagulants should be administered. For the prevention of secondary myocardial infarction, however, the value of aspirin is less clear and if, for example, atrial fibrillation is present, warfarin would be preferable. These statements concerning aspirin and warfarin may well be modified as more trial data become available. A regimen of a very low dose aspirin plus a very low dose warfarin regimen has not as yet been shown to be either effective or safe.

In regard to other antiplatelet agents, dipyridamole has a potential antithrombotic role when added to warfarin among patients with prosthetic heart valves. Platelet antiaggregants alone or in any combination are no substitute for warfarin, however.

The non-steroidal anti-inflammatory arthritic drugs that have mild antiplatelet action may be used in conjunction with warfarin without incurring an increased risk of bleeding. This is also true of calcium channel blockers that minimally impair platelet aggregation.

OVERLAPPING HEPARIN AND WARFARIN

When patients are being switched from heparin to warfarin, conventional wisdom dictates that the drugs be overlapped for two days because of the one-to-two-day delay in the peak prothrombin time response. Further elucidation of the pharmacologic nature of both compounds provides additional support for maintaining this overlap and perhaps even increasing its duration.

Although heparin administration frequently depresses the plasma concentration of antithrombin III, the effect of that depression is debatable during heparin therapy,[6] since the consequent decrease in the antithrombin III concentration will be more than offset by the increased reaction rate induced by the drug. When heparin therapy is terminated in the absence of other antithrombotic agents, however, patients with a heparin-induced decrease in antithrombin III can be considered to be in a potentially hypercoagulable state for approximately three days, until the plasma antithrombin III level has returned to normal. This is a second reason for overlapping the anticoagulants for at least that period of time.[8]

In addition, the warfarin-induced depression of protein C occurs within the first 12 to 24 hours of drug administration at about the same rate as factor VII depression. The depression of protein C while factors X, IX, and II are still near normal levels may also represent a thrombotic risk and is further reason for overlapping the two drugs for several days.

Lastly, in view of work in animals indicating that warfarin has a delayed, additive antithrombotic effect six days after drug administration,[7] some physicians may wish to extend the period of overlap to five to six days--an approach that has anecdotal support in the clinical literature.[8,9] If such an extended overlap is planned, it rarely prolongs the hospital stay.

HYPERTENSION

Blood pressures significantly in excess of 160 systolic and 90 diastolic incur the risk of cerebral hemorrhage and all reasonable efforts need be undertaken to reduce such elevations toward these bench mark values. In this regard, it should be appreciated that cerebral hemorrhage in hypertensive patients does not correlate well with the absolute level of the blood pressure, that isolated systolic hypertension may pose an even greater threat of cerebral hemorrhage than diastolic hypertension and that the former often proves more difficult to manage. Having acknowledged these facts, it may still be appropriate, on a benefit/risk basis, to utilize anticoagulant prophylaxis in some patients at high risk of cerebral embolism in whom hypertension cannot be totally eliminated despite optimal therapy. For these patients physicians would be well advised to consider utilizing the lowest of the 3 therapeutic ranges for both heparin and warfarin, as there is a correlation between cerebral hemorrhage and the intensity of anticoagulation.

In summary, it is only by routinely considering all of these factors, in addition to drug intensity, that a new day will dawn concerning the efficacy and safety of the oral anticoagulants.

REFERENCES

1. S. Wessler, A Guide to Anticoagulant Therapy, American Heart Association, 1984.
2. S. Wessler, Is anticoagulant prophylaxis of cardiac emboli practical?, Geriatrics (in press).
3. J. G. Hall, R. M. Pauli, and K. M. Wilson, Maternal and fetal sequelae of anticoagulation during pregnancy. Am J Med 68:122(1980).
4. R. A. O'Reilly, and P. M. Aggeler, Determination of the response to oral anticoagulant drugs in man. Pharmacol Rev 22:35,1980.
5. K. Fries, F. E. Konig, and T. Reich, Einfluss der Marcoumar-Therapie bei voll gestillten kindern, Schweiz Med Wochen Schr, 87:615(1957).
6. E. Marciniak, and J. P. Gockerman, Heparin-induced decrease in circulating antithrombin III, Lancet 2:581(1977).
7. S. Wessler, S. N. Gitel, H. Bank, U. Martinowitz, and R. C. Stephenson, An assay of the antithrombotic action of warfarin: its correlation with the inhibition of stasis thrombosis in rabbits, Thromb Haemost 40:486(1978).
8. J. G. Domenet, D. W. Evans, and H. Stephenson, Anticoagulants in congestive heart failure, Brit Med J, 2:866(1966).
9. W. W. Coon, and P. W. Willis III, Thromboembolic complications during anticoagulant therapy, Arch Surg 105:209(1972).
10. The Working Group on Hypertension in the Elderly. Statement on hypertension in the elderly, JAMA, 256:70(1986).

ORAL ANTICOAGULANT THERAPY AND SKIN NECROSIS:

SPECULATIONS ON PATHOGENESIS

Carl G. Becker

Professor of Pathology
Cornell University Medical College
New York, New York

Warfarin or coumadin induced necrosis of the skin was first recognized in 1952[1] and since that time, several hundred cases have been described.

The lesions may appear anywhere during the first through tenth day of therapy but they usually involve dependent tissues and or adipose areas with thights, breasts, buttocks, genitalia and lower extremities most frequently involved[2,3,4]. The initial lesion is edematous and erythematous, with petechial hemorrhage, and central ischemic necrosis following. Thrombosis of venules and capillaries with or without an inflammatory cell infiltrate has been observed microscopically (see reference 3 for review of literature pertinent to microscopic morphologic changes). It is of interest that thrombi are not described in arteries and arterioles, particularly in light of recent demonstrations of protein C deficiency (heterozygous) in a number of patients who developed skin necrosis in association with warfarin therapy[5,6], since deficiencies of protein C and of protein S have both been associated with venous rather than arterial thrombosis[7,8,9,10]. Thrombosis of veins and venules in warfarin induced skin necrosis may be a function of slower flow and reduced sheer stress in this portion of the vascular tree, and thus explain the increased frequency of lesion development in dependent regions. However, local vascular factors, especially those associated with endothelial cells have not been studied. These factors might include such things as regional differences in endothelial cell expression of thrombomodulin or other endothelial cell associated proteins that could modulate hemostatic function.

Approximately, 75% of reported cases of warfarin produced skin necrosis have occurred in women with a mean age of 53[2]. The reasons for this association are unknown but will be speculated upon below with the goal of possibly identifying those patients who are at especial risk.

A number of conditions have been associated with warfarin induced skin necrosis. Heterozygous deficiency of protein C has been demonstrated in a number of cases. The relatively rapid fall in protein C and protein S relative to the procoagulant Vitamin K dependent proteins following loading doses of coumadin or warfarin resulting in a transient state favoring a thrombotic event provides a partial explanation for the association of protein C deficiency with the development of this lesion[11],[12]. Although, a recent report describes low levels of protein C antigen in eleven of thirteen patients who had developed skin necrosis in association with warfarin therapy[13], it is not at present known if all patients who develop this lesion are deficient in protein C. Further, several types of deficiencies of protein C activity have been described. These include deficiency of protein C antigen and anticoagulant activity, deficiency of amidolytic activity relative to antigen concentration, deficiency of anticoagulant activity relative to decreased amidolytic activity and normal antigen concentration, and reduced anticoagulant activity relative to normal amidolytic activity and antigen concentration[12]. The frequency of these individual abnormalities of protein C in the population and their frequency of association with the development of skin necrosis has yet to be determined and requires both greater availability and simplification of methods necessary to measure these differences. It may prove that only certain of these abnormalities will be associated with the development of skin necrosis.

Theoretically, deficiency of protein S might also predispose to the development of warfarin induced skin necrosis since it has been associated with venous thrombosis. However, no cases have been reported, perhaps because deficiency of protein S appears to be less serious than deficiency of protein C with respect to venous thrombosis. Recently, a protein of apparent molecular weight of 138,000 has been described in plasma that binds protein S and enhances the anticoagulant activity of activated protein C[14]. Protein S binding protein was also observed to enhance the rate of factor Va inactivation by activated protein C and protein S. It is conceivable that deficiencies of this newly described protein could also contribute to the development of venous thrombosis and skin necrosis, but no data concerning this is yet available.

Even if it is assumed that most or all patients who develop skin necrosis in association with warfarin are deficient in protein C function, it remains to be explained why some patients who have previously developed skin necrosis in association with warfarin therapy have not developed it when therapy was initiated on subsequent occasions or why other patients with known deficiency of protein C have never developed the lesion. Clearly, other factors must contribute to the liklihood of lesion development even when protein C deficiency exists. This is not surprising since patients with known protein C deficiency may also escape development of venous thrombosis.

Other conditions associated with the development of warfarin induced skin necrosis include trauma, including surgical trauma, prosthetic heart valves, infection, pregnancy, abortion, cholestasis, and cancer[2],[15],[16]. All of these are conditions that would contribute to activation or amplification of pathways of coagulation or inflammation through a number of different mechanisms and could provide an initiating stimulus that in the presence of protein C deficiency could result in skin necrosis. These cases may provide clues to other endogenous and exogenous factors that could either provide triggering stimuli or contribute to failure of modulation of pathways of coagulation and inflammation.

As mentioned above, skin necrosis appears to occur much more commonly in women. It has been demonstrated that the estrogenic component of birth control pills stimulate a reduction in the activity of antithrombinIII[17]. In the presence of a deficiency of protein C, and estrogen induced deficit in antithrombin III activity would superimpose an acquired defect on a genetic one. Thus either oral contraceptives or the peri and post menopausal use of estrogens might render some women more susceptible to the development of skin necrosis. Obtaining a history of use of these compounds might be important in predicting risk and determine therapeutic strategies. It has recently demonstrated that circulating levels of protein C can be linearly related to both skin fold thickness and to use of oral contraceptives. In this study, protein C antigen was higher in 24 women using oral contraceptives than in 24 women of the same age and degree of obesity who were not using oral contraceptives. In the pooled data for all, there was an increase in protein C, measured by electroimmunoassay, of about 1% for each 1.0 mm increase in skin fold thickness[18]. The question arises as to whether obesity and/or female sex hormones cause an increased need for protein C for some adaptive reason, e.g. pregnancy, and whether under these circumstances heterozygous deficiency of protein C becomes more severe with respect to maintaining the balance between anticoagulant and procoagulant activities of blood. In this construction the special susceptibility of women to skin necrosis becomes more understandable. The vulnerability of adipose tissue to lesion development may also be related to this phenomenon, but such a relationship would be predicated on a special need of veins and venules in adipose tissue for anticoagulant activity.

Many of the patients described in reports of warfarin induced skin necrosis were suffering from other serious illnesses that provided initial stimulus for thrombus formation. It can be imagined that many were also receiving a number of other drugs. The contribution of these to induction of skin necrosis is not addressed in the available literature. However, like the rôle of estrogenic hormones, it should be considered. Solutions of sodium lactate in concentrations similar to those in Ringer's lactate have been shown to be thrombogenic in vivo in the stasis assay developed by Wessler and colleagues[19,20]. The questions arise as to how many of the reported patients received Ringer's lactate and whether this provided a thrombogenic stimulus capable of triggering events leading to skin necrosis. Similarly, many of the reported patients were infected and presumably treated with antimicrobials. Tetracycline is commonly used in the treatment of malignant pleural effusions, presumably because it serves as a stimulant of local inflammation and fibrogenesis. The mechanism is unknown, but given the degree of overlap in mediator pathways it might also directly or indirectly activate coagulation pathways. The thrombogenic stimulus may be minimal, but in the presence of protein C deficiency it might be enough to trigger the onset of skin necrosis. The same logic may apply to other antimicrobials, but at present most of those in current use have not been assayed for subtle effects on major mediator pathways. Another substance that could, paradoxically, contribute to induction of warfarin induced skin necrosis is heparin. Heparin can potentiate activation of plasminogen by tissue plasminogen activator and urokinase type plasminogen activator. Heparin is known to interfere with the capacity of fibrin to stimulate activity of tissue plasminogen activator[21]. Since many of the patients who developed skin necrosis in association with oral anticoagulants were also receiving or had recently recieved heparin, the question arises as to whether at certain concentrations and at specific times heparin can contribute to lesion induction. Hall, et al have described skin necrosis following heparin therapy in three patients, only one of whom had received coumadin. In these patients skin necrosis developed at sites of heparin injection[22].

Substances that can trigger cellular relase mechanisms should also be considered in this context. For example, morphine and synthetic opiates can trigger release of mediators from tissue mast cells[23]. Since these cells can also release activators of components of the intrinsic pathway of coagulation[24], it is conceivable that such drugs could also contribute indirectly to induction of skin necrosis in the presence of oral anticoagulants. Again, this is an unexplored possibility.

Cigarette smoking may also contribute to lesion induction in warfarin

associated skin necrosis. Constituents of cigarette smoke capable of
activating Factor XII dependent pathways in vitro[25] and in vivo[26], stimulating interleukin-1 release from human monocytes[27] triggering immediate
cutaneous hypersensitivity reactions in humans[28,29,30], presumably IgE
mediated, and others capable of activating the alternative pathway of the
complement system have been described [31,32,33]. Since any of these functions
could serve directly or indirectly to participate in induction of warfarin
associated skin necrosis it is possible that active or passive exposure to
cigarette smoke is a significant environmental risk factor for lesion
induction.

It has recently been demonstrated that immune complexes can stimulate
tissue factor expression by human umbilical vein endothelial cell monolayers and that this expression is enhanced in the presence of platelets [34].
From this data and from clinical observations relating diseases like
systemic lupus erythematosus to thrombotic disease, it is reasonable to
hypothesize that the presence of underlying, immune complex mediated
diseases might predispose to the development of skin necrosis in association with oral anticoagulants. The preponderance of such diseases among
females may in some way or ways be related to the apparent preponderance
of skin necrosis among females. The multiple known mechanisms by which
monocytes can be stimulated to express procoagulant activity, often
requiring T lymphocytes [35], make it possible that diseases associated with
cell mediated immunity could also contribute to enhanced susceptibility
to warfarin associated skin necrosis.

Finally, the rôle of stasis as a predisposing factor to the development of skin necrosis should be examined further. It is conceivable that
reduction in blood flow consequent to chilling might contribute to the
development of skin necrosis, and perhaps attention should be paid to
avoiding chilling of the skin of patients during the induction phase of
oral anticoagulant therapy. Similarly, constricting items of clothing
might also contribute to stasis and hence to lesion induction. This
raises the question of whether tight elastics in undergarments might be
related to the increased frequency of skin necrosis in breasts and
buttocks and other adipose areas.

Although much of the above might be best described as advised speculation, it is aimed at trying to identify conditions that might make some
patients more at risk of developing skin necrosis than others. The rarity
of the lesion relative to the total number of patients treated with oral
anticoagulants, and the fact that even in the presence of deficiencies of
protein C it may not occur, indicate that other additional factors must
be involved in lowering the threshold for the event.

Successful strategies for prevention of recurrence of skin necrosis
by combining therapy with heparin and lower initial doses of warfarin, or
both of the above with administration of fresh frozen plasma to compensate
for transient severe protein C and S deficiencies during the induction
phase have been described. These strategies may be especially applicable
to those patients who may be at greater risk of developing this lesion
for reasons discussed herein.

REFERENCES

1. H. Verhagen, Local haemorrhage and necrosis of the skin and under-
    lying tissues during anticoagulant therapy with Dicumarol or
    Dicumacyl, Acta Med Scand 148:453 (1954).
2. J. R. Horn, L. H. Danziger, and R. J. Davis, Warfarin induced skin
    necrosis: Report of four cases, Am J Hosp Pharm 38:1763 (1981).

3. J. Koch-Weser, Coumarin necrosis, Ann Int Med 68:1365 (1968).

4. A. C. Weinberg, G. Lieskovsky, W. G. McGehee, and K. G. Skinner, Warfarin necrosis of the skin and subcutaneous tissue of the male external genitalia, J Urology 130:352 (1983).

5. A. W. Broekmans, R. M. Bertina, andE. A. Loeliger, Protein C and the development of skin necrosis during anticoagulant therapy, Thrombosis and Haemostasis 49:251 (1983).

6. W. G. McGehee, T. A. Klotz, D. J. Epstein, and S. I. Rapaport, Coumarin necrosis associated with hereditary protein C deficiency, Ann Intern Med 101:59 (1984).

7. A. W. Broekmans, J. J. Veltkamp, and R. M. Bertina, Congenital protein C deficiency and venous thromboembolism. A study of three Dutch families, N Engl J Med 309:340 (1983).

8. C. T. Esmon, Protein C: Biochemistry, physiology, and clinical implications, Blood 62:1155 (1983).

9. J. H. Griffin, B. Evatt, and T. A. Zimmerman, Deficiency of protein C in congenital thrombotic disease, J Clin Invest 68:1370 (1981).

10. P. C. Comp, and C. T. Esmon, Recurrent venous thromboembolism in patients with a partial deficiency of protein S, N Engl J Med 311:1525 (1985).

11. S. Vigano, P. M. Manucci, S. Solinas, B. Botasso, and G. Mariani, Decrease in protein C antigen and formation of an abnormal protein soon after starting oral anticoagulant therapy, Br J Haematol 57:213 (1984).

12. S. Vigano-D'Angelo, P. C. Comp, C. T. Esmon, and A. D'Angelo, Relationship between protein C antigen and anticoagulant activity during oral anticoagulation and in selected disease states, J Clin Invest 77:416 (1986).

13. V. Rose, H. C. Kwaan, K. Williamson, D. Hoppensteadt, J Walenga, and J. Fareed, Protein C antigen deficiency and warfarin necrosis, Am J Clin Path 86:653 (1986).

14. F. J. Walker, Identification of a new protein involved in the regulation of the anticoagulant activity of activated protein C, J Biol Chem 261:1094 (1986).

15. V. Hofmann, and P. G. Frick, Repeated occurrence of skin necrosis twice following coumarin intake and subsequently during decrease of Vitamin K dependent coagulation factors associated with cholestosis, Thrombosis and Haemostasis 48:245 (1982).

16. R. N. Everett, and F. L. Jones, Jr., Warfarin-induced skin necrosis: A cutaneous sign of malignancy? Postgrad Med 79:97 (1986).

17. S. N. Gitel, R. C. Stephenson, and S. Wessler, The activated factor X-antithrombin III reaction rate: A measure of the increased thrombotic tendency induced by estrogen containing oral contraceptives, Haemostasis 7:10 (1978).

18. T. W. Meade, Y. Sterling, H. Wiekes, and P. M. Mannucci, Effects of oral contraceptives and obesity on protein C antigen, Thrombosis and Haemostasis 53:198 (1985).

19. S. Wessler, Unpublished observation.

20. S. Wessler, S. M. Reimer, and M. D. Sheps, Biologic assay of thrombosis-inducing activity in human serum, J Appl Physiol 14:943 (1960).

21. P. Andrade-Gordon, and S. Strickland, Interaction of heparin with plasminogen activators and plasminogen: Effects on the activation of plasminogen, Biochem 25:4033 (1986).

22. J. C. Hall, D. McConahay, D. Gibson, J. Crockett, and R. Conn, Heparin necrosis. An anticoagulation syndrome, JAMA 244:1831 (1980).

23. R. Levi, A. A. Chenouda, J. P. Trzeciakowski, Zhao-Gui Guo, L. M. Aarronson, R. D. Luskind, C. H. Lee, W. Gay, V. A. Subramanian, J. C. McCabe, and J. C. Alexander, Dysrhythmias caused by histamine release in guinea pig and human hearts, Klin Wochenschr 60:965 (1982).

24. H. L. Meier, A. P. Kaplan, L. M. Lichtenstein, S. D. Revak, C. G. Cochrane, and H. H. Newball, Anaphylactic release of a pre-kallikrein activator from human lung in vitro, J Clin Invest 72:574 (1983).

25. C. G. Becker, and T. Dubin, Activation of factor XII by tobacco glycoprotein, J Exp Med 146:457 (1977).

26. L. Dillon, F. Glenn, and C. G. Becker Induction of acalculous cholecystitis and pneumonitis in dogs following inhalation of constituents of cigarette smoke condensate, Am J Path 109:253 (1982).

27. T. Francus, L. C. Thompson, B. Y. Rubin, M. K. Crow, G. W. Siskind, and C. G. Becker, Tobacco glycoprotein is a potent inducer of IL-1 production. (Manuscript in preparation.)

28. C. G. Becker, T. Dubin, and H. P. Wiedemann, Hypersensitivity to tobacco antigen, Proc Natl Acad Sci 73:1712 (1976).

29. T. Francus, G. W. Siskind, and C. G. Becker, Role of antigen structure in the regulation of IgE isotype expression, Proc Natl Acad Sci 80:3430 (1983).

30. R. F. Kein, and C. G. Becker, Selective expression of IgE reactive with tobacco glycoprotein in human sera, Fed Proc 45:225 (1986).

31. A. Firpo, M. J. Polley, and C. G. Becker, The effect of tobacco derived products on the human complement system, (Abstract) Immunobiology 164:318 (1984).

32. R. R. Kew, B. Ghebrehewet, and A. Janoff, Cigarette smoke can activate the alternative pathway of complement in vitro by modifying the third component of complement, J Clin Invest 75:1000 (1985).

33. A. Firpo, F. Field, D. Wellner, F. Infante, C. G. Becker, and M. J. Polley, On the chemical characterization of a low molecular weight component of cigarette smoke which activates the alternative pathway of complement, (Abstract) in: "Complement: Laboratory and Clinical Research. XIIth International Complement Workshop," ed., J. S. Cooper, S. Karger, Basel, p. 25, (1985).

34. S. H. Tannenbaum, R. Fink, and D. B. Cines, Antibody and immune complexes induce tissue factor production by human endothelial cells, J Immunol 137:1532 (1986).

35. T. S. Edgington, H. Helin, S. A. Gregory, G. Levy, D. S. Fair, and B. S. Schwartz, Cellular pathways and signals for the induction of biosynthesis of initiators of the coagulation protease cascade by cells of the monocytic lineage, in: "Mononuclear Phagocytes," R. van Furth ed., Martinus Nijhoff, boston pp 687-696 (1985).

CLINICAL TRIALS IN MYOCARDIAL INFARCTION AND CORONARY HEART DISEASE

Lewis H. Kuller

University of Pittsburgh
Graduate School of Public Health
Department of Epidemiology
Pittsburgh, PA

The relationship between thrombosis, coronary atherosclerosis and myocardial infarction has evolved over many years.[1] There has been considerable controversy about the specific role of thrombosis in both myocardial infarction and sudden death,[2] as well as the importance of vessel wall, platelet interactions in the evolution of atherosclerosis. The interaction of vessel wall injury, platelets and hyperlipidemia in the development of the atherosclerotic plaque and complications seems to be a most plausible hypothesis.

Clinical pathological studies have also documented the importance of thrombosis in both myocardial infarction[3] and sudden death.[2] Thrombosis as opposed to coronary artery spasm or hemorrhage or rupture of an atherosclerotic plaque probably plays the predominant role in the precipitation of both sudden death and myocardial infarction. Clinical pathological studies have also documented the relationship between the size of the myocardial infarction and subsequent damage to the left ventricular wall resulting in various manifestations of "pump failure".[4] The benefits of specific therapies aimed at either preventing or reducing the size of the thrombus have also been shown.[5,6,7] Thus, the role of anticoagulants must now be evaluated in relationship to the use of antiplatelet aggregating agents such as aspirin, intravenous streptokinase, tissue plasminogen activator, immediate coronary angioplasty[8] or bypass surgery.

Another interesting and important research finding has been the identification of specific clotting factors that appear to be related in prospective studies to the risk of myocardial infarction.[9,10,11,12] Meade, et al,[9] has demonstrated an increased risk of myocardial infarction associated with either elevated fibrinogen levels or in factor VII. The levels of these clotting factors may be related to dietary intake of fat or to other cardiovascular risk factors.[13,14,15]

The role of thrombosis in the evolution of coronary artery disease is therefore clearly established. The fundamental question is the efficacy of various interventions to reduce the risk of both the initial clinical event, be it myocardial infarction, angina pectoris or sudden death, or to modify both the short and long-term natural history of the disease.

The clinical trial is part of the evolution of epidemiological studies. These studies may be divided into three types: 1) descriptive; 2) analytical;

and, 3) experimental epidemiology or clinical trials. The descriptive epidemiological studies have noted the magnitude of the problem in the community, the populations at greatest risks and the incidence, prevalence, and mortality rates within and between populations. These descriptive studies form the basis for estimating the potential benefits of subsequent clinical trials. For example, the relatively low risks of myocardial infarction and especially sudden deaths among women under the age of 65, make it unlikely that primary prevention clinical trials, that is to prevent the initial clinical event, will be feasible unless the sample size was extremely large and the intervention very simple and safe.

The analytical epidemiology studies, as noted, have identified a multitude of risk factors for coronary artery disease and their inter-relationships. Atherosclerosis is most likely an example of what is called a common source epidemic in which the primary agent is the ingestion of saturated fat and cholesterol. The extent of the atherosclerotic disease, the host susceptibility is related to a variety of other factors, both genetic and environmental, such as elevated blood pressure, cigarette smoking, activity, behavior, and specific lipoprotein phenotypes.

The precipitation of the acute event, that is myocardial infarction, sudden death, or even angina pectoris, is a function of other risk factors which convert the underlying atherosclerotic disease into its clinical manifestations. The major pathological event is most likely thrombosis. Cigarette smoking is probably the most important precipitant of either a heart attack or sudden death.[16] There are certainly other important environmental factors with also contribute to the precipitation of myocardial infarction and sudden death. Unfortunately, the identification of these specific factors has not been very successful. If we could identify such factors and intervene either by avoiding them or by specific treatments that would prevent thrombosis and precipitation of the event, then we could substantially reduce the incidence of clinical disease.

Specific treatments aimed at either prevention or early dissolution of the thrombus would seem to have potential benefit. Analytical epidemiological studies have documented that the time from the precipitant of this acute event to death is very rapid. Most coronary heart disease deaths are still sudden and occur outside of the hospital, or in the emergency rooms among individuals who are morbund on arrival.[16] This high case-fatality outside of the hospital must be considered in the evaluation of therapeutic interventions. Treatments that are primarily aimed at the reduction of in-hospital mortality have relatively little impact on the overall community cardiovascular mortality rates.

There are two populations at risk that are candidates for prevention of heart disease deaths. First, the large number of individuals who have extensive coronary atherosclerotic disease but are asymptomatic and are at potential risk of an acute event,[17,18] especially sudden death outside of the hospital. This population can be identified from their risk factors or by specific physiological measurements such as an exercise test. The power of this risk prediction has recently been noted by the six year followup of the 356,000 men in the primary screen for the Multiple Risk Factor Intervention Trial. The six year mortality rate among men with diastolic blood pressures greater than 90, serum cholesterol greater than 245 and who were cigarette smokers at entry was 21.4/1,000, while for those with none of these risk factors, serum cholesterol less than 182, systolic blood pressure less than 120, diastolic blood pressure less than 76, non-cigarette smoker, and non-diabetic, the risk was only 0.8/1,000 over six years.[19] However, even among these very high risk individuals the coronary heart disease mortality is about 4% in six years, the potential for any intervention drug therapy such as anticoagulants would be exceedingly small because the risk for any individual person still remains relatively low. Thus, one would have to treat 100 individuals to have the potential of preventing four heart disease deaths over an approximate six year period. Modification of risk factors predominantly by non-pharmacological means is obviously preferable. Even if coronary thrombosis was the primary precipitant of death among these high risk individuals and if anticoagulation therapy was highly efficacious in preventing the acute thrombosis it is unlikely that a primary prevention trial approach would be feasible.

The addition of a positive exercise test substantially increases the mortality risk especially among these high risk individuals.[20,21] Among the hyperlipidemic individuals with a positive exercise test in the Lipid Research Clinic Mortality Followup Study, the coronary heart disease mortality was about 8-10% at the end of the eight years of followup as compared to less than 2% for those with a negative exercise test. Even, however an 8% mortality at the end of eight years is only 1% per year and would still raise substantial questions about the potential for anticoagulation therapy in a primary prevention trial. It may be possible that the combination of high risk factors such as hyperlipidemia, a positive exercise test and the identification of individuals with elevated clotting factors as reported by Meade, et al, may provide us with a population suitable for a primary prevention anticoagulant trial. At the present time, however, this would seem to be relatively unlikely. It is more likely that platelets, rather than primary clotting factors, are keys to the coronary artery thrombosis. Various approaches to preventing coronary artery thrombosis using antiplatelet aggregating agents will be utilized in the immediate future.

The second group of patients at increased risk are those who have existing clinical coronary heart disease, either myocardial infarction or angina pectoris. Many analytical epidemiological followup studies have determined both the absolute risk of recurrent events and the risk factors.[22] It is now possible to stratify the risk of subsequent disease[23] on the basis of three primary determinants; 1) the degree of left ventricular dysfunction measured either by ejection fraction or symptomatology; 2) the extent of coronary artery disease, both the number and magnitude of the stenosis and the specific arteries involved such as left main disease; and, 3) the prevalence of cardiac arrhythmias either on a standard tracing or by some monitoring technique. Abnormalities of left ventricular function related to the size of the myocardial infarction appear to be the primary determinants of survival after a heart attack. Thus, primary emphasis must be given to reducing the size of the myocardial infarction. Prevention of coronary artery thrombosis and its progression may be the most critical factor in the subsequent prevention of recurrent myocardial infarction and sudden death. Maseri, et al,[3] in a recent paper suggested an important interaction between the white thrombus, spasm, transient and persistent coronary occlusion and the formation of a red thrombus or clot leading to persistent occlusion and extension.

The risk of a subsequent coronary heart disease event among these prevalent patients with clinical coronary artery disease can be further subdivided into various time frames following their initial event. Thus, we can consider the period of hospitalization, the immediate high risk or first six months or so after the event, and the subsequent long-term mortality. The risk factors are clearly different than those for the initial clinical event. Practically all individuals who have clinical coronary artery disease have extensive coronary atherosclerosis. The risk stratification makes it possible to further identify the highest risk groups who may be more amenable to specific interventions. On the other hand, these individuals in the highest stratum of risk may have such extensive disease, especially left ventricular dysfunction, that any therapies short of cardiac replacement or an artificial heart may have minimal benefit.

The clinical trial or experimental epidemiology is probably the most important component of epidemiological studies. The clinical trial depends, as noted, on a good understanding of the biology of the disease, the risk factors, and the populations most likely to be impacted by the intervention to be tested. Clinical trials are rarely successful if the specific etiological hypotheses are not well defined prior to the beginning of the trial. The successful clinical trial depends on an estimation of the proper sample size, effective intervention that will result in a large difference in the modified variable, i.e., anticoagulation, reduction of blood lipid levels or blood pressure, between the treated and control groups, the adherence to protocol by both the treated and control groups an adequate length of followup and objective and unbiased measurements of outcome. The sample size obviously depends on the estimated difference in outcome between the treated and control group. The larger the difference expected the smaller the sample size. Thus, in a clinical trial it is useful to try to identify the highest risk groups that are most likely to develop the disease as the population for the trial. As noted, however, sometimes these high risk groups have such advanced or unusual disease that they are unlikely to benefit from specific intervention.

The previous anticoagulation studies following a myocardial infarction have been discussed numerous times in the literature and were further evaluated as part of an extensive review of secondary prevention after myocardial infarction by May, Eberlein, and Furberg.[24] They noted, as have others, that there was a tendency for anticoagulation therapy to reduce the CHD mortality in each of the five clinical trials that were reviewed, but that in none was the difference between the intervention and control statistically significant. The more detailed review by Chalmers, et al.,[25] concluded that the pooling of all randomized controlled trials gave a mean case-fatality rate of 19.6% for the controls and 15.4% for the anticoagulation group, about a 21% reduction, which by various methods of combining the data from the trials was statistically significant. They noted that five of the six randomized controlled trials reported no effect because the difference favoring anticoagulation was not statistically significant. However, the sample sizes in these negative papers was relatively small and could have easily missed the 21% reduction in the true case-fatality rate. They recommended in 1977 that all patients who present no specific contraindication should receive anticoagulation during hospitalization for infarction. Gifford and Feinstein[26] on the other hand in 1969 reviewing much the same group of papers took a much more sanguine approach to anticoagulation therapy for acute myocardial infarction. They pointed out that many of the trials, even the so-called randomized clinical trials, did not meet their methodological standards that effect the scientific comparability of the treated and controls.

Genton and Turpie[27] in 1983 also reviewed the use of anticoagulation following myocardial infarction. They noted that the rationale for the use of anticoagulation drugs in acute myocardial infarction was to "prevent extension of coronary artery thrombi and therefore decrease mortality by reducing infarct size or preventing reinfarction". They further stated "whether the data from the published trials have established a beneficial effect on mortality in the acute phase remains a matter of controversy".[27] "Perhaps a more important issue relates to the use of anticoagulation therapy in myocardial infarction is the prevention of thromboembolic complications, including systemic embolization from the left ventricular mural thrombi, venous thrombosis and pulmonary embolism".[27] Although it is probable that short-term anticoagulation therapy during hospitalization may be beneficial to reduce these outcomes, it is unlikely that the future place of anticoagulation therapy will depend on the prevention of these outcomes, rather than on the reduction and prevention of the progression of thrombus and extension of the myocardial infarction.

Since the 1982 report on secondary prevention, new therapies have continued to evolve. Thus, anticoagulation therapy must now be considered in relation to other available and proven efficacious treatment in both the short and long-term period after myocardial infarction.[24] This includes the use of antiplatelet aggregating agents,[5] which have clearly been demonstrated as effective in reducing mortality following unstable angina pectoris and probably after myocardial infarction. The use of coronary angioplasty[8] and coronary bypass surgery during the immediate period after a myocardial infarction, treatment with intravenous[28,29] streptokinase and similar therapies.[30] Also the use of beta blockers immediately after a myocardial infarction[31] and in subsequent time periods, the possible value of calcium channel blocking agents, as well as specific antiarrhythmic drugs must be included in the evaluation of the use of anticoagulants.[24] There is also evidence that specific risk factor modification, especially cessation of cigarette smoking and reduction of blood lipids may have a positive effect in reducing the subsequent morbidity and mortality after a myocardial infarction.

It is unlikely and perhaps impossible to do a new anticoagulation trial during the acute or post-hospitalization period after a myocardial infarction without considering the substantial confounding by these other interventions. The modification of the risks of mortality by these other effective agents may make it extremely difficult to identify a specific effect of anticoagulants. On the other hand, prevention of both a new thrombus and an extension of a thrombus is probably the most important factor in the risk of a subsequent event among these patients who already have angina pectoris or myocardial infarction. The test of the potential value of anticoagulants, perhaps as compared to antiplatelet aggregating agents might be a worthwhile investment.

The problems of doing such a well-designed double-blind trial are substantial. Current post-hospital case-fatality is only about 5-6% at most per year and may even be lower. Thus, the sample size for such a trial would have to be substantial; clearly in the thousands. The mortality among the 40-50% low risk individuals, that is those who do not have abnormalities of left ventricular function or frequent cardiac arrhythmias at the time of hospital discharge, may be so low as to make the sample size for such a trial too great.

The availability of new techniques to monitor the effects of anticoagulation and to reduce the likelihood of hemorrhage would enhance our ability to maximize the anticoagulation effect in the intervention as compared to the control group with a minimal loss to protocol because of bleeding and other complications. The endpoints in such a study would also be critical. Few of the secondary prevention trials demonstrate much benefit in terms of the reduction in total mortality. It is unlikely that anticoagulation therapy following a myocardial infarction or angina pectoris could substantially reduce total mortality.

The length of the study would also be of considerable importance. The risk of a recurrent event declines in relationship to the time since the primary heart attack. Thus, a short-term trial might be more feasible, but would certainly require a substantially greater sample size in order to reach the approximate number of events necessary for analysis. Long-term trials will be compromised by the evolution of new therapies over time which will impact on both the treated and control groups, and certainly confound if not destroy the entire study design.

The future of anticoagulation trials may therefore depend first on better methods of measuring new thrombi in the coronary arteries that then could be used as a surrogate measure of potential efficacy as opposed to the current emphasis on clinical cardiac endpoints, such as myocardial infarction, angina pectoris and sudden death.

The role of anticoagulation in both the treatment of the acute myocardial infarction and long-term followup will remain controversial. The key to the role of anticoagulation in myocardial infarction will be the evidence for the reduction in the progression of the coronary thrombus, a decrease in the size of the myocardial infarction and left ventricular dysfunction. The efficacy of anticoagulants versus antiplatelet aggregating agents and various platelet inhibitors, and such agents as streptokinase, must now be considered as part of the approaches to reducing the impact of coronary thrombo-embolic disease.

REFERENCES

1. R. Gorlin, V. Fester and J. A. Ambrose, Anatomic-physiologic links between acute coronary syndromes. (Editorial) Circulation 74:6 (1986).
2. M.J. Davies and A, Thomas, and acute coronary artery lesions in sudden cardiac ischemic death. N Engl J Med 310:1137 (1984).
3. A. Maseri, S. Chierchia and G. Davies, Pathophysiology of coronary occlusion in acute infarction. Circulation 73:233 (1986).
4. J. E. Saffitz, R. C. Fredrickson and W. C. Roberts, Relation of size of transmural acute myocardial infarct to mode of death, interval between infarction and death and frequency coronary arterial thrombosis. Am J Cardiol 57:1249 (1986).
5. L. A. Harker, Clinical trial evaluating platelet-modifying drugs in patients with atherosclerotic cardiovascular disease and thrombosis. Circulation 73:206 (1986).
6. E. R. Eichner, Platelets, carotids, and coronaries: Critique on anti-thrombotic role of antiplatelet agents, exercise, and certain diets. Am J Med 77:513 (1984).
7. T. L. Simon, J. H. Ware and J. M. Stengle, Clinical trials of thrombolytic agents in myocardial infarction. Ann Intern Med 79:712 (1973).
8. G. S. Reeder and R. E. Vlietstra, Coronary angioplasty: 1986. Mod Concepts Cardiovasc Dis 55:49 (1986).
9. T. W. Meade, M. Brozovic, R.R. Chakrabarti, et al., Haemostatic function and ischaemic heart disease: Principal results of the Northwick Park Heart Study. Lancet 2:533 (1986).
10. L. Wilhelmsen, K. Svardsudd, K. Korsan-Bengtsen, et al., Fibrinogen as a risk factor for stroke and myocardial infarction. N Engl J Med 311:501 (1984).
11. G. J. Miller, J. C. Martin, J. Webster, et al., Association between dietary fat intake and plasma factor VII coagulant activity - A predictor of cardiovascular mortality. Atherosclerosis 60:269 (1986).
12. T. W. Meade, D. J. Howarth, Y. Stirling, et al., Fibrinopeptide A and sudden death. Lancet 2:607 (1984).
13. T. W. Meade, R. Chakrabarti, A. P. Haines, et al., Characteristics affecting fibrinolytic activity and plasma fibrinogen concentrations. Br Med J 1:153 (1979).
14. H. L. J. Markowe, M. G. Marmot, M. J. Shipley, et al., Fibrinogen: a possible link between social class and coronary heart disease. Br Med J 291:1312 (1985).
15. C. R. M. Hay, A. P. Durber and R. Saynor, Effect of fish oil on platelet kinetics in patients with ischaemic heart disease. Lancet 1:1269 (1982).
16. L. H. Kuller, J. A. Perper, W. S. Dai, et al., Sudden death and the decline in coronary heart disease mortality. J Chron Dis (1986) (In Press).

17. V. Rissanen, Sudden coronary death and coronary artery disease. Cardiology 64:289 (1979).
18. J. A. Perper, L. H. Kuller and M. Cooper, Arteriosclerosis of coronary arteries in sudden, unexpected deaths. Circulation 52(Suppl 3):27 (1975).
19. J. Stamler, D. Wentworth and J. Neaton. Middle-aged American men at very low risk of coronary death; six-year findings on the 356,222 screenees of the Multiple Risk Factor Intervention Trial (MRFIT). Presented at the X World Congress of Cardiology, Washington, D.C., September (1986).
20. D. J. Gordon, L. G. Ekelund, J. M. Karon, et al., Predictive value of the exercise tolerance test for mortality in North American men: The Lipid Research Clinics Mortality Follow-up Study. Circulation 74:252 (1986).
21. P. M. Rautaharju, R. J. Prineas, W. J. Eifler, et al., Prognostic value of exercise electrocardiogram in men at high risk of future coronary heart disease: Multiple Risk Factor Intervention Trial Experience. J Am Coll Cardiol 8:1 (1986).
22. L. H. Kuller, Natural History of Coronary Heart Disease, in: Heart Disease and Rehabilitation, Second Edition, M. L. Pollock and D. H. Schmidt, eds., John Wiley and Sons, Inc., New York, New York, 1986.
23. The Multicenter Postinfarction Research Group, Risk stratification and survival after myocardial infarction. N Engl J Med 309:331 (1983).
24. G. S. May, K. A. Eberlein, C. D. Furberg, et al., Secondary prevention after myocardial infarction: A review of long-term trials. Prog Cardiovasc Dis 24:331 (1982).
25. T. C. Chalmers, R. J. Matta, H. Smith and A. M. Kunzler, Evidence favoring the use of anticoagulants in the hospital phase of acute myocardial infarction. N Engl J Med 297:1091 (1977).
26. R. H. Gifford and A. R. Feinstein, A criticue of methodology in studies of anticoagulant therapy for acute myocardial infarction. N Engl J Med 280:351 (1969).
27. E. Genton and A. G. G. Turpie, Anticoagulant therapy following acute myocardial infarction: Part II. Antithrombotic therapy in acute myocardial infarction. Mod Concepts Cardiovasc Dis 52:49 (1983).
28. Gruppo Italiano Per Los Studio Della Streptochinasi Nell'Infarto Miocardico (GISSI), Effectiveness of intravenous thrombolytic treatment in acute myocardial infarction. Lancet 1:397 (1986).
29. The I.S.A.M. Study Group, A prospective trial of intravenous strepto-kinase in acute myocardial infarction (I.S.A.M.): Mortality, morbidity, and infarct size at 21 days. N Engl J Med 314:1465 (1986).
30. D. O. Williams, J. Borer, E. Braunwald, et al., Intravenous recombinant tissue-type plasminogen activator in patients with acute myocardial infarction: a report from the NHLBI thrombolysis in myocardial infarction trial. Circulation 73:338 (1986).
31. S. Yusuf, R. Peto, J. Lewis, et al., Beta blockade during and after myocardial infarction: An overview of the randomized trials. Prog Cardiovasc Dis 27:335 (1985).

ANTICOAGULANTS IN ACUTE MYOCARDIAL INFARCTION

Daniel Deykin

Cooperative Studies Program (151-I)
VA Medical Center
Boston, MA

INTRODUCTION

Anticoagulants in the treatment and prevention of acute myocardial infarction were initially advocated for three potential therapeutic benefits: lowering case fatality rate by limitation of infarct size, prevention of recurrent infarction, and reduction of thromboembolic complications.[1] Despite early enthusiasm for their use, anticoagulants are now rarely employed in the in-hospital phase of management of patients with acute myocardial infarction.[2] A recent survey of the Section on Clinical Cardiology of the American College of Chest Physicians[3] revealed that fewer than 10 percent of respondents used warfarin routinely, and 65 percent rarely administered warfarin during hospitalization for acute myocardial infarction. Of those who did use warfarin, there was a clear association with the age of the physician. Only two percent of physicians under the age of 40 used warfarin routinely, whereas 25 percent of physicians over 60 favored its administration. The reasons for the striking repudiation of anticoagulant therapy relate primarily to mistrust of earlier insistence on its benefits, and apprehension over its risks. Nevertheless, recent consensus statements and editorial opinions reemphasize that there is a clear-cut role for anticoagulants in the management of acute myocardial infarction: reduction of the incidence of systemic embolization in those selectively at risk. The purpose of this report is (i) to review the evidence documenting the incidence of systemic embolism, particularly cerebral, following acute myocardial infarction, (ii) to assess the magnitude of the treatment benefit of anticoagulant therapy, (iii) to specify the risks of treatment, (iv) to assess the adequacy of our present state of knowledge: do we need more information, and if we do, can we get it? Recent reviews have been published that include extensive literature citations.[4-7] In the following presentation, I have selected articles that are particularly informative.

The Incidence of Systemic Embolization Following Acute Myocardial Infarction

The incidence of systemic emboli can be estimated from several sources of data: autopsies of patients who die following acute myocardial infarction; enumeration of clinically manifest events in survivors followed prospectively in controlled clinical trials; and documentation of strokes in a study population identified by an associated condition, such as the presence of left ventricular thrombi. It is important to recognize that the assembly of the population under study strongly influences the estimate of embolism rates in that population. Autopsy series yield higher values than other sources not only because documentation of systemic infarcts is more complete than that available in clinical studies, but also because the very nature of the population under study, those who died, culls those from the overall population most likely to have complications. Similarily, a series studied because of the presence of left ventricular thrombi will yield a higher incidence than a study of all patients with acute myocardial infarction in whom patients at low risk for peripheral embolism, such as those with inferior myocardial infarction, dilute the risk of the population with increased risk, those with anterior infarction.

Early reports of autopsies of patients with acute myocardial infarction gathered by retrospective reviews of large numbers of patients demonstrated a striking incidence of mural thrombi (approximately by 45 percent, predominantly left ventricular) and that 7 percent demonstrated associated cerebral emboli.[8,9] Autopsy data derived from the Veterans Administration large scale prospective trial of anticoagulants in the treatment of acute myocardial infarction provide similar data.[10] Of 499 patients randomly assigned to the placebo arm of the trial,[11] 56 died and 31 of these were examined at autopsy. Fifteen (48 percent) had left ventricular thrombi, two (6.5 percent) had cerebral emboli, and 5 (16 percent) had peripheral arterial thromboemboli other than cerebral infarcts.

Data derived from three large prospective clinical trials of anticoagulants in acute myocardial infarction provide well-grounded estimates of the embolic stroke rate following acute myocardial infarction in untreated patients. In the Veterans Administration Cooperative Study,[10] 16 of 499 patients not receiving anticoagulants suffered an embolic stroke (3.2 percent); in the Medical Research Council Trial[11] 18 of 715 patients (2.5 percent) had cerebral emboli, as did 9 of 391 (2.3 percent) in the Bronx Municipal Trial.[12] In the aggregate, 33 of 1605 patients (2.1 percent) suffered an embolic stroke. Information is given about other systemic emboli in the VA and MRC studies: of 1214 patients at risk, 8 (0.7 percent) experienced embolism to other systemic arteries. Therefore, the total systemic (non-pulmonary) arterial embolic burden is approximately 3 percent of all patients who experience acute myocardial infarction.

It is now clear that the risk of systemic embolism is not uniformly distributed in patients with acute myocardial infarction, but is selectively experienced by those with anterior myocardial infarctions and left ventricular mural thrombi. A major prospective study designed to identify a population at high risk for stroke following myocardial infarction demonstrated that stroke occurred exclusively in patients with large infarcts, documented by peak creatine kinase in excess of 1160 international units/liter.[13] The introduction of accurate, non-invasive techniques, particularly two-dimensional echocardiography, has clarified the population at greatest risk.[14,15] Asinger and associates[16] examined the incidence of left ventricular thrombi in 70 patients with acute myocardial infarction followed prospectively with serial echocardiograms. Thirty-five had inferior wall infarctions; none of these developed left ventricular mural thrombi. Of the 35 with anterior-wall infarction, 26 showed akinesis or dyskinesis on echocardiography. Of these, 12 developed left ventricular thrombi. Therefore, of all patients in the series, 17 percent had left ventricular thrombi. Of patients with anterior wall infarcts, 34 percent had mural thrombi, and of those with apical wall motion abnormalities, almost half had left ventricular thrombi.

Two subsequent prospective series have substantiated the incidence of left ventricular thrombi detected by serial echocardiographs. Weinreich and associates[17] studied 261 patients with acute transmural myocardial infarction. Mural thrombi were found in 46 (18 percent). Forty-four occurred in 130 patients with anterior wall infarction (34 percent), but only 2 were found in the 131 patients with inferior myocardial infarction. In this series, all patients with left ventricular thrombi had apical wall motion abnormalities. Johannessen and colleagues[18] followed 90 consecutive patients with acute transmural myocardial infarction. Of these, 15 (17 percent) developed left ventricular thrombi. These were found exclusively in the 53 patients with anterior wall infarcts (28 percent of anterior infarcts).

Two series of patients assembled by the presence of anterior wall myocardial infarction also permit estimates of the frequency of left ventricular mural thrombi following acute myocardial infarction. Keating and associates[19] reported 53 such patients followed with serial echocardiographs. All had apical wall motion abnormalities, and 17 (32 percent) had left ventricular thrombi. Nordrehaug and colleagues[20] also studied 53 patients with anterior myocardial infarction in a prospective trial of the efficacy of anticoagulants in preventing systemic emboli. Of the 21 patients receiving placebo, 7 (33 percent) developed left ventricular thrombi.

From these studies a remarkably consistent estimate of the incidence of left ventricular thrombi in acute myocardial infarction may be determined. Of all patients experiencing acute transmural myocardial infarction, approximately half will develop anterior myocardial infarctions. Left ventricular thrombi will develop in approximately 30 percent of those with anterior myocardial infarction (15 percent of the total population at risk), exclusively in areas of abnormal wall motion.

These reports also buttress the estimate of the frequency of systemic embolization derived from the early large-scale prospective trials of anticoagulants in myocardial infarction. Of the 46 patients reported who had anterior myocardial infarcts plus left ventricular thrombi who were not treated with anticoagulants, 14 (30 percent) developed systemic emboli. Assuming that left ventricular thrombi develop in 30 percent of all patients with anterior wall infarcts and that half of all patients with myocardial infarctions have anterior infarctions, then 30 percent (emboli) X 30 percent (anterior infarcts) X 50 percent (all infarcts) yields an estimate 4.5 percent of all patients with acute myocardial infarction will develop systemic embolization.

One study stands in contrast to the previous, consistent estimates. Spirito and associates[21] followed 50 patients with anterior wall myocardial infarction, using echocardiographs obtained within the first 24 hours of infarction and serially thereafter. Twenty-four patients (41 percent) developed left ventricular thrombi, and 11 of these were found in the first 24 hours. Of these patients with early left ventricular thrombi, 10 (91 percent) died during the hospitalization. Of the 13 patients who developed left ventricular thrombi after the first 48 hours, 1 experienced systemic embolic phenomena. The authors concluded that their study showed a low incidence of embolism in contrast to previous studies, but in fact their study demonstrates that in making comparisons among studies, it is crucial to examine first how the study populations were assembled. In the prior reports the first echocardiographs were performed at the earliest on the third day following the onset of infarction. Therefore, those patients with thrombi developing on the first day, associated with an extremely high mortality, would have been excluded from the studies.

Determinants of Embolization

From the forgoing discussion three determinants of systemic embolization are readily definable: anterior wall infarction, apical wall motion abnormalities, and left ventricular mural thrombi. Several authors have suggested that certain morphologic characteristics of the left ventricular mural thrombi are associated with a particularly high embolic potential.[22-24] Mobile thrombi, particularly those that are pedunculated and that protrude into the left ventricular cavity, are thought to have a greater embolic potential than those that are sessile and do not protrude. The data from which these conclusions are drawn reflect either a mixed population of patients with acute myocardial infarction combined with those with left ventricular aneurysms or patients with acute myocardial infarction receiving anticoagulants. In Weinreich's study,[17] 7 of the 18 patients with anterior myocardial infarction and left ventricular thrombi, not receiving anticoagulants, experienced peripheral emboli. The mural thrombi in 6 were sessile and non-pedunculated. It seems reasonable to infer that pedunculated mobile thrombi might be more prone to embolize than flat thrombi, but since the morphology of thrombi changes rapidly, and since there are insufficient data to state that sessile thrombi do not embolize, the morphologic appearance of a thrombus does not constitute a reason for excluding anticoagulant therapy, the critical decision to be made.

Although patients with more severe wall motion abnormalities are more at risk for mural thrombi to form than those with lesser degree of dysfunction, ejection fraction measurements do not predict which patients are selectively at risk. Weinreich[17] found that the mean ejection fraction of 29 patients with anterior wall infarcts and left mural thrombi was 37 percent, but the values ranged from 10 to 56 percent. The interval between onset of infarction and risk of embolization are inversely related. Emboli occur preferentially within the first month following infarction, with a decremental frequency therafter. In Weinreich's study[17] 7 of 17 patients with anterior infarction and with left ventricular thrombi not receiving anticoagulants had systemic emboli. Four occurred in the first week following infarction. The others occurred at 6,12, and 14 weeks after infarction. In Keating's report[19] of 6 patients who experienced emboli, 3 occurred in the first two weeks; the remaining 3 occurred 3-12 weeks later.

Efficacy of Anticoagulant Therapy

The three large prospective, randomized clinical trials of anticoagulant therapy in acute myocardial infarction[10-12] provide robust estimates of the efficacy of anticoagulants in reducing the incidence of stroke following myocardial infarction. Recent reviews summarize these studies in detail.[2-7] In the Veterans Administration Cooperative Trial,[10] the stroke rate was reduced from 3.2 percent in the control group to 0.8 percent in the treated group, a highly significant result that indicated a 75 percent treatment effect (95 percent confidence limits: 21 to 100 percent). The Medical Research Council Trial[11] reported that anticoagulants reduced the stroke rate from 2.5 percent in the control patients to 1.1 percent in the treated patients, a treatment effect of 55 percent (95 percent confidence limits: 0.5 to 100 percent). In the Bronx Municipal Trial[12] the effect of anticoagulants was to lower the stroke rate from 2.3 to 1.7 percent (95 percent confidence limits: -52 to 100 percent).

Estimates of the efficacy of anticoagulants are also available from a small number of studies in which patients were classified by the

234

presence or absence of left ventricular mural thrombi. Keating and associates[19] reported data on 53 consecutive patients with anterior myocardial infarction, all of whom were followed with two-dimensional echocardiography. Seventeen patients had mural thrombi. Of these, 10 received anticoagulants and 7 did not, at the discretion of their physicians. Remarkably, 6 of the 7 patients not receiving anticoagulants developed systemic emboli. Weinreich and colleagues[17] followed 261 consecutive patients with acute transmural myocardial infarction admitted to a single institution. Forty six developed left ventricular thrombi (44 from 130 with anterior myocardial infarcts, 2 from 131 with inferior infarcts). They were able to follow the clinical course of 43 of these patients. Twenty-five patients received anticoagulants at the discretion of their physicians; eighteen did not. Of the 25 treated patients, none developed clinically evident systemic emboli, but of the 18 patients not receiving anticoagulants, 7 experienced embolic events: 6 cerebral emboli and one to the leg (one patient with a cerebral embolus also sustained a separate leg embolus). In a small controlled prospective trial, Nordrehaug and associates[20] randomized 53 patients with suspected acute anterior wall myocardial infarction to receive either full-dose heparin followed by warfarin (26 patients) or matching placebo (27 patients). The trial was conducted for only the first 10 days after infarction. In the control group, 2 patients did not have myocardial infarctions and 2 died before echocardiographs were performed. Of the 21 survivors, 7 had mural thrombi and 1 developed a systemic embolus. Of the 26 patients receiving anticoagulants, 2 died before echocardiographic examination. Of the 24 survivors, none developed mural thrombi, and none experienced a systemic embolus.

Several papers describe patients with anterior myocardial infarction, echocardiographic documentation of left ventricular thrombi, and anticoagulant treatment, but do not yield estimates of efficacy of treatment. Asinger[16] described 35 patients with anterior wall infarcts of whom 12 developed left ventricular mural thrombi. Of those 2 died and 1 was lost to follow up. Two of the remaining 9 patients did not receive anticoagulants and 7 did. No emboli occurred in either group. Johannessen and colleagues[18] describe 53 patients with anterior wall infarction in whom echocardiographs were first performed on the fifth day following the infarction and serially thereafter. Fifteen patients developed left ventricular thrombi and were placed on anticoagulants thereafter. Five patients sustained systemic emboli: 1 on day 4, before the echocardiograph was performed, 1 before anticoagulant therapy reached effective levels, and 3 occurred while the patients were at full therapeutic levels. Visser and associates[25] described 65 patients with anterior wall infarction. All were placed on warfarin therapy from the day of admission. Eighteen patients developed left ventricular thrombi, but none suffered a systemic embolus during the ensuing 4 months. Although these studies do not allow an estimate of anticoagulant efficacy, they suggest that the earlier the treatment is started, the more effective it is likely to be. In addition, beginning therapy with oral anticoagulation alone may not provide maximum protection.

A distinction should be made between the effectiveness of anticoagulants in preventing systemic emboli and their effectiveness in preventing the formation or influencing the rate of resolution of left ventricular thrombi. While some studies show that early administration of anticoagulants prevent the formation of mural thrombi, others do not. Also, there is no agreement on whether anticoagulant therapy hastens resolution of thrombi. It is clear, however, that anticoagulants can exert a protective effect against systemic emboli without a measurable effect on the morphology of the thrombi. Again Weinreich's study[17] produces useful data. Twenty-nine of 43 patients survived more than 6 months. Repeated echocardiography showed persistent mural thrombi in 11 of 19 given anticoagulants and in 6 of 10 patients not given anticoagulants.

Table I presents a reasonable estimate of the frequency of clinical outcomes following myocardial infarction, based on available data.

Table 1. Frequences in Acute Myocardial Infarction

Outcome	Frequency
Total MI's	1000
Anterior MI	500
Wall dyskinesia	300
Left Ventricular Mural Thrombi[a]	150
Cerebral Emboli	
Without anticoagulants	40
With anticoagulants[b]	16
Fatal Bleeds[c]	0

[a]   Detected by 2-dimensional echocardiography beginning on third day post-infarction.
[b]   Assuming a 60 percent treatment effect. Anticoagulation: full dose heparin begun on admission, followed by oral anticoagulants for four months.
[c]   There is less than a 5 percent chance that the true rate of fatal hemorrhage would exceed 0.15 percent (1.5/1000).

The efficacy of anticoagulants will be determined not only by the therapeutic effect of the drugs, but also by the inclusion/exclusion criteria used to count the outcomes. Since maximum therapeutic effect requires that the anticoagulants be given at admission, if patients presenting with profound shock or intractable arrythmias are treated and counted, then the benefit of treatment will be apparently lessened, since those patients will succumb before any protective effect of anticoagulants could be expected. If they are either not treated or excluded from counting later, then the apparent benefit of anticoagulants will be enhanced, but the exclusion criteria need to be explicitly stated.

The Hemorrhagic Risk of Anticoagulant Therapy

The risk for bleeding caused by anticoagulant therapy in the short term treatment of patients with myocardial infarctions reported in the three major prospective studies was appreciable. In the Bronx Municipal Study,[12] 12.8 percent of treated patients experienced hemorrhagic complications, compared to 5.3 percent of controls. In the VA Cooperative Study[10] 2.6 percent of treated patients bled in contrast to 1.2 percent of controls. In the Medical Research Council Trial,[11] 5.0 percent of treated patients bled; 1.2 percent of controls bled. It is important to distinguish minor bleeding from major or fatal hemorrhage. In all three studies no fatal hemorragic complications and no other major hemorrhagic complications were reported. Therefore, the protective benefit of anticoagulants was accomplished at a clear cost of increased minor bleeding, but with no major hemmorhagic sequellae.

The frequency of bleeding in patients reflects a combination of patient selection (to exclude known risk factors that warrant exclusion), duration of therapy, adequacy of laboratory monitoring and intensity of therapy. Clearly as the duration of therapy increases, the risk of bleeding also increases. In short term experiments even high intensity of therapy may not be associated with increased risk of bleeding. Nordrehaug and associates[20] gave sufficient warfarin to maintain the Thrombotest assay between 5 to 10 percent of control (equivalent to an International Normalized Ratio between 5 to 2.5) to 26 patients until the 10th day of hospital admission for anterior myocardial infarction. None experienced any bleeding episodes, even though the intensity of treatment was high. After reviewing the existing literature, Hirsh, Poller and I[26] have recently recommended that if prophylactic anticoagulants are to be used to prevent systemic embolization following acute myocardial infarction, the therapeutic range should be a standard International Ratio of 2.0 - 3.0, equivalent to a rabbit brain thromboplastin ratio of 1.3 - 1.5.

Do we need more information?

Reviewing the present state of the use of oral anticoagulants in preventing systemic embolization following acute myocardial infarction presents an interesting exercise in clinical epistemology. How are therapeutic decisions made? On what basis is existing information accepted or rejected? Convincing data that support the use of anticoagulants have been published and not refuted. The risk of major bleeding is very small, yet physicians, particularly those trained within the past two decades, have rejected their use. Now that elegant non-invasive techniques are available to demonstrate the antemortem presence of left ventricular thrombi, a series of small-scale studies have reemphasized the value of anticoagulants. Recognizing the limits of their studies, authors have called for another round of large-scale trials. Thus: Keating et al.,[19] "Future studies may document the initiation of thrombus formation and show prophylactic anticoagulation in the high-risk patient to be instrumental in preventing thrombus formation altogether." Weinreich et al[17] state: "A prospective, randomized study is needed to answer definitively whether anticoagulation treatment prevents embolic complications in patients with acute myocardial infarction who develop left ventricular thrombi." Asinger and associates[16] comment, "Patients at high risk for thrombus formation can be identified early, and therapeutic intervention can be identified before left-ventricular thrombi develops. Such intervention could conceivably reduce the frequency of left-ventricular thrombi during infarction and could thus reduce the number of patients at risk for peripheral embolization... Prospective studies with randomized therapeutic anticoagulation reserved for patients with severe apical wall motion abnormalities identified with initial echocardiographic studies are needed for a further evaluation of these speculations." These calls for further studies are reinforced in recent reviews and editorials.[2-7, 27-29]

In contrast, based on their assessment of available data, Chesebro and associates[5] have made specific recommendations: "Patients at no increased bleeding risk who have suspected or definite myocardial infarction, that is anterior or involving the apex, should be started on full-dose heparin immediately upon admission to the hospital because of the demonstrated benefit in reducing the incidence of left ventricular mural thrombus and peripheral emboli.... Patients with large anterior transmural infarctions... should be placed on therapy with warfarin (prolonging the prothrombin time to 1.5 - 2.5 times the normal control) for one to three months, at which time it can be discontinued unless there is evidence of heart failure or cardiomyopathy due to coronary artery disease."

Do we need new large-scale trials? We must ask: i) What new information would they yield? ii) Would they in fact change clinical practice? iii) Can they be accomplished at this time?

All the present recommendations for the use of anticoagulants to prevent systemic embolization following myocardial infarction ultimately rest on the existing large-scale trials conducted 15 to 20 years ago. Have recent changes in therapy substantially decreased the risk of embolization? The answers are not clear. Nordrehaug, et al,[20] in discussing the results of the Timolol[30] trial indicated that in that trial, in which patients were not given anticoagulants, 19 of 753 patients (2.5 percent) of patients with anterior wall infarcts had a stroke, implying that treatment with a beta-blocker, though clearly beneficial in reducing mortality and re-infarction did not decrease the risk of stroke, but the potential additional benefits or risks of anticoagulants and beta-blockers have not been prospectively tested.

The wide-spread use of fibrinolytic agents in the early hours of evolving myocardial infarction might be expected to lyse or prevent the formation of mural thrombi. Apparently not. Sharma and associates[31] describe 30 patients with acute transmural infarction given intracoronary streptokinase (within 8 hours of the onset of symptoms) followed by full-dose heparin for 10 days. Echocardiographs were performed within the first 24 hours and at 10 days. None of the 19 patients with inferior infarctions developed left ventricular thrombi during the study. Three of the 11 patients with anterior myocardial infarctions developed left ventricular thrombi within the first 24 hours, and they persisted until the 10th day. Three of the remaining 8 patients developed mural thrombi between the first and 10th day. Therefore, a total of 6 of 11 patients with anterior myocardial infarction developed left ventricular thrombi despite intracoronary streptokinase and full-dose heparin. In a preliminary report,[32] a subset of patients in the Thrombolysis in Myocardial Infarction (I) trial was described. The incidence of left ventricular thrombi in patients receiving either streptokinase or recombinant tissue plasminogen activator did not differ from that seen in a concomitant group of patients with acute myocardial infarction not receiving fibrinolytic therapy. In contrast, Eigler and colleagues[33] reported a series of 22 patients with acute myocardial infarction of whom 12 presented within 3 hours after the onset of symptoms, and therefore, received intravenous streptokinase. Ten presented later than 3 hours (mean 5.9 range 3 to 14) and who therefore, did not. Of those receiving streptokinase 1 developed left ventricular thrombi in contrast to 7 of 10 who did not receive thrombolytic. On balance, currently available evidence does not suggest that routine use of thrombolytic agents in the near future will obviate the development of left ventricular thrombi in patients with extensive anterior wall damage.

The patient population to be studied in any putative new clinical trials might differ from the previous cohorts in that they may have received fibrinolytic therapy, but the basic question posed by the trials would be the same: Can early, routine administration of anticoagulant therapy prevent systemic emboli in those at risk? The definition of those at risk would be more refined by the advent of echocardiography, but the screening process would be more complex. All patients with transmural myocardial infarction would first be sorted into those with inferior and anterior myocardial infarctions. The decision to anticoagulate would have to precede the determination of left ventricular thrombi by echocardiography, since the determination of whether or not anticoagulants would prevent left ventricular thrombus formation would be one of the main treatment goals. The number of patients that would have to be screened is formidable. If we assume that all emboli arise from anterior myocardial infarctions, then a reasonable estimate of the occurence of peripheral emboli would be 8/1000 patients with anterior myocardial infarction (selected from a larger population of all patients with myocardial infarction). Further assuming a treatment efficacy of 60 percent, an alpha error estimate of 0.05 (two-tailed) and a power of 90 percent, (or beta error estimate of 10 percent) approximately 400 patients in each of the treatment arms would be needed. Allowing for a minimum of 25 percent drop-outs, a total of 1000 patients with anterior myocardial infarction would be needed for an individual trial. This would necessitate screening at least 2000-3000 patients with acute myocardial infarction.

We must ask whether a new trial, if positive, would change clinical practice. It is difficult to imagine that such a trial would substantially enhance the estimate of anticoagulant efficacy, nor would it demonstrate a lower incidence of bleeding than that already known. What a trial could accomplish is either to redocument the benefit of anticoagulants in the present era of more complex treatment of myocardial infarction or to discount their utility. The question would be directly aimed at systemic embolization, not at over-all mortality, avoiding the anti-anticoagulant bias engendered by that controversey.[2] Whether or not a positive outcome would change practice cannot be predicted in advance.

The possibility that the presently occurring morbidity from peri-infarction emboli, now constituting 15 percent of all embolic strokes,[34] may yet be substantially reduced, makes the conduct of a new trial potentially attractive.

We come to a final question: Can we in fact conduct a trial of anticoagulants in the present therapeutic climate? The advocacy of competing therapies imposes real constraints. Aspirin prophylaxis against myocardial infarction has been endorsed in the lay press by government officials. Protocols for coronary artery by-pass graft surgery, percutaneous transluminal coronary angioplasty, and for fibrinolytic therapy call for routine use of aspirin. Since it is unwise to give full-dose anticoagulants to patients receiving aspirin,[35] these protocols are incompatible with anticoagulant therapy trials. Excluding patients on these protocols, however, seriously compromises the availability of patients for a new anticoagulant trial. Furthermore, since other modes of therapy including vasodilators, angiotensin-converting enzyme inhibitions and antiarrhythmic agents are also being studied in patients with acute myocardial infarction, we should acknowledge that there is, ultimately, a limit to the number of trials to which patients with acute myocardial infarctions may be subjected.

CONCLUSION

Most clinicians under the age of 60 have abandoned a mode of therapy that has been demonstrated to be effective and relatively safe. New, non-invasive diagnostic techniques that depict the presence of left mural thrombi in patients with acute myocardial infarction have rekindled enthusiasm for anticoagulants, leading to calls for new clinical trials. Whether or not new clinical trials will change practice, or whether or not they can be undertaken in an environment of competing therapeutic strategies is uncertain. Since the incidence of peri-infarction cerebral embolization remains substantial, the effect needed to undertake a reassessment of the utility of anticoagulants seems clearly warranted.

ACKNOWLEDGEMENT

This work was supported by the Medical Research Service of the Veterans Administration.

REFERENCES

1. I. S. Wright, C. D. Marple, and D. F. Beck, Report of the committee for the evaluation of anticoagulants in the treatment of coronary thrombosis with myocardial infarction, Am. Heart J. 36:801 (1948).
2. J. R. A. Mitchell, Anticoagulants in coronary heart disease - retrospect and prospect, Lancet 1:257 (1981).
3. J. E. Dalen, R. J. Goldberg, J. M. Gore, and J. Struckus, Therapeutic interventions in acute myocardial infarction. Survey of the ACCP Section on Clinical Cardiology, Chest 86:257 (1984).
4. R. J. Goldberg, J. M. Gore, and J. E. Dalen. The role of anticoagulant therapy in acute myocardial infarction, Am. Heart J. 108:1387 (1984).
5. J. H. Chesebro, M. Ezekowitz, L. Badimon, and V. Fuster, Intracardiac thrombi and systemic thromboembolism: detection, incidence, and treatment, Ann. Rev. Med. 36:579 (1985).
6. L. Resnekov, J. Chediak, J. Hirsh, and D. Lewis, Antithrombotic agents in coronary artery disease, Chest 89 (supplement 2):54S (1986)
7. R. S. Meltzer, C. A. Visser, and V. Fuster, Intracardiac thrombi and systemic embolization, Ann. Int. Med. 104:689 (1986).
8. W. B. Bean, Infarction of the heart. III. Clinical course and morphological findings, Ann. Int. Med. 12:71 (1938).
9. H. K. Hellerstein, and J. W. Martin, Incidence of thrombo-embolic lesions accompanying myocardial infarction, Am. Heart J. 33:443 (1947).
10. Anticoagulants in acute myocardial infarction: results of a cooperative clinical trial, JAMA 225:724 (1973).
11. Assessment of short-term anticoagulant administration after cardiac infarction. Report of the working party on anticoagulant therapy in coronary thrombosis to the Medical Research Council, Br. Med. J. 1:335 (1969).
12. A. Drapkin and C. Merskey, Anticoagulant therapy after acute myocardial infarction. Relation of therapeutic benefit to patient's age sex, and severity of infarction, JAMA 222:541 (1972).
13. P. L. Thompson and J. S. Robinson, Stroke after acute myocardial infarction: relation to infarct size, Br. Med. J. 2:457 (1978).
14. A. N. DeMaria, W. Bommer, A. Neumann, T. Grehl, L. Weinart, S. DeNardo, E. A. Amsterdam and D. T. Mason, Left ventricular thrombi identified by cross-sectional echocardiography, Ann. Int. Med. 90:14 (1979).
15. R. W. Asinger, F. L. Mikell, B. Sharma, and M. Hodges, Observations on detecting left ventricular thrombus with two dimensional echocardiography: emphasis on avoidance of false positive diagnoses, Am. J. Cardiol. 47:145 (1981).
16. R. W. Asinger, F. L. Mikell, J. Elsperger, and M. Hodges, Incidence of left ventricular thrombosis after acute transmural myocardial infarction, N. Engl. J. Med. 305:297 (1981).
17. D. J. Weinreich, J. F. Burke and F. J. Pauletto, Left ventricular mural thrombi complicating acute myocardial infarction. Long term follow up with serial echocardiographym, Ann. Int. Med. 100:789 (1984).
18. K. A. Johannessen, J. E. Nordrehaug, and G. von der Lippe, Left ventricular thrombosis and cerebrovascular accident in acute myocardial infarction, Br. Heart J. 51:557 (1984).
19. E. C. Keating, S. A. Gross, R. A. Schlamowitz, J. Glassman, J. H. Mazur, W. A. Pitt and D. Miller, Mural thrombi in myocardial infarctions. Prospective evaluation by two-dimensional echocardiography, Am. J. Med. 74:989 (1983).

20. J. E. Nordrehaug, K.-A. Johannessen, and G. von der Lippe, Usefulness of high-dose anticoagulants in preventing left ventricular thrombus in acute myocardial infarction, Am. J. Cardiol. 55:1491 (1985).

21. P. Spirito, P. Bellotti, F. Chiarella, S. Domenicucci, A. Sementa, and C. Vecchio, Prognostic significance and natural history of left ventricular thrombi in patients with acute anterior myocardial infarction: a two-dimensional echocardiographic study, Circ. 72:774 (1985).

22. H. S. Cabin and W. C. Roberts, Left ventricular aneurysm, intraaneurysmal thrombus and systemic embolus in coronary heart disease, Chest 77:586 (1980).

23. R. S. Meltzer, C. A. Visser, G. Kan, and J. Roelandt, Two-dimensional echocardiographic appearance of left ventricular thrombi with systemic emboli after myocardial infarction, Am. J. Cardiol. 53:1511 (1984).

24. J. M. Haugland, R. W. Asinger, F. L. Mikell, J. Elsperger, M. Hodges, Embolic potential of left ventricular thrombi detected by two-dimensional echocardiography, Circ. 70:588 (1984).

25. C. A. Visser, G. Kan, R. S. Meltzer, K. I. Lie, and D. Durrer. Long-term follow-up of left ventricular thrombus after acute myocardial infarction. A two-dimensional echocardiographic study in 96 patients, Chest 86:532 (1984).

26. J. Hirsh, D. Deykin, and L. Poller, "Therapeutic range" for oral anticoagulant therapy, Chest 89(Supplement 2):11S (1986).

27. J. V. Nixon, Left ventricular mural thrombus, Arch. Int. Med. 143:1567 (1983).

28. M. D. Ezekowitz, Acute infarction, left ventricular thrombus and systemic embolization: an approach to management, JACC 5:1281 (1985).

29. E. L. Kinney, The significance of left ventricular thrombi in patients with coronary heart disease: A retrospective analysis of pooled data, Am. Heart J. 109:191 (1985)

30. Norwegian Multicenter Group, Timolol-induced reduction in mortality and reinfarction in patients surviving acute myocardial infarction, N. Engl. J. Med. 304:801 (1981).

31. B. Sharma, A. Carvalho, R. Wyeth, and J. A. Franciosa, Left ventricular thrombi diagnosed by echocardiography in patients with acute myocardial infarction treated with intracoronary streptokinase followed by intravenous heparin, Am. J. Cardiol. 56:422 (1985).

32. J. Paraskos, Personal communication.

33. N. Eigler, G. Maurer, and P. K. Shah, Effect of early systemic thrombolytic therapy on left ventricular mural thrombus formation in acute anterior myocardial infarction, Am J. Cardiol. 54:261 (1984).

34. D. G. Sherman, M. L. Dyken, M. Fisher, M. J. G. Harrison, and R. G. Hart. Cerebral embolism, Chest 89(supplement 2):82S (1986).

35. J. H. Chesebro, V. Fuster, L. R. Elveback, D. C. McGoon, J.R. Pluth, F. J. Puga, R. B. Wallace, G. K. Danielson, T. A. Orszulak, J. M. Pehler, and H. V. Schaff. Trial of combined warfarin plus dipyridamole or aspirin therapy in prosthetic heart valve replacement: danger of aspirin compared with dipyridamole, Am. J. Cardiol. 51:1537 (1983).

LONG—TERM ANTICOAGULANT TREATMENT AFTER ACUTE MYOCARDIAL INFARCTION

A.W. Broekmans and E.A. Loeliger

Department of Hematology, University Hospital Leiden and
Leiden Thrombosis Centre, the Netherlands

INTRODUCTION

The results of the Dutch Sixty Plus Reinfarction Study revived the discussion on the effectiveness of long-term oral anticoagulation after myocardial infarction (1,2). This study showed that adequately maintained and sufficiently intensive oral anticoagualtion has a beneficical effect especially on the rate of fatal and nonfatal reinfarction, but also on mortality (1).

The study was reported in an era in which clinicians again were convinced that myocardial infarction is the result of thrombosis of an athero-sclerotic deformed coronary artery, hence susceptible to drugs which either dissolve a thrombus or prevent thrombosis (3). However, reports over the last 15 years have repeatedly questioned the effectiveness of oral anti-coagulants and have brought the use of oral anticoagulants in dis-repute (4-7).

Careful consideration of the studies on oral anticoagulants disclosed that insufficient anticoagulant control must be considered the main reason for anticoagulant failure (8). The lack of standardization of the pro-thrombin time resulted in studies either demonstrating no beneficial effect on recurrent myocardial infarction due to underanticoagulation or a favorable effect, however, at the cost of unacceptable high rates of bleeding complications due to overanticoagulation.

In this review we like to discuss the value of oral anticoagulant treatment in the secondary prevention of myocardial infarction. The intensity of treatment applied will be used as a guideline to assess the studies of long-term treatment in patients surviving myocardial infarction. The beneficial effects of adequately maintained oral anticoagulation will be compared with the bleeding risk associated with long-term treatment. Finally, it will be hopefully clear that oral anticoagulant therapy is not just prescribing a drug, but requires an organizational framework to fulfill the need for patient education, laboratory testing, and dosage regulation.

STANDARDIZATION OF THE PROTHROMBIN TIME IN ORAL ANTICOAGULANT CONTROL

The interpretation of clinical trials on the effect of oral antico-

Table 1 Equivalents of therapeutic range in percentages of activity
according to Quick for different thromboplastins

THROMBOPLASTIN	PERCENTAGE
Thromborel Behring	15 – 25
Ca-Thromboplastin Boehringer	25 – 35
Hepato Quick Boehringer	11 – 20
Thromboplastin-C Dade	23 – 34
Thromboplastin FS Dade	19 – 30
Diaplastin Diamed	25 – 36
Bacto-Thromboplastin Difco	15 – 25
Thrombokinase Geigy	16 – 29
Simplastin Automated Gödecke	20 – 31
Simplastin Gödecke	23 – 36
Simplastin General Diagnostics	23 – 35
Thromboplastin calcique Mérieux	26 – 37
Thrombotest Nyegaard	5 – 10
Ortho Brain Thromboplastin	20 – 29
Ca-Thromboplastin Roche	23 – 36
Neoplastine Stago	25 – 35
La Technique Biologique	18 – 28
Menschenhirnkinase	15 – 25

agulants have been hampered by the lack of standardization of the prothrombin time (8). It took a series of multicentre studies and the cooperation with the International Committee for Standardization in Haematology and the European Community Bureau of Reference to finally reach
international agreement on how to report the prothrombin time in oral
anticoagulant control. The details will be discussed by Dr. L. Poller. In
summary, the common term for the prothrombin time as measured in a patient
on long-term oral anticoagulation and normalized according to the thromboplastin calibration principle is the International Normalized Ratio
(INR) (9). The INR gives the prolongation factor of the prothrombin time as
if it had been determined with the primary International (WHO) Reference
Thromboplastin 67/40, a human brain thromboplastin. Table 1 shows, for the
majority of commercially available thromboplastins, the percentages activity according to Quick that are equivalent to 2.8-4.8 INR, the range
proven to be effective in the Sixty Plus Reinfarction Study (1).

In this context it is hardly a surprise why the often quoted study of
the Medical Research Council on short-term oral anticoagulation in patients
with acute myocardial infarction did not demonstrate significant differences between the two groups with regard to hospital mortality or myocardial
reinfarction (4). The intensity of oral anticoagulant treatment applied in
that study was 10% to 20% Thrombotest, equivalent to an INR of 2.0 to 2.8,
which reflects only mild anticoagulation (10). Recently this range was
recommended for prophylaxis of venous thrombosis(11), but it is certainly
insufficient for the prevention of arterial thrombosis. On the other hand,
a 2.5 fold prolongation of the prothrombin time as measured with the rabbit
thromboplastin most commonly used in the USA was until recently widely
recommended as upper limit of prolongation, and represents gross overanticoagulation, i.e. 10.0 INR (12).

Recently, the British Society of Hematology recommended a therapeutic
range of 3.0 to 4.5 INR for patients suffering from cardiac and arterial
thrombosis (13), almost identical to that commonly applied in the Netherlands. In other European countries consensus was reached for the same range
of INR (14).

The first study to demonstrate that intensive oral anticoagulation is needed to prevent myocardial reinfarction was the Sixty Plus Reinfarction Study (1). In six thrombosis centres, ambulant patients older than 60 years of age on anticoagulant therapy ever since their first transmural myocardial infarction, but for at least six months, were eligible for participation. Patients with bleeding problems, therapy-resistant hypertension, previous thromboembolism, atrial fibrillation, neoplastic disease, mental ilness, and patients who needed cardiac surgery were excluded.

A group of 439 patients continued oral anticoagulant therapy and another 439 received placebo. The average age of the patients was 67.6 years. The mean interval since the initial myocardial infarction was 6 years. The average follow-up was 1.5 year. The desired range for anticoagulant therapy was 5%-10% Thrombotest (2.8-4.8 INR) , which was subsequently achieved in about 70% of all prothrombin time determinations.

When analyzed for total mortality on an intention-to-treat basis there was no significant difference in outcome between the groups (table 2). During treatment, however, the difference in mortality was significant. This difference resulted from an increase in fatal myocardial infarction in the placebo-group (table 3). No significant differences were noted in mortality due to sudden death and intracranial events. No death occurred due to extracranial hemorrhage. The survival curves showed a steadily widening gap between the two groups indicating that the efficacy of anticoagulant therapy was present throughout the observation period (fig. 1). There was an unequivocal and dramatic reduction in the incidence of both fatal and nonfatal myocardial infarction in the patients treated with oral anticoagulants (table 3). This difference between the two groups remained significant, even when assessed according to intention-to-treat. The

Table 2   Sixty Plus Reinfarction Study:
           distribution of deaths between the groups

	Placebo (N=439)	Anticoagulated (N=439)	p
Intention-to-treat	69	51	0.071
Efficacy (protocol adherents)	49	28	0.017

Table 3   Sixty Plus Reinfarction Study:
           distribution of recurrent myocardial infarction
           (fatal myocardial infarction in parentheses) between the groups

	Placebo (N=439)	Anticoagulated (N=439)	p
Intention-to-treat	64 (27)	29 (11*)	0.0005
Efficacy (protocol adherents)	58 (24)	20 (4)	0.0001

* It has to be pointed out here that many of the protocol deviants suffered an increased thrombosis risk due to suspension of oral anticoagulation.

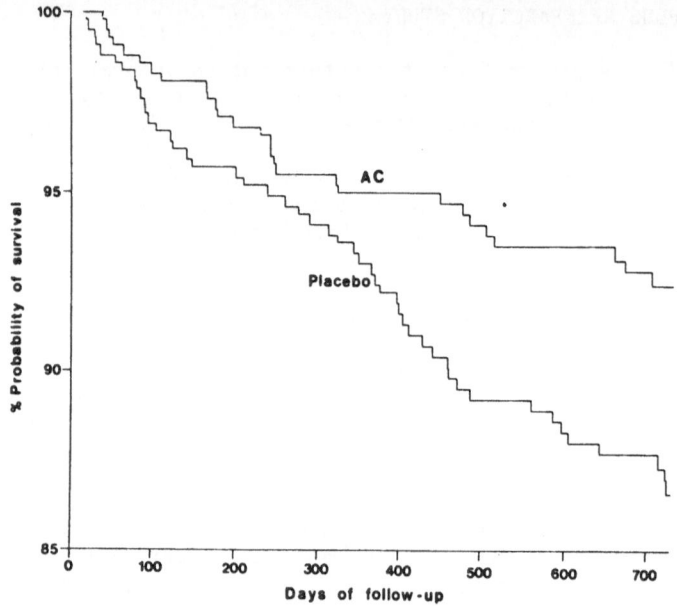

Figure 1. Sixty Plus Reinfarction Study: survival curves for the two
groups based upon deaths observed under treatement.

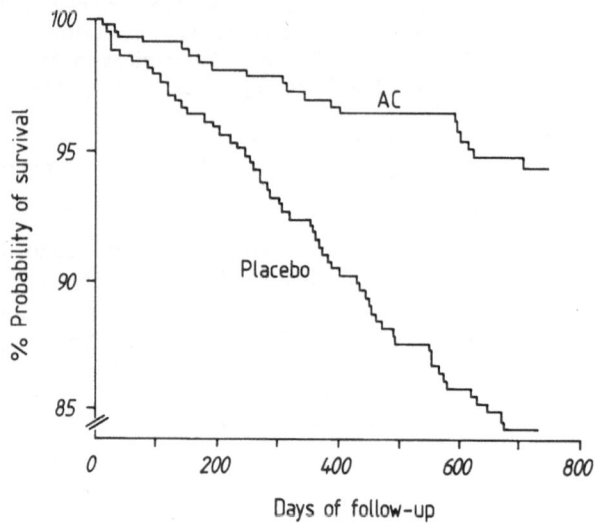

Figure 2. Sixty Plus Reinfarction Study: reinfarction-free survival curves
for the two groups based upon deaths observed under treatment.

reinfarction-free survival curves demonstrated also a steadily widening gap
(fig. 2). In addition, there was no relation between the recurrence of
myocardial infarction and either the age of the patient or the length of
oral anticoagulant treatment before entering the study. The steadiness of
the widening gap between mortality and recurrent myocardial infarction
observed in the two groups indicates that the efficacy of oral anticoagulants persisted throughout the study.

246

Subgroup analysis demonstrated moreover that patients on placebo-treatment whose first infarction occurred before the sixtieth birthday had a higher reinfarction rate than those in whom it occurred after that age was reached.

Although the results of the Sixty Plus Reinfarction Study were impressive it received criticism which can not be ignored (2,15). Most criticism concerned the time between the first infarction and entry in the study, which was in average 6 years. It is therefore not impossible that all but those patients for whom anticoagulant therapy was beneficial may have been eliminated before the start of the trial. In addition, the efficacy of oral anticoagulant treatment in patients younger than 60 years of age was not addressed.

Nevertheless, the impressive results of the Sixty Plus Reinfarction Study can be brought in proper perspective when compared with other studies on long-term treatment applying the same intensity of treatment.

PREVIOUS CLINICAL TRIALS OF LONG-TERM ANTICOAGULANT TREATMENT AFTER ACUTE MYOCARDIAL INFARCTION

Recently, three reviews dealt with the problem of efficacy of longterm therapy in patients surviving myocardial infarction (15-17). For this purpose major clinical trials were evaluated using the present epidemiological criteria for performing a study. Reasons for exclusion from the reviews were, for example, an incorrect randomization procedure, a relatively small sample size, lack of a placebo comparison group, treatment of the control group with a low dose of oral anticoagulants, or late randomization.

In two reviews the results of only three trials were included, which had randomized sufficient patients at or before hospital discharge and had an adequate group of control patients (15,16). In the literature these studies are referred to as the Medical Research Council Trial (18), Veterans Administration Cooperative Trial (19), and German-Austrian Multicenter Clinical Trial (20). The main results of these trials are summarized in table 4.

In each of these studies the rate of recurrent myocardial infarction was lower in the anticoagulated than in the control patients. However, in only the Medical Research Council Trial this difference was significant. In

Table 4: Results of some randomized clinical trials of long-term anticoagulant treatment in patients surviving acute myocardial infarction

	Medical Research Council Trial		Veterans Administration Cooperative Trial		German-Austrian Multicenter Clinical Trial	
	(N=383)	p	(N=747)	p	(N=629)	p
Mortality	21.3/14.9 *	NS	32.6/31.2	NS	10.4/12.2	NS
Recurrent infarction	39.9/20.5	<0.001	20.9/15.6	NS	8.1/ 5.0	NS
Thromboembolism	4.3/1.0	<0.05	7.7/ 3.9	< 0.05	2.3/ 0.6	NS

* Risk (%) in non-anticoagulated versus anticoagulated patients

all three studies long-term anticoagulant therapy failed to reduce the mortality rate. In the Medical Research Council Trial and the Veterans Administration Trial, however, the mortality was lower in the anticoagulated patients. Thromboembolism, which was reported as a combination of both venous and systemic thromboembolism in two trials, were effectively prevented by oral anticoagulants. In two trials the reduction of thromboembolism in the anticoagulated patients was statistically significant (18,19).

Based on the results of these trials and the bleeding risk of long-term anticoagulation the authors of one review "believe that the routine use of long-term anticoagulation therapy in survivors of acute myocardial infarction is not indicated" (16). In their opinion only patients with an increased risk for thromboembolism either systemic or venous, should be considered for chronic anticoagulation therapy.

However, in assessing the results of the aforementioned trials it is important to take into account the intensity of treatment applied. Recently, consensus was reached that for the prevention of venous thrombosis less intensive anticoagulation (2.0-3.0 INR) is required than for the prevention of arterial thromboembolism (3.0-4.5 INR) (11,13,14). The patients of the Medical Research Council Trial were in all probablility quite adequately treated with a prothrombin time aimed at 2 to 2.5 times the control value using a home made, acetone dried human brain thromboplastin (K.W.E. Denson, personal communication). This intensity is equivalent to an INR of 2.5 - 3.3. As about 20-25% of all prothrombin times were beyond this range, it means that the level of anticoagulation was sufficient intensive (18). On the contrary, the intensity of treatment applied in the Veterans Administration Trial was certainly insufficient for the prevention of recurrent myocardial infarction. In that study the prolongation of 2 to 2.5 times the control was aimed at by means of a human brain thromboplastin (19). This results in INR values of 2.0 to 2.5 or less. Finally, in the German-Austrian Clinical Trial only patients from one center received demonstrable sufficiently intensive anticoagulation (equivalent to an INR of 2.0 to 4.8); the intensity of treatment applied in the 6 other centres remained unknown (21). Under these conditions it is hardly surprising why the results of two of the three largest randomized clinical trials were disappointing.

Another way of evaluating the major clinical trials is to rely on the adequacy of oral anticoagulation. It is assumed that all comparative studies have been performed with the utmost care, although these studies did not fulfill all epidemiologal and statistical demands of the present days. Fourteen clinical trials were evaluated. A selection was made of those studies in which an apparently sufficient intensity of anticoagulation was applied. In only six studies the intensity of treatment was within an INR of 2.5 to 5.0 (1,18,22-25). Another 8 studies either over-treated or undertreated their patients, or did not provide sufficient information on the intensity of treatment (19,21,26-31).

In figure 3 the relative differences in recurrent myocardial infarction and total mortality were determined on efficacy basis. The data provided in most of the studies did not permit an intention-to-treat analysis, which would render less impressive results. The most eye catching difference between the groups of studies with sufficient intensity and the groups with inadequate or unknown intensity of treatment is that in the former the rate of recurrent myocardial infarction is likely to be lowered by two-third, and mortality accordingly, by about 40%. In the group with insufficiently defined anticoagulation there is still a trend in favor of coumarin treatment, but there is no difference in mortality.

(RECURRENT) MYOCARDIAL INFARCTIONS

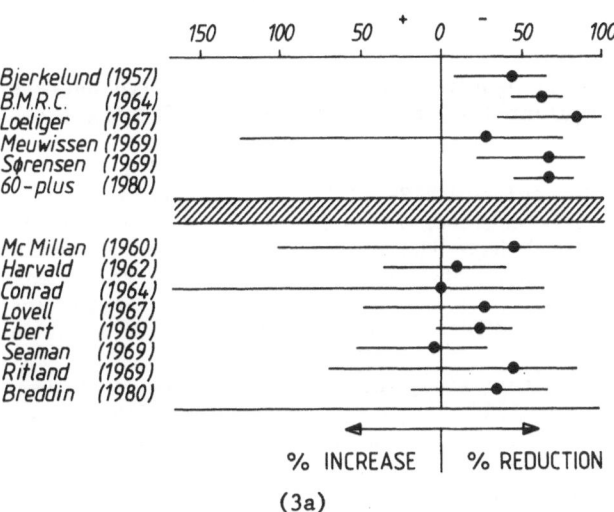

(3a)

MORTALITY

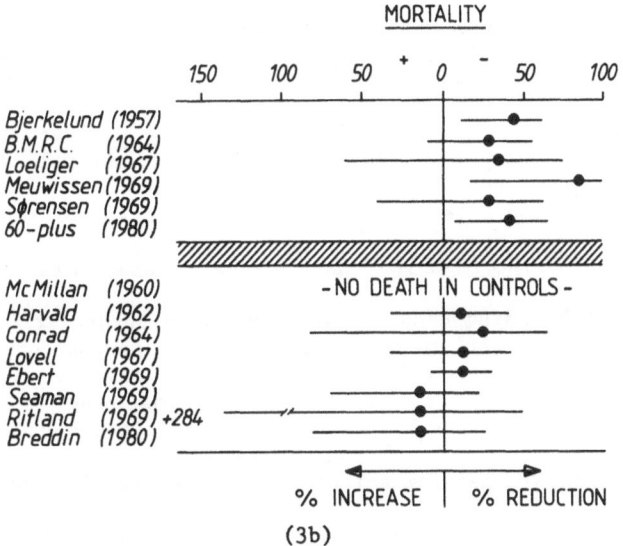

(3b)

Figure 3a and b: Results of 14 prospective comparative trials of long-term oral anticoagulation after myocardial infarction. The percentage of patients suffering form recurrent myocardial (3a) or of total mortality (3b) observed in the control group were taken as reference. The relative difference were determined mainly on an efficacy basis. 95% confidence limits are based on odds ratio considerations. The 6 trials in which levels of anticoagulation were largely inside the range of 2.5-5.0 INR are listed in the upper part of the figures, while those with prothrombin times largely outside this range or unknown are presented in the lower part.

The analysis demonstrates that the benefits of the older trials based on adequate intensity of treatment are similar to those of the Sixty Plus Reinfarction Study.

NEW CLINICAL TRIALS OF LONG-TERM ANTICOAGULANT TREATMENT

At present two major prospective and randomized clinical trials are in progress which will hopefully provide more definite answers to the dilemma of oral anticoagulant treatment in patients suffering from coronary thrombosis.

Both the Norwegian WARIS-trial (Warfarin Reinfarction Study) and the Dutch ASPECT-trial (Anticoagulants in the Secondary Prevention of Events in Coronary Thrombosis) have the same objectives and a similar design of the study. The major endpoint for the studies are total mortality, whereas recurrent myocardial infarction, bleeding complications (especially intracranial) will be regarded as important and decisive endpoints.

Eligible for the study are patients with a documented myocardial infarction who survived the hospital phase. Within three weeks after discharge from hospital the patients are randomly allocated to receive either the oral anticoagulant or the matching placebo. Dosage adjustment is made according to the prothrombin time. The desired intensity is 2.8 to 4.8 INR (10%-5% Thrombotest activity). Study treatment is given in a double blind manner.

The WARIS-trial started in January 1983 and the recruitment period ended in March 1986 (P. Smith, personal communication). During the recruitment period 1918 patients were considered for the trial and subsequently 1214 patients (63% of the patients considered) have been enrolled in the study. All patients will have a follow up period of (at least) two years.

The ASPECT-trial started in August 1986. By October 15, 1986 almost 200 patients have been enrolled. The aim is to include 4,000 patients within two years. Patients will be followed for at least one year and until the common termination date of 3 years after the start of the study.

RISK OF BLEEDING DURING LONG-TERM ANTICOAGULANT TREATMENT

The risk of bleeding complications was also subject of the Sixty Plus Reinfarction Study (1,32). In the anticoagulated group of patients the rate of bleeding was 16.6 per 100 patient-years as compared to 1.6 per 100 patientyears in the placebo group. The bleeding risk in anticoagulated patients was about ten times higher than that of placebo-treated patients.

Major extracranial bleeding episodes - defined as bleeding necessitating breaking the treatment code - were observed 4.1 times per 100 patient-years, however, none of these bleeding complications was lethal. Malignancy or other specific pathology as the source of bleeding was found in about half of the cases. Minor extracranial bleeding episodes accounted for the majority of the bleedings, 11.3 per 100 patient-years. There was no overt correlation between the incidence of bleeding and the patient's age or the duration of anticoagulant therapy before or during the trial.

The reported bleeding incidence is similar to those in other trials in which the same intensity of oral anticoagulant therapy was applied. Bjerkelund reported 12.7 bleedings per 100 patient-years, 3.6 episodes were classified as major bleeding (22).

It is obvious that overtreatment, that is too intense anticoagulation, is more damaging than beneficial. Major hemorrhages may easily induce rein-

Table 5.   Sixty Plus Reinfarction Study:
           distribution of intracranial events between the groups (fatal
           events within parentheses)

	Placeb (N=439)		Anti- coagulated (N=439)	
a. Definite diagnosis				
Intracranial hemorrhage	1*	(1)	8*	(6)
Cerebral infarction	3	(3)	0	
Cerebral tumor	1	(1)	0	
b. Non-definite diagnosis				
Death within 1 week	1	(1)	3	(3)
Persisting hemiparesis	7	(6)	0	
Transient deficit	7		1	
All intracranial events	20	(12)	12	(9)

* p   = 0.04

farction. On the other hand, moderate intensity of anticoagulation as applied for the prevention of venous thrombosis is accompanied by a relatively low bleeding incidence (33), but has scarcely any protective effect against intracardial and arterial thrombosis.

The Sixty Plus Reinfarction Study also provided important data with respect to intracranal bleeding (32). The number of definite intracranial hemorrhages was significantly higher in the anticoagulant group than in the placebo group. The rate of fatal intracranial bleeding was 0.9 per 100 patient-years. Epidemiological population studies similarly indicate a five-to-tenfold increase in the incidence of intracranial bleeding in chronically anticoagulated patients (34-36). However, in the Sixty Plus Reinfarction Study the substantial increase in intracranial bleeding complications in intensively treated out-patients was more than compensated by intracranial events in the placebo-treated patients (table 4), which was thought to be due to cerebral thromboembolism. The anticoagulated patients suffered only slightly more than half of the number of neurological events observed in the placebo group, with fewer fatalities and with a total period of neurological disability which was ten times shorter than that of the patients with neurological complications in the placebo group (32).

The risk of intracerebral bleeding is closely associated with both hypertension and age (34,35,37). In a recent study hypertension was present in 80% of the patients admitted with intracerebral hemorrhage (36). Even mild hypertension may constitute a risk factor as is suggested by sub-analysis of the intracranial events during the Sixty Plus Reinfarction Study. The blood pressure at the entry of the study was higher in the 12 anticoagulated patients (average blood pressure 155/90 mmHg) than in the 20 placebo-treated patients (average bloodpressure 145/80 mmHg) with intracranial events. It should be stressed that patients with therapy resistant hypertension were excluded from the study and that only a few patients had at the entry of the study a blood pressure exceeding 100 mmHg diastolic and 180 mmHg systolic.

It may be concluded that adequate long-term oral anticoagulant therapy as applied in the Netherlands increases the risk of intracranial and extra-cranial bleeding complications by a factor of about 10, but that this increase is by far outweighed by the beneficial effect in the prevention of venous, cardiac, and arterial thromboembolism.

ORGANIZATIONAL INFRASTRUCTURE FOR LONG-TERM ORAL ANTICOAGULANT TREATMENT

The Dutch infrastructure with a network of regionally centralized centres for the control of anticoagulant therapy in out-patients and home-patients is not a paradigm for anticoagulant control (38). It merely reflects the care needed for adequate and safe anticoagulation. Starting oral anticoagulant treatment is not simply prescribing a drug. It requires in addition patient education, accurate laboratory testing and adequate dosage regulation. An infrastructure will provide the necessary facilities: a 24-hour around-the-clock service staffed by competent and skilled laboratory personnel and by clinical consultants well trained in dosage regulation; internal and external quality assurance programs to monitor the accuracy and precision of the laboratory tests, and therapeutic quality control, that regularly reviews the levels of anticoagulation and the clinical results, including recurrences and bleeding complications.

In the last ten years the need for an organizational infrastructure for the control of oral anticoagulant therapy has been recognized in many countries. Out-patients clinics for anticoagulant control operate in Great Britain, West-Germany, Austria and Italy and even in some cities of the United States of America (39).

An organizational infrastructure will also facilitate the solution of problems already posed in 1948 by Dr Irving S. Wright "... It is not sufficient to state that a patient has received anticoagulants. Key questions which must be answered are: how much, how long, what levels of effectiveness were obtained and how consistently were these maintained? With this information, it should usually be possible to determine whether a failure was caused by drug or was the responsibility of those administering it" (40).

REFERENCES

1. Sixty Plus Reinfarction Study Research Group. A double-blind trial to assess long-term oral anticoagulant therapy in elderly patients after myocardial infarction. Lancet 1980; ii:989-94.
2. Mitchell JRA. Anticoagulants in coronary heart disease - retrospect and prospect. Lancet 1981; 1: 257-62.
3. Gorlin R, Fuster V, Ambrose JA. Anatomic-physiologic links between acute coronary syndromes. Circulation 1986; 74: 6-9.
4. Working Party on Anticoagulant Therapy in Coronary Thrombosis to the Medical Research Council. Assessment of short-term anticoagulant administration after cardiac infarction. Br Med J 1969; 1:335-42.
5. International Anticoagulant Review Group. Collaborative analysis of long-term anticoagulant administration after acute myocardial infarction. Lancet 1970; i: 203-9.
6. Merskey C, Drapkin A. Long-term anticoagulant therapy after myocardial infarction. JAMA 1974; 230:208-9.
7. May GS, Eberlein KA, Furberg CD, et al. Secondary prevention after myocardial infarction: a review of long-term trials. Prog Cardiovasc Dis 1982; 24:331-52.
8. Loeliger EA. The optimal therapeutic range in oral anticoagulation: History and proposal. Thromb Haemost 1979; 42:1141-52.

9.   International Committee for Standardization in Haematology and International Committee on Thrombosis and Haemostasis: ICSH/ICTH recommendations for reporting prothrombin time in oral anticoagulant control. Thromb Haemost 1985; 53:155-6.

10. Loeliger EA. Anticoagulant therapy in acute myocardial infarction. Am Heart J 1985; 110:1322-3.

11. Dalen JE, Hirsh J. American College of Chest Physicians and the National Heart, Lung, and Blood Institue National Conference on Antithrombotic Therapy. Arch Intern Med 1986; 146:462-72.

12. Loeliger EA, Van den Besselaar AMHP, Lewis SM. Reliability and clinical impact of the normalization of the prothrombin times in oral anticoagulant control. Thromb Haemost 1985; 53:148-54.

13. Poller L. Therapeutic ranges in anticoagulant administration. Br Med J 1985; 290: 1683-6.

14. Loeliger EA, Poller L, Samama M, et al. Questions and answers on prothrombin time standardization in oral anticoagulant control. Thromb Haemost 1985; 54:515-7.

15. Hirsh J. Effectiveness of anticoagulants. Sem Thromb Hemost 1986; 12:21-37.

16. Goldberg RJ, Gore JM, Dalen JE, Alpert JS. Long-term anticoagulant therapy after acute myocardial infarction. Am Heart J 1985; 109:616-22.

17. Leizorovicz A, Boissel JP. Oral anticoagulant in patients surviving myocardial infarction. A new approach to old data. Eur J Clin Pharmacol 1983; 24:333-6.

18. Working Party on Anticoagulant Therapy in Coronary Thrombosis to the Medical Research Council. An assessment of long-term anticoagulant administration after cardiac infarction. Second report. Br Med J 1964; 2: 837-43.

19. Ebert RV; Borden CW, Hipp HR, et al. Long-term anticoagulant therapy after myocardial infarction. Final report of the Veterans Administration Cooperative Trial. JAMA 1969; 207:2263-6.

20. Breddin K, Loew D, Lechner K, et al. The German-Austrian Aspirin Trial: A comparison of acetylsalicylic acid, placebo, and phenprocoumon in secondary prevention of myocardial infarction. Circulation 1980; 62 (suppl. V): V63-V72.

21. Breddin K, Loew D, Lechner K, et al. Secondary prevention of myocardial infarction: A comparison of acetylsalicylic acid, placebo and phenprocoumon. Haemostasis 1980; 9:325-44.

22. Bjerkelund CJ. The effect of long-term treatment with dicoumarol in myocardial infarction. Acta Med Scand 1957; 158 (Suppl. 330): 13-212.

23. Loeliger EA, Hensen A, Kroes F, et al. A double-blind trial of long-term anticoagulant treatment after myocardial infarction. Acta Med Scand 1967; 182:549-66.

24. Meuwissen OJAT, Vervoorn AC, Cohen O, et al. Double-blind trial of long-term anticoagulant treatment after myocardial infarction. Acta Med Scand 1969; 186:361-8.

25. Sørensen OH, Friis T, Jørgensen AW, et al. Anticoagulant treatment of acute coronary thrombosis. Acta Med Scand 1969; 185:65-72.

26. MacMillan RL, Brown KGW, Watt DL. Long-term anticoagulant therapy after myocardial infarction. Can Med Assoc J 1960; 83:567-70.

27. Harvald B, Hilden T, Lund E. Long-term anticoagulant therapy after myocardial infarction. Lancet 1962; ii:626-30.

28. Conrad LL, Kyriacopoulos JD, Wiggins CW, Honinck GL. Preventon of recurrences of myocardial infarction. Arch Intern Med 1964; 114:348-58.

29. Lovell RHH, Denborough MA, Nestel PJ, et al. A controlled trial of long-term treatment with anticoagulant after myocardial infarction in 412 male patients. Med J Aust 1967; 2:97-104.

30. Seaman AJ, Griswold HE, Beaume RB, Ritzman L. Long-term anticoagulant prophylaxis after myocardial infarction. N Engl J Med 1969; 281: 115-9.
31. Ritland S, Lygren T. Comparison of efficacy of 3 and 12 months' anticoagulant therapy after myocardial infarction. Lancet 1969; i:122-4.
32. Sixty Plus Reinfarction Study Research Group. Risks of long-term oral anticoagulant therapy in elderly patients after myocardial infarction. Lancet 1982;i:64-8.
33. Hull R, Hirsh J, Jay R, et al. Different intensities of anticogulation in the long-term treatment of proximal venous thrombosis. N Engl J Med 1982; 307:1676-81.
34. Whisnant JP, Cartlidge NEF, Elveback LR. Carotid and vertebral-basilar transient ischemic attacks: effect of anticoagulants, hypertension, and cardiac disorders on survival and stroke occurrence - a population study. Ann Neurol 1978; 3:107-15.
35. Furlan AJ, Whisnant JP, Elveback LR. The decreasing incidence of primary intracerebral hemorrhage: A population study. Ann Neurol 1979; 5:367-73.
36. Wintzen AR, De Jonge H, Loeliger EA, Bots GTAM. The risk of intracerebral hemorrhage during oral anticoagulant treatment: A population study. Ann Neurol 1984; 16:553-8.
37. Kase CS, Robinson RK, Stein RW, et al. Anticoagulant - related intracerebral hemorrhage. Neurology 1985; 35:943-8.
38. Loeliger EA, Van Dijk-Wierda CA, Van den Besselaar AMHP, et al. Anticoagulant control and the risk of bleeding. In: Anticoagulants and Myocardial Infarction: A Reappraisal. Ed. TW Meade. John Wiley and Sons Ltd, Chichester 1984; 135-77.
39. Errichetti AM, Holden A, Ansell J. Management of oral anticoagulant therapy. Experience with an anticoagulation clinic. Arch Intern Med 1984; 144: 1966-8.
40. Wright IS, Marple CD, Beck DF. Anticoagulant therapy of coronary thrombosis with myocardial infarction. JAMA 1948; 138: 1074-99.

FOLLOWING CORONARY THROMBOLYSIS

Sol Sherry

Department of Medicine
Thrombosis Research
Center
Temple University School
of Medicine
Philadelphia, PA

There are many aspects of the subject "following coronary thrombolysis" but probably the most important is the prevention of rethrombosis. This is an area of continuing clinical investigation, and a solution of the problem is most important for improving the efficacy of coronary thrombolysis and for clarifying the subsequent management of the patient.

The problem of rethrombosis is a complex one since multiple factors are involved initially in the thrombotic event, and a situation of high risk remains after lysis of the thrombus.

What does histological examination of the thrombus tell us? Many years ago, several investigators(Leary 1934, Clark et al 1936, Constantindes 1966, Friedman and Van den Bovenkamp 1966)pointed out that the thrombus is super-imposed on a ruptured atheromatous plaque in a coronary vessel whose over-lying intima has been torn by a crack, fissure or ulcer. A white head of platelets has filled the area of injury in a manner analogous to a hemosta-tic plug and has served to initiate fibrin formation in and around the platelet mass. A red cell-fibrin coagulum then forms on top of the platelet head and occludes the vessel.

Thus, some of the factors involved are an injury to the intima over-lying an atheromatous plaque, the strength of the thrombogenic stimulus which emanates from it, the interaction of platelets with the vessel wall, the interaction of platelets with each other, and the activation by platelets of the clotting mechanism. Each of these factors is further influenced by various accelerators and inhibitors which can modify the final response.

What is missing from this picture, however, is the dynamics of blood flow and its relationship to the thrombotic process. In the presence of a normally patent vessel, thrombogenic signals and mediators of all types, involving both platelets and the coagulation cascade, are usually either completely washed away or significantly tempered by blood rapidly flowing past the intimal injury. However, when the lumen is significantly encroached upon by an atheroma, the normal washing away effect is interfered with; blood flow through the area becomes dyskinetic with segmentation of flow rates including static zones. Therefore we must add the degree of under-lying vessel ·stenosis, and its effects on flow dynamics to our list.

Finally coronary thrombolysis adds one more factor to the equation, i.e. whether the lysis is complete or not. The fact that a vessel previously occluded is now being reperfused does not tell us whether the situation has been completely reversed to the pre-thrombotic state. As a matter of fact, there is evidence that it frequently is not. Under this circumstance, not only is the encroachment on the vessel lumen greater than the pre-thrombotic state but there is fibrin-bound thrombin exposed to the flowing blood. Thus, while the initial vascular injury may be covered over, there is now a new or additional thrombogenic stimulus.

In summary, the factors predisposing to rethrombosis include:
. An underlying vascular injury with a strong thrombogenic stimulus;
. Ability of platelets to interact with the vessel wall;
. Ability of platelets to undergo aggregation;
. Deficient local prostacylin production;
. Ability of platelets to activate clotting;
. Deficiency in coagulation inhibitors;
. High degree of underlying stenosis of the vascular lumen;
. Presence of residual clot; and
. Impaired run-off of blood flow in the area of previous thrombosis.

This constellation of factors serves to emphasize the complexity of the situation, and why no single therapeutic intervention is likely to provide an adequate solution.

Data on the frequency of reocclusion following successful thrombolysis are misleading, since anticoagulants have been administered routinely either with the thrombolytic agent or following its use. Thus anticoagulation with heparin and subsequently with oral agents probably has decreased the reocclusion rate significantly. The data are also misleading in that the timing of repeat angiograms to verify sustained patency or subsequent reocclusion has varied considerably among the reported studies.

FREQUENCY OF REOCCLUSION AFTER INTRACORONARY THROMBOLYSIS
(Presence or Absence of Reocclusion Proven by Repeat Angiogram)

STUDY	NO. REOCCLUSIONS/ NO. PATIENTS	%
STRETOKINASE		
Cribier et al	10/38	26
Rentrop et al	9/55	16
Serruys et al	7/48	15
Schwarz et al	1/18	5
Meyer et al	4/18	22
Harrison et al	7/24	29
Erbel et al	10/59	17
TOTAL	48/260	18
UROKINASE		
Cernigliari et al	7/43	16

Fig. 1

With this in mind, shown in Fig. 1 are the findings in a number of studies reporting the incidence of reocclusion as proven angiographically in vessels previously reperfused by the administration of a thrombolytic agent via an intracoronary catheter(Cribier et al 1983, Rentrop et al 1981, Serruys et al 1982, Meyer et al 1982, Erbel et al 1985, Cernigliari et al 1982). The average has been 18%.

Observations made in patients following successful reperfusion by a one hour intravenous infusion of streptokinase or a four hour infusion of rt-PA, as shown in Fig. 2, reveal a similar reocclusion rate to intracoronary thrombolysis(Spann et al 1984, Neuhaus et al 1983, Rogers et al 1983, Schroder et al 1983, Chesebro et al 1985, Gold et al 1986, Mathey et al 1985).

The overall reocclusion rate following reperfusion in all of these studies, i.e. 81 out of 445, is 18%. We can conclude from this that, at present, approximately one out of five reperfused vessels will reocclude despite conventional anticoagulant therapy and regardless of whether the thrombolytic agent is given locally or systematically.

When does the reocclusion occur?

Knowledge of the frequency of reocclusion as a function of time following reperfusion is very important information for planning an appropriate preventive approach. Here again the literature can be misleading.

For example, Gold et al(1986)in their studies of rt-PA reported that of 11 patients whose totally occluded vessel was reperfused after an intravenous infusion of rt-PA for 60-120 minutes, reocclusion occurred in 5 or 45% within one hour of cessation of the therapy. Reocclusion following streptokinase therapy also has been claimed to be most frequent shortly after reperfusion was evident. However, Rothbard and Fitzpatrick(1985)in their study of 48

FREQUENCY OF REOCCLUSION AFTER INTRAVENOUS THROMBOLYSIS
(Presence or Absence of Reocclusion Proven by Repeat Angiograms)

STUDY	NO. REOCCLUSIONS/ NO. PATIENTS	%
STRETOKINASE		
Spann et al	6/21	29
Neuhaus et al	4/24.	17
Rogers et al	4/26	15
Schroder et al	1/11	9
Chesebro et al	3/12	25
TOTAL	18/94	19
rt—PA		
Gold I (1—2 hr. inf.)	5/11	45
Gold II (4 hr. inf.)	2/13	15
UROKINASE		
Mathey	1/24	4

Fig. 2

successfully reperfused patients studied angiographically immediately and 24 hours after successful thrombolysis, claim that only 2% of patients showed worsening of stenosis and 4% worsening of flow over a 24 hour period of observation. Independently, Chesebro(1985)and associates came to a similar conclusion.

How are we to reconcile these differences?

My impression is that there are two periods of risk for reocclusion: 1) an immediate and high frequency one during or immediately after the administration of the thrombolytic agent when the flow rate is still inadequate; and 2) a later, lower and more protracted frequency of rethrombosis once reperfusion has been established and sustained.

What is the major demonstrable factor influencing rethrombosis?

Harrison et al(1984)using two independent techniques; quantitative coronary angiography and computer-based videodensitometry, analyzed the geometry of the residual lesion after reperfusion, and then correlated the information with the presence or absence of rethrombosis. Their results showed that rethrombosis is in part related to the size of the residual lumen after the establishment of reperfusion. Vessels with residual stenotic cross-sectional areas less than 0.4 mm^2 i.e. approximately 80% residual stenosis or greater, were at high risk for rethrombosis. Whereas vessels with minimal cross-sectional areas greater than 0.4 mm^2 are unlikely to rethrombose. In the study of Gold et al(1986), quantitative angiographic analysis also indicated that acute reocclusion only occurred in patients with 80% or greater residual stenosis while patients with less than 80% residual stenosis did not rethrombose on heparin anticoagulation. That a major residual stenosis is a serious risk factor for rethrombosis is agreed to by all investigators; however the degree of residual stenosis predisposing to frequent reocclusion varies with the investigator. Roger et al(1983) reports 90%, Gold et al(1986)and Harrison et al(1984) 80%, Gash et al(1986) 75% and Serruys et al(1983)58%.

What is the residual stenosis due to?

The two primary contributors to impediment to flow in the reperfused vessel are an atheromatous plaque and residual thrombus(Brown et al 1986). In the study by Gash et al(1986), residual thrombus appeared to be a more important risk factor than an atheromatous stenosis.

The elimination of these two readily demonstrable factors which contribute very significantly to the problem of rethrombosis are subject to different approaches. Relief from the anatomical obstruction caused by atheromas currently requires a mechanical or surgical approach but relief from residual thrombus has been approached in several different ways.

Let us consider each of these approaches beginning with the thrombolytic approach. As clots age, they become more resistant to lysis; serum is squeezed out as the fibrin molecules become more compacted and cross linking takes place. These changes slow the diffusion of an activator into the clot and render the fibrin substrate more resistant to lysis by plasmin. All of this is consistent with clinical experience, i.e. as thrombi or emboli age they become more resistant to lysis by thrombolytic agents. For example, Schroder et al(1983)in their original study on high dose, brief duration intravenously administered streptokinase for coronary thrombolysis, reported successful reperfusion in 75% of cases when the therapy was given in the first three hours after the onset of symptoms, and only 38% when it was started after three hours. When one reviews the current literature on intravenously administered streptokinase it is apparent that high success rates are reported when therapy is initiated early, and low success rates when several hours have passed before the therapy is begun.

Therefore, one approach to eliminating residual thrombus and obtaining maximum reperfusion is to start the therapy as quickly as possible after the onset of ischemic symptoms; at that time the clot is still soft and readily lysable and the best results are obtained in myocardial salvage. To be able to initiate therapy within the first two hours or less in the vast majority of patients will require a more efficient and effective lay education and medical system than exists today for handling patients at the onset of their ischemic event.

Another, but not mutually exclusive thrombolytic approach aimed at increasing flow by reducing the amount of residual thrombus, is to prolong the duration of therapy. In the study of Gold et al(1986), a four hour intravenous infusion of rt-PA in seven patients with an 80% or greater stenosis at the time of reperfusion, i.e. those at highest risk of rethrombosis, prevented a reocclusion during their hospital stay, whereas therapy limited to two hours in five patients with an 80% or greater stenosis at the time of reperfusion did not prevent a reocclusion in any. Taylor et al(1984), rather than giving the usual 1-1.5 million units of streptokinase over a one hour period, gave a total of 1.3 million units over a four hour period and reported a reperfusion rate as high as 82%.

To re-emphasize this point, it is likely that the early rate of rethrombosis can be reduced by initiating therapy much earlier than in the past and by treating over a longer period of time.

The antithrombotic approach is based on two considerations: 1) anticoagulant therapy can improve the efficacy of thrombolytic therapy as the success of the latter is hampered by the rate of new clotting; when clotting exceeds the rate of lysis it is responsible either for the failure of reperfusion of for early rethrombosis; and 2) anticoagulant therapy can prevent a subsequent or late reocclusion. The basic approach has been to use heparin initially followed by coumarin therapy. Since anticoagulation has been a fairly routine measure in association with thrombolytic therapy, one suspects that in its absence the incidence of rethrombosis would have been much higher.

However, the benefits of anticoagulation must be weighed against its hazards, especially since thrombolytic therapy may increase the risk of a significant bleed. Thrombolytic therapy will lyse hemostatic plugs at the site of recent invasive procedures and, when there is extensive plasma plasminogen activation, as with streptokinase, a state of inadequate hemostasis is produced. Both of the above, i.e. bleeding sites and an inadequate hemostatic mechanism, are known to be high risk factors for heparin induced bleeding complications. Indeed a large part of the 4% of serious bleeds associated with thrombolytic therapy have occurred after the therapy have occurred after the therapy has been completed and the patient placed on heparin. Therefore, one must recognize that the routine use of heparin anticoagulation following thrombolytic therapy, while necessary, already contributes significantly to the bleeding risk associated with the procedure. Thus attempts to augment anticoagulant therapy by giving heparin simultaneously with the thrombolytic agent and/or increasing the state of anticoagulation can be associated with an increased number of major bleeding episodes.

For example, Ganz et al(1984), in an attempt to increase the frequency of reperfusion and to limit rethrombosis during an evolving infarction, gave an intravenous bolus dose of heparin, 40 units per kg body weight, immediately after a 15 minute infusion of 750,000 units of streptokinase, and then gave a continuous infusion of heparin so as to maintain a partial thromboplastin time of 100 seconds or more for several days. Reperfusion was reported as high as 96% (78 of 81 patients) and reocclusion as low as 8%. However, there was a 12.3% incidence of major bleeding including a 2.5% incidence of intracranial hemorrhage. In the large I.S.A.M. study (The I.S.A.M. Study Group 1986), which evaluated the effects of a short term infusion of 1.5 million units of streptokinase on mortality and cardiac function in patients with an acute myocardial infarction, heparin, aspirin and phenprocoumon were given simultaneously with streptokinase. The incidence of hemorrhagic complications was 5.9% including a 0.5% incidence of intracranial bleeding. The control group had no intracranial bleeds and the incidence of a hemorrhagic episode was 1.5%. Certainly streptokinase is not a safe drug when used with a shotgun antithrombotic approach.

Actually one of the advantages associated with streptokinase therapy is the rapid and extensive activation of plasma plasminogen which produces an anticoagulant state: all the circulating fibrinogen is either partially or extensively degraded, very high levels of fibrinogen breakdown products are in the circulation, clotting is slow and poor, and platelet function is impaired. This state exists for several hours and avoids the necessity for the simultaneous administration of heparin or immediately upon the termination of the streptokinase infusion.

On the other hand, when circulating plasminogen is activated slowly and the proteolytic state which ensues is mild, as in the use of the highly clot selective agents, reclotting is more likely to take place. In the study of Gold et al(1986), a 60-120 minute infusion of rt-PA was associated with a 45% incidence of early rethrombosis. Unless the therapy is prolonged, large doses of heparin administered simultaneously with the thrombolytic agent will be required to prevent rethrombosis. However, the combination of a thrombolytic agent with large doses of heparin, as noted earlier, is a high risk situation for a bleeding complication; in the TIMI trial(The TIMI Study Group 1985)the incidence of bleeding complications with rt-PA was similar to that observed with streptokinase.

To my knowledge, the commonly available platelet function inhibitors have not been used alone in any study; rather, when employed, drugs like aspirin and dipyridamole have been used to supplement the action of simultaneously administered anticoagulants. Since their administration has been empirical, it is not clear whether their addition has resulted in a reduction of rethrombosis, or increased the bleeding complication rate or both.

Incidentally, there is a report of the combined use of PGE1 and streptokinase by intracoronary administration for acute myocardial infarction. Sharma et al(1986)claim that reperfusion was established in all 10 cases where it was tried; also, among 4 intracoronary streptokinase failures, the subsequent administration of PGE1, a platelet aggregation inhibitor and a vasodilator, resulted in rapid reperfusion in two. This approach merits further study but the extent of its usefulness, even is confirmed, will depend upon its successful application to systemic therapy.

The vasodilator approach is based on the view that vessel spasm as well as thrombosis underlies the pathogenesis of an acute occlusive event, and that relief of spasm along with the thrombolysis will mediate a more effective reperfusion. Maseri and associates(Hackett et al 1985)have reported that in a group of patients who failed to reperfuse on nitrates alone, combined intracoronary thrombolytic and isosorbide dinitrate therapy decreased the frequency of rethrombosis as compared to that observed with intracoronary thrombolysis alone. As with PGE1, this form of combined therapy deserves further study.

The most frequently used approach for stabilizing the reperfused vessel has been the mechanical approach i.e. to eliminate any reduced run-off either by balloon angioplasty or coronary by-pass surgery. Each of these two procedures has its advocates(Meyer et al 1982, Serruy et al 1983, Erbel et al 1985, Sutton et al 1986, Anderson et al 1986). The major questions still to be resolved are the appropriate timing of the procedure and which patients require it. At present satisfactory answers are not available. Under any circumstance, patients who have had successful thrombolysis will at some point have to undergo further study to determine whether angioplasty or surgery is indicated as part of the management of their coronary artery disease.

In summary, the problem of rethrombosis in the coronary artery following reperfusion by thrombolysis has been reviewed. Various approaches have been undertaken to limit its frequency, the most popular being a combination of anticoagulation and a mechanical procedure. Nevertheless, there is much to be learned before definitive recommendations can be made as to the best way to deal with this problem. Once it is resolved satisfactorily, other therapeutic considerations following coronary thrombolysis will fall in line, including the prevention of a subsequent episode of coronary thrombosis.

REFERENCES

Anderson, J.L., Battistessa, S.A., Clayton, P.D., Cannon III, C.Y., Askins, J.C., and Nelson, R.M., 1986, Coronary bypass surgery early after thrombolytic therapy for acute myocardial infarction. Ann. Thorac. Surg., 41: 176.

Brown, B.G., Gallery, C.A., Badger, R.S., Kennedy, J.W., Mathey, D., Bolson, E.L., and Dodge, H.T., 1986, Incomplete lysis of thrombus in the moderate underlying atherasclarotic lesion during intracoronary infusion of streptokinase for acute myocardial infarction: quantitative angiographic observations, Circulation, 73: 653.

Cenigliaro, C., Sansa, M., Campi, A., Sante Bongo, A., and Rossi, P., 1982, Intracoronary thrombolysis with urokinase in acute myocardial infarction. Effects on reperfusion and left ventricular wall motion, G. Ital. Cardiol., 12: 365.

Chesebro, J.H., Smith, H.C., Holmes, D.R., Bove, A.A., Bresnahan, D.R., Bresnahan, J.F., Gibbons, R.J., Miller, F.A., Mock, M.B., Reeder, G.S., Vliestra, R.E., and Brown, B.G., 1985. Reocclusion and clot lysis between 90 minutes, 1 day, and 10 days after thrombolytic therapy for myocardial infarction, Circulation, 72(II): III-55(Abstract).

Clark, E., Graef, I., and Chasis, H., 1936, Thrombosis of the aorta and coronary arteries, Arch. Path., 22: 183.

Constantinides, P., 1966, Plaque fissures in human coronary thrombosis, J. Atherscler. Res., 6: 1.

Cribier, A., Berland, J., Champoud, O., Moore, N., Behar, P., and Letac, B., 1983, Intracoronary thrombolysis in evolving myocardial infarction. Sequential angiographic analysis of left ventricular performance, Br. Heart J., 50: 401.

Erbel, R., Pop, T., Henkel, B., Schreiner, G., Rupprecht, H.-J., Henrichs, K.-J., and Meyer, J., 1985, Immediate angioplasty after reperfusion in acute myocardial infarction, Circulation, 72(II): III-223(Abstract).

Friedman, M., and Van den Bovenkamp, G.J., 1966, The pathogenesis of coronary thrombus, Amer. J. Path., 48: 19.

Ganz, W., Geft, I., Shah, P.K., Lew, A.S., Rodriguez, L., Weiss, T., Maddahi, J., Berman, D.S., Charuzi, Y., and Swan, H.J., 1984. Intravenous streptokinase in evolving myocardial infarction. Am. J. Cardiol., 53: 1209.

Gash, A.K., Spann, J.F., Sherry, S., Belber, A.D., Carabello, B.A., McDonough, M.T., Mann, R.H., McCann, W.D., Gault, J.H., Gentzler, R.D., and Kent, R.L., 1986. Factors influencing reocclusion after coronary thrombolysis for acute myocardial infarction, Am. J. Cardiol., 57: 175.

Gold, H.K., Leinbach, R.C., Garabedian, H.D., Yasuda, T., Johns, J.A., Grossbard, E.B., Palacios, I., and Collen, D., 1986, Acute coronary reocclusion after thrombolysis with recombinant human tissue-type plasminogen activator: Prevention by a maintenance infusion, Circulation, 73: 347.

Hackett, D., Davies, G., Chierchia, S., and Maseri, A., 1986, Streptokinase and nitrates increase the frequency of coronary reperfusion in acute myocardial infarction, J. Am. Coll. Cardiol., 7(2) (Supplement A): 220 A (Abstract).

Harrison, D.G., Ferguson, D.W., Collins, S.M., Skorton, D.J., Ericksen, E.E., Kioschos, J.M., Marcus, M.L. and White, C.W., 1984, Rethrombosis after reperfusion with streptokinase: importance of geometry of residual lesions, Circulation, 69: 991.

Leary, T., 1934, Experimental arteriosclerosis in the rabbit compared with human (coronary) arteriosclerosis, Arch. Path., 17: 453.

Mathey, D.G., Schofer, J., Sheehan, F.H., Becher, H., Tilsner, V., and Dodge, H.T., 1985, Intravenous urokinase in acute myocardial infarction. Am. J. Cardiol., 55: 878.

Meyer, J., Merx, W., Schmitz, H., Erbel, R., Kiesslich, T., Dorr, R., Lambertz, H., Bethge, C., Krebs, W., Bardos, P., Minale, C., Messmer, B.J., and Effert, S., 1982, Percutaneous transluminal coronary angioplasty immediately after intracoronary streptolysis of transmural myocardial infarction, Circulation, 66: 905.

Neuhaus, K.L., Tebbe, U., Sauer, G., Kreuzer, H. and Kostering, H., 1983, High dose intravenous streptokinase in acute myocardial infarction. Clin. Cardiol., 6: 426.

Rentrop, P., Blanke, H., Karsch, K.R., Kaiser, H., Kostering, H. and Leitz, K., 1981, Selective intracoronary thrombolysis in acute myocardial infarction and unstable angina pectoris, Circulation, 63: 307.

Rogers, W.J., Mantle, J.A., Hood, W.P., Baxley, W.A., Whitlow, P.L. Reevers, R.C., and Soto, B., 1983, Prospective randomized trial of intravenous and intracoronary streptokinase in acute myocardial infarction, Circulation, 68: 1051.

Rothbard, R.L., and Fitzpatrick, P.G., 1985, Comparison of residual coronary artery stenosis and flow immediately and 24 hours after successful thrombolysis, Circulation, 72(II): III-55 (Abstract).

Schroder, R., Biamino, G., Enz-Rudiger, L., Linderer, T., Bruggemann, T., Heitz, J., Vohringer, H.-F., and Wegscheider, K., 1983, Intravenous short-term infusion of streptokinase in acute myocardial infarction. Circulation, 63: 536.

Schwarz, F., Schuler, G., Katus, H., Hofmann, M., Manthey, J., Tillmanns, H., Mehmen, H.C., and Kubler, W., 1982, Intracoronary thrombolysis in acute myocardial infarction: Duration of ischemia as a major determinant of late results after recanalization. Am. J. Cardiol., 50: 933.

Serruys, P.W., Wigns, W., Van den Brand, M., Ribeiro, V., Fioretti, P., Simoons, M.L., Kooijman, C.J., Reiber, H.J.C., and Hugenholz, P.G., 1983, Is transluminal coronary angioplasty mandatory after successful thrombolysis? Quantitative coronary angipgraphic study. Br. Heart J., 50: 257.

Sharma, B., Wyeth, R.P., Lane, G.E., Giminez, H.J., Hutchins, S.W., and Franciosa, J.A., 1986, Combined intracoronary prostaglandin El and streptokinase in acute myocardial infarction, J. Am. Coll. Cardiol, 7(2) (Supplement A): 208 A (Abstract).

Spann, J.F., Sherry, S., Carabello, B.A., Denenberg, B.S., Mann, R.H., McCann, W.D., Gault, J.H., Gentzler, R.D., Belber, A.D., Maurer, A.H., and Cooper, E.M., 1984, Coronary thrombolysis by intravenous streptokinase in acute myocardial infarction. Acute and follow-up studies, Am. J. Cardiol., 53: 655.

Sutton, J.M., Taylor, G.J., Mikell, F.L., Moses, H.W., Korsmeyer, C.,
    Dove, J.T., Batchelder, J.E., Wellons Jr., H.A., and Schneider, J.A.,
    1986, Thrombolytic therapy followed by early revascularization for
    acute myocardial infarction, Am. J. Cardiol., 57: 1227.
Taylor, G.J., Mikell, F.L., Moses, H.W., Dove, J.T., Batchelder, J.E., Thull,
    A., Hansen, S., Wellons Jr., H.A., and Schneider, J.A., 1984, Intra-
    venous versus intracoronary streptokinase therapy for acute myocardial
    infarction in community hospitals. Am. J. Cardiol., 54: 256.
The I.S.A.M. Study Group, 1986, A prospective trial of intravenous
    streptokinase in acute myocardial infarction (I.S.A.M.). Mortality,
    morbidity and infarct size at 21 days. N. Engl. J. Med., 314: 1465.
The TIMI Study Group, 1985, The thrombolysis in myocardial infarction
    (TIMI) trial, N. Engl. J. Med., 312: 932.

ARTERIAL THROMBOEMBOLISM:

VALVULAR HEART DISEASE AND PROSTHETIC HEART VALVES

James E. Dalen

Professor of Medicine
University of Massachusetts at Worcester
Worcester, MA

Systemic embolism has long been recognized as a major complication of valvular heart disease, specifically mitral valve disease. In the absence of mitral valve disease or atrial fibrillation (AF), clinically detectable systemic emboli are uncommon in patients with isolated aortic valve disease (1).

MITRAL STENOSIS

Systemic emboli occur in patients with mitral stenosis (MS) due to the formation of clots within the left atrium. Systemic embolism is unrelated to the severity of MS; systemic embolism including cerebral embolism may be the first symptom of MS in a previously asymptomatic patient (2).

In patients in whom the diagnosis of MS is established, approximately 20% have a history of systemic embolism (3-5). At postmortem examination, the incidence of systemic embolism is much higher, in the range of 40% (6-7). In patients with unoperated MS, systemic embolism is a major cause of death. In a 10 year follow-up of patients with unoperated MS, Rowe et al (8) found that 19% of deaths were due to systemic embolism. Olesen (9) found that 22% of all deaths in patients with MS were due to thromboembolism.

As noted, the incidence of systemic embolism in patients with MS is unrelated to the severity of the lesion. The two factors that are associated with the incidence of systemic embolism in patients with MS are age and the presence of AF. The impact of age and the presence of AF were made clear in a study of 737 patients with MS reported by Coulshed et al (3). As shown in Table 1, in patients younger than 35, the incidence of systemic embolism was 5% in those in NSR, but 27% in those with AF. In patients over age 35, the incidence of systemic embolism was 11% in those with NSR, and 32% in those with AF.

Table 1. INCIDENCE OF SYSTEMIC EMBOLISM IN 737 PATIENTS WITH MS*

AGE (YR)	RHYTHM	NUMBER	% WITH EMBOLI
<35	Normal sinus rhythm	197	5
>35	Normal sinus rhythm	195	11
<35	AF	51	27
>35	AF	294	32

*Coulshed et al, reference #3

The size of the left atrium as detected by echocardiography is related to the probability of AF; as the left atrium enlarges, the probability of AF increases (10). However once AF is present, the size of the left atrium is unrelated to the probability of systemic embolism.

The presence of paroxysmal or chronic AF in a patient with MS is an indication for chronic anticoagulation with warfarin. The therapeutic range recommended by the ACCP/NHLBI National Conference on Antithrombotic Therapy (1) is warfarin sufficient to prolong the prothrombin time to 1.2 to 1.5 times control using rabbit brain thromboplastin (standardized INR=2.0-3.0). Longterm anticoagulation with warfarin should also be considered in patients with MS who are in NSR, but older than age 35. If systemic embolism occurs in patients with MS, full dose warfarin therapy sufficient to prolong the prothrombin time to 1.5 to 2.0 times control (INR=3.0 to 4.5) should be given.

MITRAL REGURGITATION

The incidence of systemic embolism in patients with mitral regurgitation (MR) is somewhat lower than in patients with MS (11). However when chronic MR is complicated by AF, the risk of systemic embolism approaches that of MS. In a study by Coulshed et al (3), shown in Table 2, the incidence of systemic embolism in patients with chronic MR increased from 8% for those in NSR to 22% in those with AF. Systemic embolism is uncommon in patients with acute MR because AF is uncommon.

Table 2. SYSTEMIC EMBOLISM IN MITRAL VALVE DISEASE

	#	Incidence Systemic Embolism (%)		
		NSR	AF	TOTAL
Mitral Stenosis	737	8%	32%	19%
Mitral Insufficiency	102	8%	22%	16%

*Coulshed et al, reference #3

As with MS, chronic anticoagulation with warfarin is indicated when MR is complicated by AF. In the absence of a history of systemic embolism, the dose of warfarin should be sufficient to prolong the prothrombin time to 1.2 to 1.5 times control (rabbit brain thromboplastin). Full dose warfarin, sufficient to prolong the prothrombin time to 1.5 to 2.0 times control (INR = 3.0-4.5) should be given if systemic embolism is documented.

MITRAL VALVE PROLAPSE

Most patients, with mitral valve prolapse (MVP) are asymptomatic and cardiovascular complications are rare. However, there is significant evidence that otherwise unexplained cerebral ischemic events, particularly transient ischemic events, do occur in some patients with MVP (12-17).

The recommendations of the ACCP/NHLBI National Conference on Antithrombic Therapy (18) for the prevention of systemic embolism are shown in Table 3. No therapy is indicated in patients with asymptomatic, uncomplicated MVP. In patients with a history of unexplained TIA's, ASA 1 gram/day is indicated. If TIA's recur despite ASA, low intensity warfarin sufficient to prolong the prothrombin time to 1.2-1.5 control (INR = 2.0-3.0) is indicated. Low intensity warfarin is also indicated if MVP is complicated by AF or significant MR. Full dose warfarin (protime 1.5-2.0 times control) should be reserved for patients with MVP complicated by documented systemic embolism.

Table 3. RECOMMENDED ANTITHROMBOTIC THERAPY IN PATIENTS WITH
MITRAL VALVE PROLAPSE

ACCP/NHLBI NATIONAL CONFERENCE ON ANTITHROMBOTIC THERAPY (18)

Patient Status	Recommended Therapy
Asymptomatic	None
Unexplained TIA's	ASA 1 gram/d
Recurrent TIA's, despite ASA	Warfarin, protime 1.2-1.5 times control (INR = 2.0-3.0)
AF and/or significant MR	Warfarin, protime 1.2-1.5 times control (INR=2.0-3.0)
History of systemic embolism	Warfarin, protime 1.5-2.0 times control (INR = 3.0-4.5)

MITRAL ANNULAR CALCIFICATION

Mitral annular calcification (MAC) is a common condition in the elderly, particularly in women (19). MAC may be associated with MS, MR and conduction disorders, but it remains uncomplicated in most patients. Several reports have indicated that there may be an increased incidence of thromboembolism and calcific emboli in this disorder (20-22).

In asymptomatic patients with MAC without AF, antithrombotic therapy is not indicated. When MAC is complicated by AF, low intensity warfarin (prothrombin time 1.2 to 1.5 times control) is indicated. If systemic embolism (as opposed to calcific embolism) occurs, full dose warfarin is recommended (1).

MECHANICAL PROSTHETIC HEART VALVES

Patients with mechanical prosthetic heart valves are at particular risk of systemic emboli. Emboli may originate as left atrial thrombi, particularly when AF is present, and they may originate as thrombi that may form on the mechanical valve. In the absence of antithrombotic therapy, the risk of systemic embolism is extreme; ranging from 30 to 69% in one year (23-26).

Systemic emboli are more common in patients with mitral prostheses, due to the frequency of AF, and in patients with valves that have exposed metal struts (27).

In patients with mechanical mitral prosthetic valves who are treated with chronic warfarin, the annual incidence of systemic embolism is 6 to 10% (28-29). The rate of embolism in patients with mechanical prosthetic valves in the aortic position is approximately 1-4% per year (30).

Given the high incidence of systemic embolism in patients with mechanical prosthetic valves, it is recommended that they receive full dose warfarin therapy sufficient to prolong the prothrombin time to 1.5

to 2.0 times control using rabbit brain thromboplastin (INR=3.0-4.5). If emboli occur despite full dose warfarin, dipyridamole (400 mgm/d) should be added to the regimen. If bleeding occurs while on full dose warfarin, the dose of warfarin should be lowered to prolong the prothrombin time to 1.2 to 1.5 times control, and dipyridamole (400 mgm/d) should be added (27).

BIOPROSTHETIC VALVES

The primary advantage of bioprosthetic valves is that they are less thrombogenic than mechanical valves. The annual rate of embolism in patients with bioprosthetic valves in the mitral position is 1.4 to 5.4% (2). Most emboli in patients with bioprosthetic valves in the mitral position occur in patients with AF, those who have a prior history of systemic embolism or were noted to have clot in the left atrium at the time of surgery (27). Several reports (31,32) have noted an increased incidence of emboli in the first three months after surgery.

The incidence of emboli in patients with bioprosthetic valves in the aortic position is much lower because of the low incidence of AF and left atrial clot.

The ACCP/NHLBI National Conference on Antithrombotic Therapy (18) recommended that patients with bioprosthetic valves in the mitral position should be treated with less intense warfarin (prothrombin time 1.2 to 1.5 times control using rabbit brain thromboplastin) for three months after surgery. In patients with AF, a history of systemic embolism or clot in the left atrium, less intense warfarin should be administered chronically.

In patients with bioprosthetic valves who are in NSR and do not have a history of systemic embolism or clot in the left atrium, warfarin therapy is not indicated. One study has suggested that aspirin, .5 gm/d may be beneficial in such patients (33).

CONCLUSIONS

In patients with valvular heart disease, those who are at the greatest risk of systemic embolism are those with mitral valve disease, particularly when it is complicated by chronic or paroxysmal AF. Long term treatment with less intense warfarin (prothrombin time 1.2 to 1.5 times control) offers the potential to prevent systemic embolism in these patients.

All patients with mechanical prosthetic valves are at risk of systemic embolism and require full dose warfarin therapy (protime 1.5 to 2.0 times control using rabbit brain thromboplastin). The risk of embolism in patients with bioprosthetic valves is dependent upon associated risk factors, rather than the bioprosthetic valve itself. Antithrombotic therapy is not required unless AF is present, there is a history of systemic embolism or clot was present in the left atrium at the time of surgery.

REFERENCES

1. Levine HJ, Pauker SG, Salzman EW: Antithrombotic therapy in valvular heart disease. Chest 89, Feb. Supplement, 36S, 1986.
2. Dalen JE: Mitral stenosis. In: Dalen JE, Alpert JS, eds. Valvular Heart Disease, Second Edition, Boston, MA: Little, Brown and Co., 49:1986.

3. Coulshed N, Epstein EJ, McKendrick CS, Galloway RW, Walker E: Systemic embolism in mitral valve disease. Br Heart J 32:26, 1970.
4. Ellis LB, Harken DE: Arterial embolization in relation to mitral valvuloplasty. Am Heart J 62:611, 1961.
5. Bannister RG: The risks of deferring valvotomy in patients with moderate mitral stenosis. Lancet 2:329, 1960.
6. Weiss S, Davis D: Rheumatic heart disease. III. Embolic manifestations. Amer Heart J 9:45, 1933.
7. Graham GK, Taylor JA, Ellis LB, Greenberg DJ, Robbins SL: Studies in mitral stenosis. Arch Int Med 88:632, 1951.
8. Rowe JC: The course of mitral stenosis without surgery: Ten- and twenty-year perspectives. Ann Intern Med 52:741, 1960.
9. Olesen KH: The natural history of 271 patients with mitral stenosis under medical treatment. Br Heart J 24:349, 1962.
10. Sherrid MV, Clark RD, Cohn K: Echocardiographic analysis of left atrial size before and after operation in mitral valve disease. Am J Cardiol 43:171, 1979.
11. Wood P: Diseases of the heart and circulation. Philadelphia: JB Lippincott Co, 1956.
12. Barnett HJM: Transient cerebral ischemic: pathogenesis, prognosis and management. Ann R Coll Physicians Surg Can 7:153, 1974.
13. Barnett HJM, Jones ME, Boughner DR, Kostuk WJ: Cerebral ischemic events associated with prolapsing mitral valve. Arch Neurol 33:777, 1976.
14. Hirsowitz GS, Saffer D: Hemiplegia and the billowing mitral leaflet syndrome. J Neurol Neurosurg Psychiatry 41:381, 1978.
15. Saffro R, Talano JV: Transient ischemic attack associated with mitral systolic clicks. Arch Intern Med 139:693, 1979.
16. Hanson MR, Hodgman JR, Conomy JP: A study of stroke associated with prolapsed mitral valve. Neurology 23:341, 1978.
17. Barnett HJM, Boughner DR, Taylor DW: Further evidence relating mitral valve prolapse to cerebral ischemic events. N Engl J Med 302:139, 1980.
18. ACCP-NHLBI National Conference on Antithrombotic Therapy. Dalen JE, Hirsch J, editors. Chest 89, February Supplement, 1986.
19. Pape LA: Pathogenesis and etiology of valvular heart disease. In: Dalen JE, Alpert JS, eds. Valvular Heart Disease, Second Edition, Boston, MA: Little, Brown and Co., 1, 1986.
20. Guthrie JJ, Fairgrieve JJ: Aortic embolism due to a myxoid tumor associated with myocardial calcification. Br Heart J 25:137, 1963.
21. Fulkerson PK, Beaver BM, Auseon J, Graber HL: Calcification of the mitral annulus: etiology, clinical associations, complications and therapy. Am J Med 66:967, 1979.
22. Kalman P, DePace NL, Kotler MN, et al: Mitral annular calcification and echogenic densities in the left ventricuar outflow tract in association with cerebral ischemic events. J Cardiovasc Ultrasonogr 1:155, 1982.
23. Duvoisin GE, Brandenburg RO, McGoon DC: Factors affecting thromboembolism associated with prosthetic heart valves. Circulation Supplement 1:70, 1967.
24. Akbarian M, Austen WG, Yurchak PM, Scannell JG: Thromboembolic complications of prosthetic cardiac valves. Circulation 37:826, 1968.
25. Stein DW, Rahimtoola SH, Kloster FE, Selden R, Starr A: Thrombotic phenomena with nonanticoagulated, composite-strut aortic prostheses. J Thoracic Cardiovasc Surg 71:680, 1976.
26. Bjork VO, Henze A: Management of thromboembolism after aortic valve replacement with the Bjork-Shiley tilting disc valve. Scand J Thorac Cardiovasc Surg 9:183, 1975.
27. Stein PD, Collins JJ Jr, Kantrowitz A: Antithrombotic therapy in mechanical and biological prosthetic heart valves and saphenous vein bypass grafts. Chest 89, February Supplement 46S, 1986.

28. Starr A, Grunkemeier G, Lambert L, Okies JE, Thomas D: Mitral valve replacement. Circulation 54:47 (Suppl III), 1976.
29. Salomon NW, Stinson EB, Griepp RB, Shumway NE: Mitral valve replacement: long-term evaluation of prosthesis-related mortality and morbidity. Circulation 56:94, 1977.
30. Edmunds LH: Thromboembolic complications of current cardiac valvular prostheses. Ann Thorac Surg 34:96, 1982.
31. Ionescu MI, Smith DR, Hasan SS, Chidambaram M, Tandon AP: Clinical durability of the pericardial xenograft valve: Ten years experience with mitral replacement. Ann Thorac Surg 34:265, 1982.
32. Oyer PE, Stinson EB, Griepp RB, Shumway NE: Valve replacement with the Starr-Edwards and Hancock prostheses: comparative analysis of late morbidity and mortality. Ann Surg 186:301, 1977.
33. Nunez L, Gil Aguado M, Larrea JL: Prevention of thromboembolism using aspirin after mitral valve replacement with porcine bioprosthesis. Ann Thorac Surg 37:84, 1984.

CLINICAL TRIAL DILEMMAS AND CEREBROVASCULAR DISEASE

Lewis H. Kuller

University of Pittsburgh
Graduate School of Public Health
Department of Epidemiology
Pittsburgh, PA

The death rate due to stroke in the United States and other countries has declined substantially in the past forty years.[1,2] This decline has been accentuated since the introduction of specific antihypertensive therapy. The decrease has been noted in many countries, and apparently is a combination of not completely understood lifestyle factors, which have impinged on the prevalence and type of hypertensive disease and risk of stroke and the efficacy of the treatment of hypertensive disease.

Longitudinal studies in Olmstead County, Minnesota,[3] by the Mayo Clinic Group, has documented a decline in the incidence of stroke. There is, however, relatively little evidence that either the acute case-fatality or the long-term survival after stroke has changed substantially in the past years.

The role of anticoagulation therapy in the treatment and prevention of stroke has been controversial.[4,5,6,7] There appears to be a consensus that anticoagulation therapy in patients who have had a completed stroke is unlikely to be beneficial and may be potentially hazardous. The primary role of anticoagulation therapy appears to be in the prevention of stroke among patients with transient cerebral ischemia.[8] There are only four randomized trials of anticoagulation therapy among patients with transient cerebral ischemia.[8] These studies were primarily done in the early to middle 1960s, involved relatively few patients, were usually not blinded, and generally suggested that anticoagulation therapy was effective in decreasing the frequency of transient cerebral ischemia and possibly in the prevention of cerebral infarction but not mortality.

In 1977 the first randomized controlled trial of aspirin in cerebral ischemia were reported.[8,9,10] Five major trials have now been published relating the use of aspirin to the prevention of stroke or recurrent transient ischemic attack (TIA) among patients with either stroke or transient cerebral ischemia on admission to the study. In general, these studies have suggested that aspirin therapy reduces the frequency of recurrent transient cerebral ischemia and may have a beneficial effect on stroke,[11,12,13] but not on total mortality.

One trial has attempted to evaluate the efficacy of anticoagulation therapy versus antiplatelet therapy in individuals who were initially on anticoagulation therapy following transient cerebral ischemia.[14] In this study in Sweden, 135 patients who had been treated for two months with anti-coagulation therapy following their transient cerebral ischemic attack were randomized into a continuing anticoagulation treatment and to antiplatelet therapy. They were followed for twelve months. There were no significant differences between the two groups, three strokes occurring among the aspirin group and one in the anticoagulation group. The number of recurrent TIAs were somewhat higher in the aspirin group, while myocardial infarctions occurred more often in the anticoagulation group. A further two-year followup noted that TIA or cerebral infarctions occurred in eight patients during anticoagulation treatment, as opposed to 22 patients treated with aspirin, while there were two lethal hemorrhages on the anticoagulation therapy. The authors concluded that short-term anticoagulation treatment during the first critical period, perhaps 3-12 months after the initial ischemic symptoms is preferable followed by safer but less effective anti-platelet drugs as a long-term prophylaxis in patients with transient cerebral ischemia.

The Mayo Clinic Group,[4] after reviewing the data on the treatment of transient cerebral ischemia proposed: 1) "that the majority of patients with vertebral-basilar TIA should be treated medically; 2) if a skilled surgeon and an experienced angiographer are available, patients with typical carotid TIA who are suitable medical risks should have angiography followed by carotid endarterectomy if an appropriate lesion is found; and, 3) non-operated patients with TIA, of less than two months duration, are treated with three months of Warfarin therapy, unless contra-indicated before aspirin is begun. Non-operated patients with continuing TIAs of two or more months duration are treated with aspirin, unless there has been a recent increase in the frequency, duration, or severity of TIA. Under these circumstances Warfarin therapy is advised for three months before aspirin is started. Aspirin therapy should then be continued until the patient has been free of TIA for at least one year. No treatment is advised for non-operated patients whose last episode of TIA was longer than 12 months ago".

Several recent papers have questioned the value of extracranial carotid endarterectomy.[15,16,17,18] Specifically, there has been concern about the risk benefits of the surgical procedure. The potential high morbidity and mortality of the surgical procedure has raised serious questions about the benefits of the surgical procedure.[19,20] In spite of the lack of clinical trials to demonstrate clear efficacy of this procedure,[8] the number of carotid endarterectomies has continued to increase substantially in the United States.[18] Furthermore, there are very wide variations in the reported morbidity and mortality following the procedure.[21] Several investigators have suggested that the procedure is unlikely to be beneficial unless the operative and post-operative morbidity/mortality from the surgical treatment is less than three percent.[18]

A study in Rochester, Minnesota reported that among 130 patients with transient cerebral ischemia that were not treated,[22] 13% had a stroke within one month, 15% in three months, 23% at one year, and 43% by five years of followup. Among those treated with anticoagulants, only 4% had had a stroke within the first month, 9% by one year, and 21% by five years. The risk of stroke was much greater among the patients with TIA than would be expected in the general population. Among the 122 patients with carotid TIA there were 48 strokes and among the 64 vertebral-basilar TIAs there were 31 strokes. The net probability of stroke occurrence was somewhat higher in those with vertebral-basilar as opposed to carotid artery TIA.

The high frequency of stroke noted in the first few months after the initial TIA may be due to an ascertainment bias. The TIA patients were identified both from clinical records of patients reporting only TIA, and from stroke patients who reported prior TIA. Thus, the probability of being identified as a stroke first with history of TIA is inversely related to between initial TIA and stroke. Furthermore, individuals with TIA and no subsequent clinical disease are clearly much less likely to be identified especially if they did not seek care at the time of their TIA.

Heyman[23] studied 390 patients with TIA admitted to Duke University Hospital. Of the 390 patients, 324 (83%) had arteriographic studies. Ulcerations and obstructive lesions were present in 217 and 159 of these had endarterectomy. There were 69 strokes during the five-year followup, but 23 or one-third occurred during the initial hospital admission as a complication of arteriography or endarterectomy 16 or spontaneous 7 patients. At the end of five years the cumulative rate of stroke was 22.7% and of myocardial infarction or sudden death 21%. Risk factors for stroke included diabetes mellitus, elevated blood pressure, prior myocardial infarction and prior stroke.

Mohr, et al.[24] on the other hand, noted that only 10% of strokes are proceeded by transient ischemic attacks because of the low incidence of large artery atherothrombotic stroke. Other studies previously reviewed have noted a much higher frequency of TIA prior to stroke. Case-selection and criteria for TIA diagnosis clearly effect the importance of TIA prior to stroke. Specific treatment of TIA might be beneficial to the individual patient, but could have relatively little effect on the overall stroke rates in a community.

The preliminary report from the Pilot Stroke Data Bank[25] noted that among 1158 strokes, 708 (61%) were cerebral infarction, of which 172 (15%) were atherosclerotic, 200 (17%) embolic, 100 (9%) lacunae and 236 (20%) etiology unproven. Also, 220 (19%) of the 1158 were classified as TIA.

The Harvard Cooperative Stroke Registry reported that embolism accounted for 31% of the 694 strokes. Of the 215 patients with embolism, 34% had atrial fibrillation and 25% valvular heart disease. The high frequency of atrial fibrillation prior to stroke has recently been reviewed.[27] The prevention of cerebral embolism by anticoagulants or other antithrombo-embotic therapy is obviously of considerable importance and may rival the interest in the treatment of TIA.

The development of new non-invasive techniques to measure carotid artery disease has made it possible to evaluate the natural history of carotid artery disease among patients with TIAs, carotid bruits or completely asymptomatic individuals.[28] Several recent studies have clearly documented that carotid artery stenosis of less than 75% is rarely associated with subsequent stroke.[29,30,31] The risk of stroke even among patients with greater than 75% stenosis or even total carotid occlusion is relatively low. Hennerici,[32] for example, recently reported on 49 asymptomatic individuals with internal carotid artery occlusion, 43 uni-lateral and 6 bilateral, that during an estimated 31 month followup there were 23 deaths, 47%, 13 of the deaths were from cardiac causes, 5 from stroke and 5 from other causes. There were 8 (16%) ipsilateral strokes over the six years of followup with all of the strokes occurring within the first two years.

A recent extensive Canadian study of patients initially identified with carotid bruit also showed that the risk of stroke was relatively low even among individuals with greater than 75% carotid stenosis.[29] During a 42 month followup about 20% of those with 75% or greater stenosis had a cerebral ischemic event, TIA or stroke, for those with 30-74% stenosis about 8% and less than 30% stenosis about 4%. The incidence of cardiac ischemia was directly related to degree of carotid stenosis. Furthermore, the incidence of cerebral ischemia was much higher in those with prior cardiac disease and with progression of carotid stenosis. All of the strokes were preceeded by transient cerebral ischemia and it did not seem worthwhile to treat the asymptomatic individual with extensive carotid artery stenosis until TIA had occurred. The risk of stroke among these patients was substantially less than that for a cardiac event, similar to the results of the Hennerici study.[31,32] Prospective followup studies of patients with carotid bruit have also documented the high risk of cardiac rather than cerebrovascular disease.

In the previously described study by Heyman of TIA patients,[23] the risk of cardiac disease was directly related to the extent of carotid disease. Patients without obstructive or ulcerated lesions in the carotid arteries had a five year cumulative rate of myocardial infarction or sudden death of only 5%, while those with carotid lesions had a 29.5% rate of cardiac events. There was no difference in the rate of myocardial infarction or sudden death among patients treated medically or surgically.

Several studies have now noted a much higher prevalence of coronary artery disease determined at angiography among patients with carotid artery disease.[33] In a recent study Hertzer, et al.,[33] performed coronary angiography on 506 patients with extracranial cerebrovascular disease. Severe surgically correctable coronary artery disease were documented in 37% of patients previously suspected of having coronary disease and 16% of asymptomatic individuals. The presence of coronary artery disease was greater in men and diabetics.

Extensive carotid artery stenosis is a marker of a diffuse vascular disease including both coronary and peripheral vascular disease.[34] It is unlikely that any non-specific therapy not aimed at reducing the complications of atherosclerotic disease including the prevention of thrombosis will reduce the overall mortality among such patients.

The frequency of stroke is relatively low compared to that of coronary artery disease and it would not seem logical to emphasize therapy predominantly for stroke in such patients without considering their high risk of both coronary artery and peripheral vascular disease.

The increase use of procedures such as ultrasound, and doppler flow studies to measure the prevalence of carotid artery disease among selected patients, especially those with carotid bruit, individuals undergoing coronary bypass surgery and those with other manifestations of vascular disease, as well as patients with transient cerebral ischemia will provide a very large pool of potential high risk patients and therapeutic dilemma.

The risk of stroke is relatively low among patients with asymptomatic carotid bruit and as noted even in those individuals with relatively severe carotid stenosis. Several authors have noted the substantial risk of carotid artery surgery. In Cincinnati, between 1980-83, the number of carotid endarterectomies rose 74% with a combined stroke or death rate of 6.5%. Aysmptomatic carotid artery disease was the indication for 50% of the endarterectomies during both time periods.[20] Dyken[21] has also noted the remarkable increase in the frequency of endarterectomy in the United States and the approximate 2% mortality following the surgical procedure. The prevalence of asymptomatic carotid bruit in the older, at-risk population, may be as high as 20%.[16,35] Among 20 million people 65 years of age or older, 4,000,000 may have bruit, 60-70% of such individuals will have at least 50% carotid artery stenosis, 2,000,000. However, a large number of individuals will have carotid stenosis without symptoms or bruit. The exact percentage has not been determined in any random sample of the elderly. Our recently completed study of a sample of asymptomatic individuals over 60 years of age with systolic hypertension, systolic blood pressure greater than 160 and diastolic less than 90, demonstrated that the prevalence of flow significant carotid stenosis, an internal carotid to common carotid artery peak blood flow velocity ratio of equal to or greater than 1.4 was about 56%. Clearly there is a high pool of potentially detectable patients at high risk of clinical vascular disease, especially myocardial infarction and sudden death. As noted, the risk of stroke is relatively low and specific surgical treatment is not going to be a satisfactory solution to the problem.

There is a major need at the present time to evaluate specific therapies for individuals with asymptomatic carotid artery disease, especially those with at least 50 or perhaps 75% carotid artery stenosis. Will antiplatelet aggregating agents, low dose anticoagulants or therapy aimed at reduction of the progression of atherosclerosis by either dietary or pharmacological means to decrease low density lipoprotein cholesterol (LDL) or raise high density lipoprotein cholesterol (HDL) be beneficial. Decreased cigarette smoking or treatment of hypertension may be the best approach to reducing the risk of vascular disease. The needs for such a study are apparent considering the growing frequency of diagnostic techniques and the increasing prevalence of surgical procedures in the United States. The treatment of these patients is currently based on opinion rather than on sound scientific evidence.

It is unlikely that new clinical trials to test the efficacy of anticoagulants versus antiplatelet aggregating agents or surgical techniques specifically to prevent stroke will be feasible given the low risk of disease and polarization of views about the efficacy of specific therapies.

It would seem more realistic to consider trials to decrease vascular disease and possibly total mortality. With possibly a 15-20% risk of vascular disease within three years as noted in the study of Chambers, et al.,[30] individuals with at least 30% stenosis of a carotid artery, the sample size would not have to be excessive or the time period very lengthy.

Several studies suggest that anticoagulation therapy followed by antiplatelet aggregating agents is highly effective in reducing the risk of both stroke and recurrent transient ischemic attack, especially within the first few months after a TIA. A primary emphasis should be on the improved identification of TIA. The primary risk of such treatment is unwanted bleeding, the proper control of the anticoagulants becomes a primary concern.

The clinical trials represent the cornerstone for good scientific practice in medicine. The current treatment of carotid artery disease, TIA and embolism strongly suggest the need for new clinical trials and that a more systematic approach to therapy is indicated. Much of therapy is currently based on the art rather than on the science of medicine.

REFERENCES

1. National Center for Health Statistics, Advanced report of final mortality statistics, 1984. NCHS Monthly Vital Statistics Report 35:5 (1986).
2. P. K. Whelton, Declining mortality from hypertension and stroke. S Med J 75:33 (1982).
3. W. M. Garraway, J. P. Whisnant, A. J. Furlan, Et al., The declining incidence of stroke. N Engl J Med 300:449 (1979).

4. B. A. Sandok, A. J. Furlan, J. P. Whisnant and T. M. Sundt, Jr., Guidelines for the management of transient ischemic attacks. Mayo Clin Pro 53:665 (1978).

5. L. H. Kuller, The transient ischemic attack, in: Curr Concepts of
    Cerebrovascular Disease - Stroke IX:23, W. K. Hass, ed., American
    Heart Association, New YOrk (1974).
6. C. H. Millikan and F. H. McDowell, Treatment of transient ischemic
    attacks. Stroke 9:299 (1978).
7. E. Genton, H. J. M. Barnett, W. S. Fields, et al., XIV. Cerebral
    ischemia: The role of thrombosis and antithrombotic therapy.
    Stroke 8:150 (1977).
8. C. H. Millikan, Treatment of occlusive cerebralvascular disease, in:
    "Cerebrovascular Survey Report for the National Institute of
    Neruological and Communicative Disorders and Stroke", F. McDowell
    and L. R. Caplan, eds., (Revised 1985).
9. J. A. Byer and J. D. Easton, Therapy of ischemic cerebrovascular
    disease. Ann Intern Med 93:742 (1980).
10. J. P. Kistler, A. H. Ropper and R. C. Heros, Therapy of ischemic
    cerebral vascular disease due to atherothrombosis. N Engl J Med
    311:100 (1984).
11. M. L. Dyken, Assessment of the role of antiplatelet aggregating agents
    in transient ischemic attacks, stroke and death, in: Curr Concepts
    of Cerebrovascular Disease - Stroke, O. M. Reinmuth, ed., American
    Heart Association, New York (1979).
12. H. J. M. Barnett, J. W. D. McDonald and D. L. Sackett, Aspirin -
    effective in males threatened with stroke. Stroke 9:295 (1978).
13. M. L. Dyken, Editorial: Transient ischemic attacks and aspirin, stroke
    and death; negative studies and type II error. Stroke 14:2 (1983).
14. J. E. Olsson, C. Brechter, Backlund H, et al., Anticoagulant vs anti-
    platelet therapy as prophylactic against cerebral infarction in
    transient ischemic attacks. Stroke 11:4 (1980).
15. W. S. Fields, V. Maslenikow, J. S. Meyer, et al., Joint study of
    extracranial arterial occlusion. V. Progress report of prognosis
    following surgery or nonsurgical treatment for transient cerebral
    ischemic attacks and cervical carotid artery lesions. JAMA 211:
    1993 (1970).
16. L. H. Kuller and K. C. Sutton, Carotid artery bruit: Is it safe and
    effective to auscultate the neck? Stroke 15:944 (1984).
17. H. J. M. Barnett, F. Plum and J. N. Walton, Carotid endarterectomy -
    an expression of concern. Stroke 15:941 (1984).
18. M. L. Dyken and R. Pokras, The performance of endarterectomy for
    disease of the extracranial arteries of the head. Stroke 15:948
    (1984).
19. J. D. Easton, D. G. Sherman, Stroke and mortality rate in carotid
    endarterectomy: Two hundred twenty-eight consecutive operations.
    Stroke 8:565 (1977).
20. T. G. Brott, R. J. Labutta and R. F. Kempczinski, Changing patterns
    in the practice of carotid endarterectomy in a large metropolitan
    area. JAMA 255:2609 (1986).
21 L. G. Slavish, G. G. Nicholas and W. Gee, Review of a community
    hospital experience with carotid endarterectomy. Stroke 15:956
    (1984).
22. J. P. Whisnant, N. E. F. Cartlidge and L. R. Elveback, Carotid and
    vertebral-basilar transient ischemic attacks: Effect of anti-
    coagulants, hypertension, and cardiac disorders on survival and
    stroke occurrence--a population study. Ann Neurol 3:107 (1978).
23. A. Heyman, W. E. Wilkinson, B. J. Hurwitz, et al., Risk of ischemic
    heart disease in patients with TIA. Neurology 34:626 (1984).
24. J. P. Mohr, Transient ischemic attacks and the prevention of strokes.
    (Editorial) N Engl J Med 299:93 (1978).
25. S. C. Kunitz, C. R. Gross, A. Heyman, et al., The Pilot Stroke Data
    Bank: Definition, design, and data. Stroke 15:740 (1984).
26. J. P. Mohr, L. R. Caplan, J. W. Melski, et al., The Harvard Cooperative
    Stroke Registry: A prospective registry. Neurology 28:754 (1978).

27. P. Sandercock, J. Bamford, C. Warlow, R. Peto, Is a controlled trial of long-term oral anticoagulants in patients with stroke and non-rheumatic atrial fibrillation worthwhile? Lancet 1:788 (1986).

28. J. R. Crouse, G. H. Harpold, F. R. Kahl, et al., Evaluation of a scoring system for extracranial carotid atherosclerosis extent with B-mode ultrasound. Stroke 17:270 (1986).

29. B. R. Chambers and J. W. Norris, Outcome in patients with asymptomatic neck bruits. N Engl J Med 315:860 (1986).

30. G. O. Roederer, Y. E. Langlois, K. A. Jager, et al., The natural history of carotid arterial disease in asymptomatic patients with cervical bruits. Stroke 15:605 (1984).

31. M. Hennerici and W. Rautenberg. Letter to the Editor. N Engl J Med 311:1123 (1984).

32. M. Hennerici, H. B. Hulsbomer, W. Rautenberg and H. Hefter, Spontaneous history of asymptomatic internal carotid occlusion. Stroke 17:718 (1986).

33. N. R. Hertzer, J. R. Young, E. G. Beven, et al., Coronary angiography in 506 patients with extracranial cerebrovascular disease. Arch Intern Med 145:849 (1985).

34. N. R. Hertzer, E. G. Beven, J. R. Young, et al., Incidental asymptomatic carotid bruits in patients scheduled for peripheral vascular reconstruction: Results of cerebral and coronary angiography. Surgery 96:535 (1984).

35. B. R. Chambers and J. W. Norris, Clinical significance of asymptomatic neck bruits. Neurology 35:742 (1985).

ATRIAL FIBRILLATION AND STROKE:

THE VIEW FROM CARDIOLOGY

James E. Dalen

Professor of Medicine
University of Massachusetts at Worcester
Worcester, MA

More than 90% of all systemic emboli, including cerebral emboli, originate as intracardiac thrombi. The cardiovascular disorders that predispose to intracardiac thrombi are valvular heart disease, prosthetic heart valves, myocardial infarction and atrial fibrillation (AF) (1).

It is now clear that the most important of these disorders is atrial fibrillation. The incidence of atrial fibrillation in six series (2-7) totalling more than 1000 patients with systemic embolism (2-7) is shown in Table 1. Note that the average incidence of AF in these patients was 57% as compared to a 24% incidence of myocardial infarction.

Table 1. INCIDENCE OF ATRIAL FIBRILLATION AND MYOCARDIAL INFARCTION
IN PATIENTS WITH SYSTEMIC EMBOLISM

REPORT	# PATIENTS WITH SYSTEMIC EMBOLISM	AF	MYOCARDIAL INFARCTION
		(%)	(%)
Abbott et al (2)	313	74	33
Szczepanski (3)	260	51	17
Green et al (4)	149	49	17
Silvers et al (5)	106	75	22
Lorentzen et al (6)	130	37	24
Satiani and Evans(7)	122	43	25
	1080	(57%)	(24%)

In a review of systemic embolism at the Massachusetts General Hospital from 1937 to 1979, Abbott et al (2) compared the profile of patients with systemic embolism during three different time periods: 1937-1953, 1954-1963, and 1963-1979. As shown in Table 2, the average age increased from 52 in 1937-1953 to 70 in 1964 to 1979. The percent of patients with rheumatic heart disease decreased from 46% in 1937-1953 to 20% in 1963-1979 while the percent of patients with coronary artery disease increased from 38% in 1937-1953 to 68% in 1964-1979. The

incidence of AF in these patients with systemic embolism was nearly
constant over this 40 year period; 80% in 1937-1953, 75% in 1954-1963,
and 74% in 1963-1979. As the prevalence of rheumatic heart disease has
declined, and as our population has grown older, coronary artery disease
has become the commonest cause of AF.

Table 2. SYSTEMIC EMBOLISM AT THE MASSACHUSETTS GENERAL HOSPITAL,
1937-1979

	1937-1953	1954-1963	1964-1979
# Patients	200	260	313
Average Age	52	63	70
Type Heart Disease (%)			
Rheumatic Heart Disease	46	36	20
Coronary Disease	38	52	68
Myocardial Infarction	16	26	33
Atrial Fibrillation	80	75	74

*Abbott et al, reference #2

In a clinical series of 230 patients with AF, Hurst et al (8) noted
that 46% had coronary artery disease, as compared to a 20% incidence of
valvular heart disease. The findings of a postmortem series of 333
patients who had been in AF prior to death was essentially the same; 51%
had coronary artery disease, and 30% had valvular heart disease (9) as
shown in Table 3.

Table 3. UNDERLYING HEART DISEASE IN PATIENTS WITH
ATRIAL FIBRILLATION

	CLINICAL SERIES* N = 230	POSTMORTEM SERIES** N = 333
Coronary Artery Disease	46%	51%
Valvular Heart Disease	20%	30%
Hypertension	11%	10%
Other Heart Disease	15%	4%
No Heart Disease Detected	8%	5%

*Hurst et al, reference #8
**Hinton et al, reference #9

In the clinical series by Hurst et al (8), all but 8% of the
patients with AF had evidence of organic heart disease. In the
postmortem series (9), only 5% of the patients had no evidence of heart
disease. The commonest cause of AF at the present time is non-valvular
heart disease; that is heart disease other than valvular heart disease.

The high incidence of systemic embolism in patients with mitral
valve disease complicated by AF has long been recognized (10). In
addition, the impact of AF on the incidence of systemic embolism in
patients with prosthetic heart valves is also well recognized (11).
However, the importance of AF in patients without valvular heart disease
is not as well documented (12).

A very important study of patients with AF who had postmortem
examination at the Massachusetts General Hospital was reported by Hinton
et al (9). The incidence of systemic embolism at postmortem in patients
who had been in normal sinus rhythm prior to death was 7%. The incidence
of systemic embolism in patients with mitral valve disease with AF was
41%. However, the incidence of systemic embolism in patients with CAD

complicated by AF was essentially the same; 35% as shown in Table 4. These findings indicate that AF, rather than the type of heart disease is the critical risk factor for systemic embolism.

Table 4. POSTMORTEM INCIDENCE OF SYSTEMIC EMBOLISM IN PATIENTS
WITH ATRIAL FIBRILLATION

TYPE HEART DISEASE	#	INCIDENCE EMBOLISM
Mitral Valve Disease (MVD)	70	41%
Coronary Artery Disease (CAD)	171	35%
CAD and MVD	26	35%
Controls, NSR	58	7%

*Hinton et al, reference #9

The impact of non-valvular AF, that is AF without valvular heart disease, on the incidence of systemic embolism is well illustrated by data from the Framingham Study. Wolf et al (13) reported the incidence of stroke during a follow-up of 24 years. The observed incidence of stroke was compared to the predicted rate based on age and blood pressure. As shown in Table 5, in patients without AF or valvular heart disease, the observed rate of stroke was the same as predicted. However, in patients with AF and valvular heart disease, the observed rate of stroke was 17 times greater than predicted on the basis of age and blood pressure. The critical finding was that the rate of stroke in patients with AF without valvular heart disease was more than five times greater than predicted. It is clear that patients with non-valvular AF are at increased risk of embolic stroke. This risk has been estimated to be 5% per year (14).

Table 5. AF AND STROKE, THE FRAMINGHAM STUDY*

GROUP	PERSON-YEARS OBSERVED	EXPECTED** RATE STROKE	OBSERVED RATE	RELATIVE RISK
No AF, No RHD	109,51	3.1	2.9	.93
AF, RHD	154	2.6	45.4	17.5
AF, no RHD	481	7.4	41.4	5.6

*Wolf et al, reference #13
**Expected on basis of age, blood pressure

Further evidence of the importance of non-valvular AF is provided by the study of patients with thyrotoxicosis. In the past, it was believed that patients with thyrotoxicosis complicated by AF were not at risk of systemic embolism. Three reports (15-17) of the incidence of systemic embolism in patients with thyrotoxicosis are summarized in Table 6. Note that the incidence of AF in these patients with thyrotoxicosis ranged from 10 to 28%. The incidence of systemic emolism in patients with thyrotoxicosis who had AF ranged from 10 to 40%. The majority of the emboli were strokes.

Identification of patients at risk of systemic embolism offers a significant opportunity to prevent cerebral embolism since 70% of all systemic emboli enter the cerebral circulation. Nearly one-fifth of all ischemic strokes are due to cerebral embolism (14). Non-valvular AF is the underlying cause of more than one-half of all cerebral emboli (14).

Table 6.   THYROTOXICOSIS, AF, AND SYSTEMIC EMBOLISM

REPORT	# PATIENTS WITH THYROTOXICOSIS	% IN AF	% EMBOLISM IN PATIENTS WITH AF
Bar-Sela et al, (15)	142	21	40
Yuen et al, (16)	210	10	24
Stafforth, et al (17)	845	28	10
Totals	1197	(24%)	(14%)

If chronic anticoagulation with warfarin is effective in preventing systemic embolism in patients with non-valvular AF, we can expect a significant reduction in the number of ischemic strokes. Clinical trials to assess the risks and benefits of chronic anticoagulation in patients with non-valvular AF are currently in progress in the United States and in Europe.

REFERENCES

1. Dalen JE. Systemic Embolism. In: Rippe JM, Irwin RW, Alpert JS, Dalen JE, eds. Intensive Care Medicine, Little, Brown, Boston, 1985, 209.
2. Abbott WM, Maloney RD, McCabe CC, Lee CE, Wirthlin LS: Arterial embolism: A 44 year perspective. Am J Surg 143:460, 1982.
3. Szczepanski KP: Results of surgical treatment of arterial embolism. Scand J Thorac Cardiovasc Surg 13:71, 1979.
4. Green RM, DeWeese JA, Rob CG: Arterial embolectomy before and after the Fogarty catheter. Surgery 77:24, 1975.
5. Silvers LW, Royster TS, Mulcare RJ: Peripheral arterial emboli and factors in their recurrence rate. Ann Surg 192:232, 1980.
6. Lorentzen JE, Roder OC, Hansen HJB: Peripheral arterial embolism. Acta Chir Scand 502:111, 1980.
7. Satiani B, Evans WE: Immediate prognosis and five year survival after arterial embolectomy following myocardial infarction. Surg Gynecol Obstet 150:41, 1980.
8. Hurst JW, Paulk EA Jr, Proctor HD, Schlant RC: Management of patients with atrial fibrillation. Am J Med 37:728, 1964.
9. Hinton RC, Kistler JP, Fallon JT, Friedlich AL, Fisher CM: Influence of etiology of atrial fibrillation on incidence of systemic embolism. Am J Cardiol 40:509, 1977.
10. Levine HJ, Pauker SG, Salzman EW: Antithrombotic therapy in valvular heart disease. Chest 89, Feb. Supplement 36S, 1986.
11. Stein PD, Collins JJ Jr, Kantrowitz A: Antithrombotic therapy in mechanical and biological prosthetic heart valves and saphenous vein bypass grafts. Chest 89, Feb. Supplement 46S, 1986.
12. Dunn M, Alexander J, de Silva R, Hildner F: Antithrombotic therapy in atrial fibrillation. Chest 89, Feb. Supplement 68S, 1986.
13. Wolf PA, Dawber TR, Thomas HE Jr, Thomas E Jr, Kannell WB: Epidemiologic assessment of chronic atrial fibrillation and risk of stroke: The Framingham study. Neurology 28:973, 1978.
14. Sherman DG, Dyken ML, Fisher M, Harrison MJG, Hart RG: Cerebral embolism: Chest 89, Feb. Supplement 82S, 1986.
15. Bar-Sela S, Ehrenfeld M, Eliakim M: Arterial embolism in thyrotoxicosis with atrial fibrillation. Arch Intern Med 141:1191, 1981.
16. Yuen RWM, Gutteridge DH, Thompson PL, Robinson JS: Embolism in thyrotoxic atrial fibrillation. Med J Aust 1:630, 1979.
17. Staffurth JS, Gibberd MC, Fui SNT: Arterial embolism in thyrotoxicosis with atrial fibrillation. Br Med J 2:688, 1977.

ATRIAL FIBRILLATION AND STROKE: THE VIEW FROM NEUROLOGY

David G. Sherman

Department of Medicine(Neurology)
University of Texas Health Science Center
San Antonio, Texas

INTRODUCTION

Atrial fibrillation is the most frequent cardiac disorder associated with ischemic stroke. Most, but certainly not all strokes in patients with atrial fibrillation, are due to an embolus dislodged from a left atrial thrombus. A large number of these patients also have cerebrovascular disease that may be responsible for their stroke. Thus the diagnostic dilemma in these patients is to determine which potential stroke mechanism is in fact responsible for their stroke. Once the mechanism is determined a course of rational, if not scientifically proven, therapy can be instituted. What follows is a summary of our current criteria for the diagnosis of cardiogenic brain embolism, observations on the nature of stroke in patients with nonvalvular atrial fibrillation (NVAF), and some recommendations regarding the anticoagulant management of these patients.

CARDIOGENIC BRAIN EMBOLISM: DIAGNOSIS

About 15% of all ischemic strokes are due to a cardiogenic embolus. The fraction is somewhat higher in young individuals with stroke accounting for 25% of strokes in this group. One-third of patients with stroke or transient ischemic attack(TIA) have a possible cardiac source of emboli. The cardiac source established in half of these patients will be the likely cause of their stroke while the other half will be found to have a vascular lesion that could also have accounted for the focal ischemic event.(1,2) The determination as to whether a stroke or TIA was caused by a cardiogenic embolus rather than by some other mechanism is based on clues obtained from the history, physical examination and ancillary studies. Generally the issue is whether the stroke is due to large or small vessel atherosclerotic disease, the most common cause of stroke and TIA, or caused by a suspected or unsuspected cardiac disorder.(3)

Certain features are suggestive of, but not diagnostic of, a cardiogenic brain embolus. Prior TIAs are uncommon in cardiogenic embolus occurring in only about 10% of these patients. In contrast, about 40% of patients with a stroke due to atherosclerotic vascular disease will have a preceeding TIA.(4) A sudden onset, while awake, of a focal neurologic deficit is typical of a cardiogenic embolism. While a similar onset can occur with an atherothrombotic stroke, a more typical onset is on awakening with a neurolgic deficit that stutters over the next few hours until it finally reaches its maximal level of severity. Loss of consciousness at onset should also raise suspicions of a cardiogenic embolus.(5) A seizure at onset, though traditionally considered to be suggestive of a cardiogenic embolus, has not proven to be valuable in substantiating a cardiac origin for the patient's stroke.(4,5) A prior or coexistent systemic embolus is rare, seen in 2.3% of patients, but when present is strong evidence for a cardiogenic embolus. The vast majority, about 80%, of cardioembolic strokes are localized to the middle cerebral artery circulation. Emboli so frequently lodge in a branch of the middle cerebral artery that clinical presentations such as the sudden onset of a Wernicke's aphasia should alert the physician to the possibility of a cardiogenic thrombus as the source of the stroke. Ischemia at the basilar artery bifurcation, the "top of the basilar" syndrome, territory or the posterior cerebral artery distribution is also commonly due to a cardiogenic embolus.(6) The lacunar syndromes resulting from occlusion of the small penetrating arteries supplying the internal capsule are rarely due to a cardiogenic embolus. The large, so called, "giant lacunes" may occur when an embolus occludes the proximal middle or posterior cerebral artery where these tiny vessels arise. The common lacunar syndromes are pure motor hemiplegia, pure sensory stroke and dysarthria-clumsy hand occurring in a patient with hypertension. Thus a highly suggestive, but by no means specific, clinical presentation for a cardioembolic stroke would be a patient with atrial fibrillation or some other known cardiac disorder who suffers the sudden onset while awake of a TIA or stroke in the cortical middle or posterior cerebral artery territories.

     Computed tomography (CT) may provide evidence favoring a cardiogenic brain embolus. A CT scan done within the first few hours following a stroke is generally normal and serves primarily to exclude intracerebral or other intracranial bleeding and to identify disorders such as brain neoplasms that may mimick stroke or TIA. One may rarely see a small vascular density representing the embolus within the cerebral artery. The scarred remains of prior embolic strokes may also be detected incriminating the heart as the possible source of the stroke. One of the most suggestive CT findings of cardiogenic embolus however is the detection of a hemorrhagic infarct. These infarcts appear as mottled areas of increased density within the region of infarction. Five to fifteen percent of cardiogenic brain embolic infarctions will develop into hemorrhagic infarctions. It may be difficult to differentiate a hemorrhagic infarct from a resolving intracerebral hematoma on CT scan. The presumed mechanism and management implications of hemorrhagic infarction are discussed further in the section on antithrombotic therapy of cardiogenic embolus.

NONVALVULAR ATRIAL FIBRILLATION

     The term nonvavular atrial fibrillation (NVAF) describes a group of individuals with atrial fibrillation not associated with mitral stenosis. Such individuals are generally first recognized to have NVAF during their early 60's with the majority having associated hypertension or ischemic heart disease.(7-10) The prevalence of NVAF increases progressively with advancing age after the age of 55. Two to five percent of the general population over age 60 are affected with this abnormal cardiac rhythm. While it has been long recognized that atrial fibrillation associated with mitral stenosis was an important risk factor for stroke, it is only in recent years that NVAF has come to be recognized as an important risk factor for stroke.(7,11-16) About one-third of individuals with NVAF will suffer a stroke during their life-time.(8,11,13,15) This represents an average annual stroke incidence of 5%. If one surveys all patients with ischemic stroke about 15% are associated with atrial fibrillation.(17-22)

In older patients with stroke i.e. those over 75 years old, the fraction with atrial fibrillation progressively increases occurring in 25- 40% of these cases.

The mere association of NVAF does not guarantee that the NVAF caused the stroke. These patients often have other vascular and cardiac abnormalities that might also have caused the patient's stroke. Clinical and autopsy studies suggest that 50-70% of ischemic strokes in these patients are due to embolization of fragments of left atrial thrombi. (17,19,23,24) The obvious implication of these observations is that one must keep an open mind regarding the presumed stroke pathophysiology and search for vascular or other cardiac lesions that may have produced the patient's stroke.

Risk Factors for Stroke

It is commonly assumed that among those individuals with NVAF there are those with greater or lesser degrees of stroke risk. The most frequently cited potentially important risk factors are the duration of the atrial fibrillation and accompanying cardiac abnormalities. Recent onset atrial fibrillation is presumed to carry an increased risk for stroke based on the observation that of those patients suffering a stroke, NVAF is generally first recognized at the time of the patient's stroke.(8,20,23) Presumably the onset of atrial fibrillation leads to stasis and thrombus formation within the atrium especially the appendage. This thrombus is most friable when recently formed before becoming organized and adherent to the atrial wall. Similar reasoning has been used to incriminate intermittent or paroxysmal atrial fibrillation as a feature carrying increased stroke risk. The increased risk for stroke within days following cardioversion of the unanticoagulated patient with atrial fibrillation also supports this contention.(26) Congestive heart failure conveys an increased risk for embolic stroke in patients with NVAF.(7,11)

One of the more sobering observations with stroke due to NVAF is that it tends to be large and functionally devastating unheralded by a warning TIA. At least half of patients experiencing stroke from NVAF either die or are severely disabled as a consequence of their stroke.(8,13,23,27) No more than 1 in 20 of these patients will be alerted by a prior TIA to the impending stroke.(8) What possible explanation can there be for this tendency of NVAF to produce large strokes rather than TIAs or small strokes? It may be that the fibrillating atrium allows thrombus to form and propagate relatively undisturbed isolated within the atrial appendage. The fragments of this thrombus may be of sufficient size to occlude a major cerebral artery producing a large and disabling or fatal stroke. In contrast the turbulent rush of blood past a diseased heart valve or arterial wall sweeps small loosely attached platelet-fribrin thrombi into the circulation before they have the opportunity to enlarge.

Antithrombotic Therapy

What if any therapy can prevent strokes in patients with NVAF is unknown. Chronic anticoagulation reduces embolic stroke in individuals with mitral stenosis and atrial fibrillation. This observation has led some physicians to chronically anticoagulate selected patients with NVAF considered at increased risk of stroke. Others, driven by fear of potential bleeding complications, prescribe low dose warfarin, aspirin or no antithrombotic therapy pending the results of appropriate clinical trials addressing this issue.

The occurrence of an embolic stroke in a patient with NVAF necessitates a decision regarding anticoagulation. There is a risk of recurrent embolus in such an individual. This risk is on the order of 10-20% in the year following the stroke.(8,13,20,22,23,27) The period of maximal risk is within the first few days such that about 12% of patients with a cardiogenic embolus will suffer a recurrence within the first two weeks. Studies of immediate anticoagulation following cardioembolic stroke suggest that the risk of recurrence can be reduced to one-third.(23,28-33) However, this potential benefit of immediate anticoagulation must be weighed against the increased risk of hemorrhage, particularly brain hemorrhage in those patients. Some reports of immediate anticoagulation have not noted an increased risk of worsening brain hemorrhage.(23,29,34-37) Others have found complications of brain hemorrhage in up to 16% of patients.(22,28,31-33) Given the increased risk for brain hemorrhage in some unselected series of patients, some have addressed the issue of whether or not it is possible to identify a subgroup of patients with an unacceptable increased risk for brain hemorrhage with immediate anticoagulation. The goal of such identification is to provide guidelines as to which patients can be safely anticoagulated following an embolic stroke. In hopes of discovering features conveying undue risk of brain hemorrhage, some 62 cases of hemorrhagic brain infarction were accumulated by the Cerebral Embolism Study Group.(38,39) A number of potentially relevant factors were examined including patient age, nature of any associated cardiac disease, hypertension, level of anticoagulation, CT appearance and infarct size. A consistent finding was that those patients with large cerebral infarcts were much more likely to undergo hemorrhagic tranformation of their infarct. This observation has been made in other clinical and autopsy studies.(33,36,40-42) It was noted that some 10-15% of cardioembolic strokes were destined to undergo hemorrhagic transformation. This hemorrhagic transformation most often takes place without any clinical worsening by the patient. If, however, the patient had been anticoagulated at the time of the embolic stroke or was anticoagulated immediately following their stroke and developed a hemorrhagic infarct, there was a much greater risk for clinical worsening and death from an intracerebral hemorrhage. Thus patients with clinical or CT evidence of a large brain infarct are at particularly increased risk for developing a hemorrhagic infarct whether anticoagulated or not. Should they, however, be anticoagulated their risk for worsening brain hemorrhage increases considerably. From these observations arose the first caution about the use of immediate anticoagulation following embolic stroke. Namely, that immediate anticoagulation should be avoided in patients with large embolic brain infarcts.

In addition to the finding that large infarcts were more prone to hemorrhagic transformation, an interesting observation was made relevant to the timing of hemorrhagic transformation. The presumed sequence of events leading to a hemorrhagic infarction are as follows. An embolus lodges in a cerebral artery occluding its lumen and producing ischemia and infarction in the brain already deprived of blood flow. With the passage of time, generally from several hours to a couple of days, the embolus lyses allowing portions of the ischemic brain to be reperfused. It is at this time that blood may extravasate through ischemic vessel walls into the areas of brain infarction producing a hemorrhagic infarct. The timing of these events is relevant to the decision about when anticoagulants can be safely begun in these patients. Serial CT scans in these patients suggest that within the first 6 hours following a cardioembolic stroke 90% of the 10-15% of embolic strokes destined to undergo hemorrhagic transformation will appear normal or have low density nonhemorrhagic infarcts.(38) Over the next 24-36 hours however, 90% of those destined to undergo hemorrhagic transformation will have done so. The therapeutic implications of these observations are obvious. One cannot rely on a CT scan done within the first few hours following an embolic stroke to reliably exclude those patients at risk for developing hemorrhagic transformation of their infarct. One can however be reasonably assured that a CT scan done around 36-48 hours following the embolic stroke will identify the vast majority of those patients whose brain infarction is destined to undergo hemorrhagic transformation. Other factors that have been suggested as being associated with increased risk of brain hemorrhage with anticoagulation are sustained hypertension (BP>180/110) and the use of bolus heparin therapy.

Based on the above observations the following recommendations have been proposed as guides to the immediate anticoagulation of a cardioembolic stroke. If a cardioembolic etiology is presumed for a stroke, anticoagulation should be initially delayed. A CT scan should be obtained 36-48 hours following the stroke and examined carefully for evidence of hemorrhagic infarction. If present anticoagulants should be delayed for at least 7-10 days. If the CT scan does not reveal evidence of hemorrhagic infarction the size of the infarction must be considered. Due to the risk of hemorrhagic transformation of large infarcts, anticoagulation should be delayed for at least 7-10 days. In addition, patients with blood pressures persistantly elevated above 180/110 should have anticoagulants delayed regardless of the infarct size. Patient with small or medium sized infarcts without hypertension and with no evidence of hemorrhage by CT scan by 36-48 hours can be anticoagulated with hopefully minimal risk of a major brain bleed and the benefit of a reduced risk for recurrent embolic stroke.

SUMMARY

In summary NVAF is an important risk factor for stroke identifying a population at a six fold increased stroke risk. When stroke occurs it tends to be large and without a preceding TIA. These patients commonly have other cardiovascular disorders that must be considered as a potential cause of brain ischemia. The appropriate management of these patients to prevent cardioembolic stroke is unknown and must be individualized pending appropriate clinical trials. Following a cardioembolic stroke anticoagulation should be considered only in patients with small or moderate sized infarcts who have no evidence of hemorrhagic infarction on a CT scan and delayed until 36-48 hours post stroke onset.

REFERENCES

1. Hachinski VC, Rem JA, Boughner DR, Barnett HMJ. The common coincidence of carotid and cardiac lesions. In: Stober T, Schimrigk K, Ganten D, Sherman D, eds. CNS Control of the Heart. Boston, Martinus Nijhoff Pub. 1986 pp 215-220.

2. Bogousslavsky J, Hachinski VC, Boughner DR, Fox AJ, Vinuela F, Barnett HJM. Cardiac and arterial lesions in carotid transient ischemic attacks. Arch Neurol 1986;43:223-228.

3. Cerebral Embolism Task Force. Cardiogenic brain embolism. Arch Neurol 1986;43:71-84.

4. Caplan LR, Hier DB, D'Cruz I. Cerebral embolism in the Michael Reese stroke registry. Stroke 1983;14:530-536.

5. Ramirez-Lassepas M, Cipolle RJ, Bjork RJ, Kowitz JJ, Weber JC, Stein SD. Does cardioembolic stroke have a neurologic profile? In: Stober T, Schimrigk K, Ganten D, Sherman D, eds. CNS Control of the Heart. Boston, Martinus Nijhoff Pub. 1986 pp 211-214.

6. Fisher CM. Posterior cerebral artery syndrome. Can J Neurol Sci 1986;13:232-239.

7.   Brand FN, Abbott RD, Kannel WB, Wolf PA: Characteristics and prognosis of lone atrial fibrillation: 30 year follow-up in the Framingham study. JAMA 1985;254:3449-3453.

8.   Sherman DG, Goldman L, Whiting RB, et al: Risk of thromboembolism in patients with atrial fibrillation. Arch Neurol (Chicago) 1984;41:708-710.

9. Martin A: Atrial fibrillation in the elderly. Brit Med J 1977;1:712-716.

10. Svareborg A: Seventy-year old people in Gothenburg: A population study in an industrialized Swedish city. Acta Med Scand (suppl) 1977;611:5-37.

11. Wolf PA, Dawber TR, Thomas HE, Kannel WB: Epidermiologic assessment of chronic atrial fibrillation and risk of stroke: The Framingham study. Neurology (Minneap) 1978;28:973-977.

12. Takahashi N, Seki A. Imataka K, et al: Clinical features of paroxysmal atrial fibrillation: An observation of 94 patientts. Jap Heart J 1981;22:143-149.

13. Fisher CM: Reducing risks of cerebral embolism. Geriatrics 1979;34:59-66.

14. Aberg H: Atrial fibrillation. Acta Med Scand 1969;185:373-379.

15. Hinton RC, Kistler P, Fallon JR, et al: Influence of etiology of atrial fibrillation on incidence of systemic embolism. Amer J Cardiol 1977;40:509-513.

16. Fairfax AJ, Lambert CD, Leatham A: Systemic embolism in chronic sino-atrial disorder. New Eng J Med 1976;295:190-192.

17. Britton M, Gustafsson C: Nonrheumatic atrial fibrillation as a risk factor for stroke. Stroke 1985;16:182-188.

18. Lovett JL, Sandok BA, Giuliani ER, Nasser FN: Two-dimensional echocardiography in patients with focal cerebral ischemia. Ann Intern Med 1981;95:1-4.

19. Olsen TS, Skriver EB, Herning M: Cause of cerebral infarction in the carotid territory: Its relation to the size and the location of the infarct and to the underlying vascular lesion. Stroke 1985;16:459-465.

20. Wolf PA1, Kannel WB, McGee DL: Duration of atrial fibrillation and imminence of stroke: The Framingham study. Stroke 1983;14:664-667.

21. Harrison MJG, Marshall J: Atrial fibrillation. TIAs and completed strokes. Stroke 1984;15:441-442.

22. Kelley RE, Berger JR, Alter M, Kovacs AG: Cerebral ischemia and atrial fibrillation: Prospective study. Neurology (Minneap) 1984;34:1285-1291.

23. Hart RG, Coull BM, Hart D: Early recurrent embolism associated with nonvalvular atrial fibrillation. A retrospective study. Stroke 1983;14:688-693.

24. Mohr JP, Caplan LR, Melski JW, et al: The Harvard Cooperative Stroke Registry: A prospective registry. Neurology (Minneap) 1978;28:754-762.

25. Josrgensen L, Torvik A: Ischemic cerebrovascular diseases in an autopsy series. J Neurol Sci 1966;3:490-509.

26. Bjerkeland CJ, Orning OM: The efficacy of anticoagulant therapy in preventing embolism related to D.C. electrical conversion of atrial fibrillation. Amer J Cardiol 1969;23:208-216.

27. Sage JI, Van Uitert RL: Risk of recurrent stroke with atrial fibrillation: Difference between rheumatic and atherosclerotic heart disease. Stroke 1983;14:537-540.

28. Shields RW Jr, Laureno R, Lachman T, et al: Anticoagulant-induced hemorrhage in acute cerebral embolism. Stroke 1984;15:426-437.

29. Furlan AJ, Cavalier SJ, Hobbs RE, et al: Hemorrhage and anticoagulation after nonseptic embolic brain infarction. Neurology 1982;32:280-282.

30. Koller RL: Recurrent embolic cerebral infarction and anticoagulation. Neurology 1982;32:283-285.

31. Bass E: Anticoagulation in cedrebral embolism. Can J Neurol Sci 1983;10:32-36.

32. Calandre L, Ortego JF, Berbemo F, et al: Anticoagulation and hemorrhagic infarction in cerebral embolism secondary to rheumatic heart disease Arch Neurol 1984;41:1153-1154.

33. Martias-Guiu J, Alvarez J, Davalos A, et al: Heparin therapy for stroke. Neurology 1984;34:1619-1620.

34. Cerebral Embolism Study Group: Immediate anticoagulation of embolic stroke: A randomized trial. Stroke 1983;14:668-676.

35. Lodder J, van der Lugt PJM: Evaluation of the risk of immediate anticoagulant treatment in patients with embolic stroke of cardiac origin. Stroke 1983;14:42-46.

36. Lodder J: CT-detected hemorrhagic infarction: Relation with the size of the infarct, and presence of midline shift. Acta Neurol Scand 1984;70:329-335.

37. Martin GJ, Biller J: Nonseptic cerebral emboli of cardiac origin. Arch Intern Med 1984;144:1997-1999.

38. Cerebral Embolism Study Group: Timing of hemorrhagiic transformation of cardioembolic stroke. In: Stober T, Schimrigk K, Ganten D, Sherman D, eds. CNS Control of the Heart. Boston, Martinus Nijhoff Pub. 1986 pp229-232.

39. Cerebral Embolism Study Group: Brain hemorrhage in embolic stroke. In: Stober T, Schimrigk K, Ganten D, Sherman D, eds. CNS Control of the Heart. Boston, Martinus Nijhoff Pub. 1986 pp 249-253.

40. Cerebral Embolism Study Group. Immediate anticoagulation of embolic stroke: Brain hemorrhage and management options. Stroke 1984;15:779-789.

41. Bingham WF: Treatment of mycotic antracranial aneurysms. J Neurosurg 1977;46:428-437.

42. Drake ME, Shin C: Conversion of ischemic to hemorrhagic infarction by anticoagulant administration: Report of two cases with evidence from serial computed tomographic brain scans. Arch Neurol 1983;40:44-46.

CARDIAC EMBOLIC STROKE: ANTICOAGULATING THE ELDERLY

Stanford Wessler

Department of Medicine
New York University School of Medicine
New York, New York

SCOPE OF THE PROBLEM

Stroke remains the third commonest cause of death in the United States. Cerebral infarcts from cardiac emboli represent a progressively increasing percentage of strokes, as non-traumatic cerebral hemorrhages secondary to hypertension continue to decline. In no age group is this increase in cerebral infarction from cardiac emboli more apparent than in the elderly. 75 per cent of individuals over age 85 are not in nursing homes;[1] yet an increasing number of these individuals remain at risk of premature death or disability from an embolic stroke.

In 1981 there were 164,000 deaths from stroke and an additional 1,870,000 stroke survivors.[2] It has been estimated that approximately 15 per cent of these strokes were caused by cardiac emboli.[2-4] Some clinical surveys demonstrate an incidence as high as 23%[5] and necropsy data suggest that cardiac emboli to the brain may be even more frequent.[6,7] If, however, anticoagulant prophylaxis could prevent even one-half of the 15 per cent of strokes referable to cardiac sources, then over 12,000 lives would be saved annually and 140,000 additional individuals would be spared disabling, neurologic deficits. Such results would compare favorably with the benefits achieved in the United States from either the prevention of poliomyelitis by vaccination or of rheumatic heart disease by penicillin.

At the present time convincing clinical trials are lacking to justify, by themselves, the widespread administration of anticoagulant prophylaxis to achieve these goals in the elderly. Some experienced clinicians believe the available data are sufficiently strong to recommend prospective anticoagulation among subsets of cardiac patients;[4] whereas others, examining the same information base, prefer delaying such a broad prophylactic recommendation until more convincing evidence of anticoagulant efficacy becomes available.[7]

The physician, therefore, is confronted by a not unusual dilemma in clinical medicine, wherein a therapeutic decision must be implemented or withheld based on incomplete information--a situation not unlike that described by Samuel Butler when he wrote in 1912: "Life is the art of drawing sufficient conclusions from insufficient premises".[8]

Many of these cardiac embolic strokes occur among the elderly. It has been estimated, for example, that 5 per cent of patients over age 70 have atrial fibrillation;[9] and in one report strokes among fibrillators averaged 20 per cent per year throughout a nine-year observation period.[10] These percentages take on even greater meaning when the over-age 85 group that is today just over 2 million, is projected to rise to over 5 million in less than 15 years.

AN APPROACH TO PROPHYLAXIS

One may begin by acknowledging that at least 4 propositions appear to be accepted by the majority of knowledgeable investigators familiar with the area under review. (1) Clinically apparent cardiac emboli to the brain occur among only an exceedingly small percentage of the vast number of patients with heart disease; this remains true even among those subsets of patients with the types of cardiac pathology most prone to cerebral embolism. (2) Cardiac cerebral emboli are usually unheralded by any prodromata including transient ischemic attacks. (3) These emboli, frequently causing large infarcts, are often associated with extensive edema that can itself produce damaging mass pressure effects on adjacent non-infarcted cerebral tissue. (4) Recurrence is common and most frequent in the days to weeks immediately following the initial insult.

Several therapeutic implications can be derived from these 4 propositions. First, one must be prepared (even after a careful preselection among the most stroke-susceptible cardiac lesions) to treat several hundred patients to prevent one stroke. Accordingly, the benefit/risk ratio as well as the benefit/cost ratio must be readily acceptable for the population to receive therapy. Second, large infarcts, with their inherent risk of extensive cerebral edema, may preclude secondary anticoagulant prophylaxis. Finally, because recurrence rates are high, therapy will be prolonged if not indefinite, unless the cardiac lesion responsible for embolization is actually eliminated.

It is only in the past decade, and particularly in the last 5 years, that critical information has become available in 3 areas that has offered new dimensions to the use of anticoagulants in both the primary and secondary prevention of stroke from cardiac emboli and particularly so in the elderly. These areas are : (1) cardiac imaging and the epidemiologic identification of embolus-prone cardiac populations, (2) the relation of computed tomography and nuclear magnetic imaging to the pathology of cerebral infarction, and (3) improvements in the benefit/risk ratio of anticoagulant prophylaxis.

CRITERIA FOR ANTICOAGULATION AFTER CEREBRAL INFARCTION

Until the advent of the widespread availability of CT scanning, the prompt antemortem distinction between cerebral hemorrhage and infarction was fraught with uncertainty. Today, it is possible, through CT, to identify immediately and with remarkable assurance symptomatic cerebral bleeding outside an infarcted area no matter what the cause, and eliminate these patients from further consideration for anticoagulation. However, in contrast to this early identification of hemorrhage, it is during the fourth to eighth day after ictus that CT may reach its greatest sensitivity in recognizing infarction.[11] MRI, although it can easily identify a lesion on day one, cannot discriminate well between hemorrhage and infarction in the first 48 to 72 hours. Therefore, at the present time, the clinician can choose between 2 approaches: (1) perform MRI first to demonstrate a lesion, followed promptly by CT only to rule out hemorrhage if a lesion is seen; or (2), perform a CT scan initially which, if negative in the presence of a typical stroke syndrome, is diagnostic of an infarct, since extensive hemorrhage or a large tumor have been ruled out. For pragmatic reasons the latter alternative is probably preferable.

In so far as the distinction between hemorrhage beyond or within the infarcted area is concerned, CT has also been decisive. Of comparable importance has been the capacity of CT to distinguish, within the infarcted area, between isolated petechial, confluent petechial and gross or massive hemorrhage. Petechial hemorrhage within the infarct, as identified by CT, is not aggravated by anticoagulants.

Whether and when to initiate anticoagulant therapy after a cerebral infarction has occurred are particularly controversial. Such controversy can be minimized, however, by recalling some of the pertinent changes in the brain that result from vascular occlusion. In the early stages of infarction the involved tissue is edematous occupying an increased volume. This usually begins to recede within one to two weeks of stroke onset. But, if the infarct is large, the swollen tissue may cause narrowing of an adjacent ventricle and may even produce herniation and secondary brain stem hemorrhage.[12] Following vascular occlusion the infarcted area frequently contains focal or confluent petechial hemorrhages. At autopsy infarcts may be entirely ischemic, but more usually will reveal slight, moderate or extensive hemorrhage. Even when severe, these hemorrhages differ pathologically and by CT from the massive cerebral hemorrhage due to rupture of a small intracerebral artery, as in hypertensive disease. As noted from the CT data, petechial hemorrhage within necrotic brain tissue, is part and parcel of the cerebral necrotic process and is not aggravated by anticoagulant therapy.[12,13]

The proportion of patients with cerebral infarction in whom no vascular occlusion can be demonstrated at necropsy is disturbingly high and cannot be ascribed to venous obstruction or undisclosed disease of the arteries in the neck. There are, fortunately, instances in which a simple straightforward pathogenetic mechanism is demonstrable, as when an occlusion of a single large cerebral artery is associated with a cerebral infarct in its precise area of distribution and each is of a similar age. Although such cases form only a small minority, they do establish the pathological characteristics of infarction so that an infarct can be recognized in the absence of vascular disease. It has been reported that hemorrhages are found almost exclusively in infarcts that are embolic in origin;[14] but such an exclusive relationship between emboli and hemorrhagic infarcts is not a uniform opinion.[12,13] Since the spontaneous lysis of coronary artery thrombi is a well documented finding,[15,16] there is no reason to discriminate a priori against similar phenomena occurring within intracerebral arteries. For it is possible (though as yet unproven) that a thrombus may form and persist long enough to produce an infarct (in minutes) and then be lysed before it can undergo organization.

Since the bleeding occurs from numerous capillaries within a zone of necrotic brain, hemorrhages are multiple and petechial or appear as a confluence of petechial hemorrhages. In gross cerebral hemorrhage, a phenomenon characteristically related to hypertensive rather than atherosclerotic disease, the bleeding occurs most often from a single large vessel, often an artery, with the formation of a mass of relatively pure blood passing into and excavating essentially normal brain tissue, the latter altered only secondarily by the hemorrhage.

Most of these pathologic observations and interpretations, made in an era preceding CT and MRI, have been confirmed by the latter techniques and nothing found by them has contradicted any of these pathologic findings.

Minute petechial hemorrhages, in fact, that are beyond CT resolution have been recognized at autopsy. Although cerebral angiography can identify some cerebral artery occlusions, this is not invariably the case and when occlusions are found the distinction between embolus and thrombus is not always apparent. Finally, cerebral angiography is not itself without risk.

As a result of this analysis, combining clinical, CT and pathologic observations, it becomes difficult to escape the conclusion that it is the cerebral infarct recognized by CT, rather than the vascular occlusion, that provides the key piece of information in deciding whether anticoagulants should even be considered for patients with a clinical stroke.[17]

Accordingly, following a stroke, it can be recommended that 2 CT scans be obtained: the first on day 1 or 2, the second between days 5 and 7. If the patient is neither obtunded nor showing evidence of clinical deterioration and if there is no hemorrhage outside the infarcted area; then the patient becomes a <u>potential</u> candidate for anticoagulation.[17] In the overwhelming majority of these patients a lumbar puncture is not only unnecessary, but represents a potential site for bleeding, if anticoagulants are administered.[18]

Such recommendations are not likely to be readily acceptable to all physicians. There are those who, in selected stroke patients, would opt for earlier anticoagulation after one CT scan, because they believe that in these patients the risk of worsening the infarct is negligible, whereas if anticoagulants are administered promptly, the likelihood of a second thromboembolic episode is diminished. Although this is a tenable position from a safety point of view, it must be recognized that prompt anticoagulation would be unlikely to prevent a second embolization within 2-4 days after the first, because studies in animals have demonstrated that it may take 3-4 days for partial adherence of a freshly formed bland thrombus to the endothelial wall to occur and 8-12 days for organization of the lesion to become extensive.[19,20] Even at that time a thrombus may be pedunculated and susceptible to fragmentation so that the threat of embolization may persist unpredictably for weeks or longer. There is another group of physicians who prefer to wait 2 or more weeks after infarction to initiate anticoagulant prophylaxis, because of concern that even a 7-day delay may be inadequate to provide assurance that anticoagulants will not seriously augment intra-infarct hemorrhage.[21] Finally, there are still others who believe it is inappropriate, on the basis of current knowledge, to anticoagulate patients with stroke and atrial fibrillation unless they also have rheumatic heart disease.[7] At present, physicians must make their own decisions as to which of these options is most prudent: there is still a role here for clinical judgment, and the same physician might, for different patients, choose different times at which to initiate prophylaxis or to forego anticoagulation altogether.

Using the CT-diagnosed infarct as the basis for considering anticoagulation may concern some who would question whether this approach should include acute strokes originating in the carotid and basilar-vertebral systems, whether the concept should apply to strokes secondary to hemorrhage in a cerebral artery placque, or to the lacunar infarcts usually seen in hypertensive patients. For any of these patients in whom emboli presumably did not come from the heart, however, there exists still another indication for anticoagulation as long as the patient is sufficiently incapacitated by the stroke as to be limited to a bed or a bed and chair existence, if only for days to weeks. This indication is the risk of venous thromboembolism. The incidence of deep venous thrombosis among stroke patients, as demonstrated by ^{125}I fibrinogen limb scans, has been reported as high as 53 percent[22] and among this group anticoagulants can prevent pulmonary emboli.[23]

RISK FACTORS

Additional concerns that affect benefit/risk ratios particularly applicable to the elderly in both short and long-term anticoagulant prophylaxis after embolic stroke need also to be addressed.

Hypertension

In further consideration of hypertension as a risk factor for cerebral hemorrhage beyond what has already been stated at this symposium, two additional observations are warranted. One is that transient elevations of blood pressure may accompany acute cerebral infarction; the other that normotensive individuals may develop hypertension months to years after initiation of prophylaxis. These observations provide not only an additional reason for delaying the administration of anticoagulation after acute infarction, but also stress the importance of periodic evaluation, especially in the elderly, so that if hypertension develops, attempts can be initiated to treat it effectively.

Aspirin

Many patients who sustain a cardiac embolic stroke are already on a maintainance dose of aspirin for a variety of other conditions including cardiovascular disease. If anticoagulants are to be administered, aspirin should be discontinued. Since the aspirin effect on platelets is irreversible, since the half life of the platelet is approximately 4 days, and since anticoagulants and aspirin together represent an increased risk of bleeding, these observations provide still another reason for delaying the initiation of anticoagulant therapy until after the second CT scan 5-7 days following stroke onset.

Falls Among The Elderly

Falls among the elderly in the absence of anticoagulants are a major health hazard. Of the 11,600 individuals killed by falls in the U.S. in 1984, 58% occurred in those over age 75.[24] One-half of the fatalities were from concussion or cerebral hemorrhage. The remainder of the deaths were from pulmonary embolism, bronchopneumonia or respiratory failure. Osteoporosis, to cite one risk factor, is responsible for 1.2 million fractures in the U.S. annually, more than a quarter of a million of which are hip fractures. By extreme old age one of every three women and one of every six men will have had a hip fracture **and these are fatal in 12 to 20 percent of cases.**[25] Several analyses have been published indicating that falls among the elderly appear to result from the accumulated effect of multiple specific disabilities some of which are remedial.[26] Particular steps that families of patients or patients themselves can take to minimize the likelihood of falling have been published.[27,28]

The unanswered question is whether a low-dose warfarin regimen would, in actual fact, facilitate or aggravate a cerebral hemorrhage secondary to a fall. Each physician must resolve this dilemma based on his evaluation of the likelihood of a major head injury from a fall against the likelihood of a cerebral embolism. For example, if the patient is not a frequent faller and one who could be helped to avoid falling, such patients, if they have a prosthetic heart valve or atrial fibrillation, should be anticoagulated. Part of the periodic reevaluation which involves blood pressure determinations, should also include the evaluation of the likelihood of a patient

REGIMEN	HEPARIN (u/24h)	WARFARIN (PT RATIO) US	INR
LOW	10-20,000	1.3-1.7	2.0-3.5
MEDIUM	24-50,000	1.6-1.9	3.0-4.2
HIGH	60-80,000	1.8-2.1	3.9-5.0

falling. Tests to determine the risk of a fall have also been published.[26] Ironically, low-dose warfarin may be desirable prophylaxis, if the fall results in a hip fracture instead of a cerebral hemorrhage. Lethal pulmonary embolism is not a rare complication of hip fracture and warfarin in low doses may prevent this untoward outcome.[29]

Age and Sex

It has not been established that either age or sex, per se, represent an increased risk of hemorrhage, provided the patient is hemostatically competent and the anticoagulant regimens are prudent.

ANTICOAGULANT REGIMENS

And, finally, we come to anticoagulant regimens. What dose can be recommended for patients 5-7 days after a cerebral infarct? What dose can be suggested for long-term maintenance or for patients, particularly among the elderly, for the primary prevention of cardiac embolization?

The figure lists 3 regimens of increasing intensity that appear to have some general acceptance. The low dose schedules for heparin range from 10 to 20,000 units per 24 hours and for warfarin, using rabbit thromboplastin the ratios are from 1.3-1.7. The medium and high intensity ranges are also shown without overlap for heparin and with overlap for warfarin. One can discard immediately the high dose ranges for both drugs as being too likely to lead to major hemorrhage. Among the group of elderly individuals under discussion, a question can be raised as to whether the intermediate range should also be excluded at least as a broad recommendation.

The clinical trials at McMaster University,[30] strongly suggest that 20,000 units of heparin per 24 hours are approximately equipotent with a prothrombin time ratio of 1.3 Both drugs have efficacy against recurrent venous thromboembolism and incur only occasional minor bleeding. Although not yet fully supported by clinical trials, it can be suggested on the basis of current evidence that, for the prevention of embolic stroke in the elderly patient, the anticoagulant regimen should begin with subcutaneous heparin 10,000 units twice daily, overlapped with warfarin maintained at a prothrombin time ratio range between 1.3-1.5. If the ratio dropped to 1.2 there would still be some antithrombotic effect and if the ratio rose to 1.6 it would be unlikely for a major hemorrhage to develop. The regimen just mentioned would probably offer an 80% chance of preventing cardiac embolic stroke while being essentially devoid of a major coumarin-induced hemorrhage. Increasing warfarin intensity to the intermediate range would increase the antithrombotic potency of the drug, but it would also increase the likelihood of a major hemorrhage. In short, if cardiac emboli cannot be prevented by a low-dose anticoagulant regimen, the drug should perhaps not be employed on a wide scale for the prevention of cardiac embolic stroke among the elderly.

REFERENCES

1. Population estimates and projections. U.S. Dept. Commerce, Bureau of the Census Series P-25 #965(1985).

2. M. L. Dyker, P. A. Wolf, H. J. M. Barnett, et al: Risk factors in stroke. A statement for physicians by the subcommittee on risk factors and stroke of the stroke council. Stroke 15:1105(1984).

3. G. J. Martin, J. Biller, Nonseptic cerebral emboli of cardiac origin. Arch Int Med 144:1997(1984).

4. Cerebral Embolism Task Force: Cardiogenic brain embolism. Arch Neurol 43:71(1986).

5. P. A. Wolf, W. Kannel, D. L. McGee, et al: Duration of atrial fibrillation and imminence of stroke: The Framingham Study. Stroke 14:664(1983).

6. A. Torvik, L, Jorgensen: Thrombotic and embolic occlusions of the carotid arteries in an autopsy material. Part I, Prevalence, location and associated diseases. J Neurol Sci 1:24(1964).

7. I. Starkey, C. Warlow: The secondary prevention of stroke in patients with atrial fibrillation. Arch Neurol 43:66(1986).

8. S. Butler: The Note-books of Samuel Butler, London, A C Fifield, p 11(1912).

9. A. J. Moss: Atrial fibrillation and cerebral embolism. Arch Neurol 41:707(1984).

10. J. Sage, R. Van Uitert: Risk of recurrent stroke in patients with atrial fibrillation and non-valvular heart disease. Stroke 14:537(1983).

11. J. K. Campbell, O. W. Houser, J. C. Stevens, H. W. Wahner, H. L. Baker, W. N. Folger: Computed tomography and radionuclide imaging in the evaluation of ischemic stroke. Radiology 126:702(1978).

12. I. Feigen, G. W. Budzilovich: The general pathology of cerebrovascular disease. In: Handbook of Clinical Neurology vol 11, Vinken P.J. Bruyn G. W. eds. North Holland Publishing Co. Amsterdam, pp 128(1972).

13. A. M. Hakim, A. Ryder-Cooke, D. Melanson: Sequential computerized tomographic appearance of strokes. Stroke 14:893(1983).

14. M. Fisher, R. D. Adams: Observations on brain embolism with special reference to the mechanism of hemorrhagic infarction. J Neuropathol Exp Neurol 10:92(1950).

15. F. Khaja, J. A. Walton Jr., J. F. Brymer, et al. Intracoronary fibrinolytic therapy in acute myocardial infarction. Report of a prospective randomized trial. N Engl J Med 308:1305(1983).

16. K. P. Rentrop, F. Feit, H. Blanke, et al. Effects of intracoronary streptokinase and intracoronary nitroglycerin infustion on coronary angiographic patterns and mortality in patients with acute myocardial infarction. N Engl J Med 311:1457(1984).

17. S. Wessler, Is anticoagulant prophylaxis of cardiac emboli practical? Geriatrics (in press).

18. Health and Public Policy Committee, American College of Physicians. The diagnostic spinal tap. Ann Int Med 104:880(1986).

19. H. M. Marin, M. Stefanini: Experimental production of phlebothrombosis. Surg Gynec Obst 110:263(1960).

20. S. Wessler: Thrombosis in the presence of vascular stasis. Am J Med 33:648(1962).

21. C. R. Hornig, W. Dorndorf, A. L. Agnoli: Hemorrhagic cerebral infarction--a prospective study. Stroke 17:179(1986).

22. C. P. Warlow, D. Ogston, A. S. Douglas: Deep venous thrombosis of the legs after strokes. Part I. Incidence and predisposing factors, Lancet 1:1178(1976).

23. A. T. Miyamoto, L. S. Miller: Pulmonary embolism in stroke: prevention by early heparinization of venous thrombosis detected by iodine-125 fibrinogen leg scans. Arch Phys Med Rehab 61:584(1980).

24. National Safety Council Accident Facts, p 83 (1985).
25. S. R. Cummings, J. L. Kelsey, M. C. Nevitt, K. J. O'Dowd. Epidemiology of osteoporosis and osteoporotic fractures. Epidemiol Rev 7:178(1985).
26. M. E. Tinetti, T. F. Williams, R. Mayewski: Fall risk index for elderly patients based on number of chronic disabilities. Am J Med 80:429 (1986).
27. D. Allen: Falls--big worry for the elderly. Family Safety 38:23(1979).
28. M. Peszczynski: Why people fall. Am J Nursing 65:86(1965).
29. R. A. Nishimura, M. D. McGoon, C. Shub, et al. Echocardiographically documented mitral-valve prolapse. Long-term follow-up of 237 patients. N Engl J Med 313:1305(1985).
30. R. Hull, T. Delmore, C. Carter, et al: Adjusted subcutaneous heparin versus warfarin sodium in the long-term treatment of venous thrombosis. N Engl J Med 306:189(1982).

ANTICOAGULANTS FOR THE TREATMENT OF TRANSIENT ISCHEMIC ATTACKS

Fletcher H. McDowell

The Burke Rehabilitation Center
785 Mamaroneck Avenue
White Plains, NY   10605

Anticoagulants as a treatment for Transient Ischemic Attacks were originally suggested over 30 years ago. After 30 years of study and many clinical reports covering their use plus several specifically conducted studies to evaluate their effectiveness, there is no unanimity of opinion now whether or not they are a useful treatment for the prevention of recurrent transient ischemic attacks and whether they reduce the possibility of stroke in the future (6,11,23,47).

Until the advent of data suggesting that aspirin or agents which prevent platelet aggregation were effective in reducing the frequency of transient ischemic attacks and subsequent stroke, anticoagulants were considered, despite the lack of absolute certainty of effectiveness, the therapy of choice for patients with transient ischemic attacks. Even today, often coumadin anticoagulants are given on a regular basis to individuals who are having transient ischemic attacks, especially during the period of their evaluation.

A review of the basis of the problem of whether or not coumadin anticoagulants are useful for the treatment of transient ischemic attacks follows, and some conclusions about the matter are made.

The problem is complicated in a number of ways. First, there has been no unanimity of opinion on a precise definition of a transient ischemic attack. Second, there has been no unanimity of opinion on the natural history of transient ischemic attacks, whether all patients who have them, go on to have subsequent stroke or whether they represent in a large portion of patients, a benign phenomenon. Third, over the past 30 years, there have been changing concepts about the causation of transient ischemic attacks which have affected evaluation of anticoagulants. Fourth, there has been no uniform methodology for the study of the effects of anticoagulants. Fifth, there is no clear understanding of how Coumadin anticoagulants stop TIA, if they do. Sixth, all reports on the use of anticoagulants in the treatment of patients with TIA have flaws, and they are difficult to compare one to another. Seventh, statistical evaluation of the results of treatment has varied in quality and quantity. Eighth, it has been rare in studies that the effects of Coumadin anticoagulants on reduction of transient ischemic attacks and subsequent stroke have been separated from the complications of using anticoagulants which have some evidence of being preventable.

It is not clear when the concept of transient ischemic attacks developed. It was after the early papers of Millikan and Miller Fisher, that the concept of ischemia was added to the observation that patients frequently had transient attacks of what resembled small strokes prior to a permanent neurological deficit. It is however interesting that the concept of premonitory symptoms suggesting cerebral infarction was recognized and written about in textbooks of neurology such as Gowers as early as 1893 when he stated in his Manual of Diseases of the Nervous System (25), "In thrombosis from atheroma on the other hand, the premonitory symptoms are frequent. They depend on the interference with the supply of blood due to the disease of the vessels. They may exist for months before onset or only for a few hours. The most common symptoms are dull general headache, giddiness, tingling, numbness, slight weakness in one half of the body, sometimes limited to a single limb and often but not always, corresponding in seat the subsequent paralysis. Less commonly, there is defective articulation or some mental change, failure of memory or irritability due to the general malnutrition of the brain that is produced by widespread arterial disease. In all cases, their presence is far more significant than their absence."

This description by Gowers covers most of the recognized clinical points of what we now believe constitute a transient ischemic attack and also highlight one of the most likely reasons for their occurrence. J. Ramsey Hunt, in his article, written in 1914 on The Relation of Carotid Occlusion to the Cause of Stroke also noted (28), "that is important also to note that the visual disturbance and vascular changes in the optic nerve may precede other organic cerebral symptoms, the collateral circulation failing to develop in the distribution of the ophthalmic artery. Unilateral headaches and vertigo, especially assuming the upright posture, epileptic attacks, failing memory, attacks of threatened hemiplegia, cerebral intermittent claudication are some of the vascular symptoms that should suggest the possibility of carotid obstruction."

Wilson, in his textbook on Neurology noted that (56), "Promontory signs lacking in embolism are often conspicuous in thrombotic cases more so than hemorrhagic, days or weeks before and they may give the observer and inkling of what is likely to occur. Here comprised headache, not infrequently on the same side as the commencing damage, vertigo, defective memory, transient confusion of thought and more specifically heaviness or momentary weakness, numb feeling or other paresthesia in the limb or limbs that are on the verge of becoming involved." Whether such symptoms constitute minor antecedent or merely indicate general vascular trouble is immaterial. They are the straws which show how the intracranial wind is blowing.

The older writers on cerebral vascular disease recognized that fleeting attacks of symptoms suggested the possibility of developing stroke as long as one hundred or more years ago. Attention was again called to the occurrence of these attacks in the early 50's by Miller Fisher and it was first suggested by Millikan that anticoagulants might be useful in stopping these attacks and preventing stroke.

Most of the studies of transient ischemic attacks in the past have have not had a consistent definition of what symptoms constitutes one of these attacks. This has made comparison of one study to another difficult. In some studies the diagnostic criteria were exacting while in others patients were included who by present standards probably did not have transient ischemic attacks. Currently accepted criteria for the diagnosis of a transient ischemic attack usually include the following (6,10,31,41): First there is virtually always a sudden onset of a focal neurological deficit developing over a matter of minutes, and usually

CAROTID SYSTEM TIA

Rapid Onset 2-3 min.

Duration 2-30 min.

SYMPTOMS

Unilateral weakness - arm, face, leg

Unilateral numbness - arm, face, leg

Dysphasia or Dysarthria

Transient monocular visual loss

FIGURE 1

lasting no more than 20 to 30 minutes, with a swift return to normal function. By general agreement, the duration of neurologic disability, is not longer than 24 hours. If it lasts longer than this, the patient is believed to have had a mild permanent stroke. Two types of transient ischemic attacks are recognized, those that are associated with alterations in the circulation in the part of the brain supplied by the carotid arteries and those that are caused by alterations in the circulation in areas of the brain supplied by the vertebral and basilar artery system. For the patient who is having symptoms due to alterations in the circulation in the brain supplied by the carotid artery, as seen in Figure 1, the most common history is one of the sudden onset of weakness or paralysis on one side of the body, most often in an upper extremity, or the occurrence of clumsiness in performance of skilled movements in the extremities on the same side. Frequently, patients will be aware of a droop of the face on one side. Often they may complain of loss of feeling or numbness in the face or arm with paresthesias on one side of the body. The most reliable evidence of a transient ischemic attack is a history of motor impairment. Usually a patient is quite aware of this because it generally interferes with the skilled movements of a hand, and the usual dexterity in manipulating objects. If the cerebral flow is decreased in the dominant cerebral hemisphere, the patient will almost invariably have some transient word finding difficulty or more obvious evidence of dysphasia. In some patients, the symptoms of transient ischemia will consist only of loss of vision or reduced vision in one eye and they may report that they have had painless unilateral blindness lasting five to ten minutes with normal vision reappearing rather rapidly. Homonymous visual field defects are rarely noticed by the patient. All of the clinical phenomena are reported as a decrease or absence of function coming on all at once with no suggestion of slow progression.

For those patients who have transient ischemic attacks due to changes in blood flow in the brain supplied by the vertebral basilar arteries, the onset, as with other transient ischemic attacks, is swift and the episode rarely lasts more than 30 minutes. With transient ischemic attacks in the areas of the brain supplied by the vertebral and basilar artery, the range of symptomatology is wider and at times a little less definite, as seen in Figure 2, generally, the most commonly reported symptoms are a deficit in motor performance with weakness or clumsiness of arms or legs or a brief loss of postural tone. There may be combinations of weakness of an arm on one side, along with weakness of a leg on the other, or the patient may actually become briefly quadriplegic. The episodes of sensory loss can represent a variety of combinations of numbness or paresthesia in both

VERTEBRAL BASILAR SYSTEM TIA

Rapid onset 2-5 min.

Duration   2-30 min

SYMPTOMS

Unilateral, bilateral or shifting weakness

and sensory loss, ataxia, imbalance,

dysequilibrium, Dysarthria

Homonymous visual loss or blindness

Diplopia

Combinations of the above

FIGURE 2

arms, both legs, the face on one side and the arm or leg on the other side
or all four extremities. There may be loss of vision with complete
blindness to partial blindness in both fields of vision. Usually the
visual field defects are homonymous. With brainstem ischemia, the patient
may complain of double vision, difficulty with maintaining equilibrium and
occasionally vertigo without the sensation of nausea. Patients may report
difficulty with enunciation and problems with swallowing. These criteria
while generally accepted now were not universally adhered to.

It is generally accepted that a diagnosis of a transient ischemic
attacks caused by cerebral blood flow changes in the brain supplied by the
vertebral or basilar artery should not be made unless the symptoms consist
of more than brief episodes of dizziness. There should be other evidence
of brainstem ischemia such as diplopia, weakness or sensory loss before a
definite diagnosis can be made.

Virtually all diagnoses of transient ischemic attacks are made from
the history obtained from the patient. It is extremely rare for a
physician to actually observe a patient having an attack because of their
short duration and the often minimal symptoms and signs which accompany
the attack. Careful inquiry therefore is necessary to make an accurate
diagnosis.

PREVALENCE OF TIA AMONG PATIENTS WITH STROKE

4-75% reported

1/3-1/2 of all patients

PREVALENCE OF TIA IN POPULATION STUDIES

1 per 1,000 to 63 per 1,000

FIGURE 3

The prevalence of transient ischemic attacks has been under study for 30 years and there still is no agreement on the exact percentage of the population who have these attacks. The reported percentage of patients who have had transient ischemic attacks before major strokes, varies widely, the range is from 4% to 75%, Figure 3. Studies indicate that one third to one half of the patients will have had some symptoms prior to their stroke which could be construed as being a transient ischemic attack. The frequency of transient ischemic attacks is clearly age related and the highest incidence occurs in individuals over 65 years of age.

Originally, it was believed that transient ischemic attacks invariably were followed within a relatively short period of time, by an ischemic stroke. Careful follow-up of patients who have had transient ischemic attacks reveal that the natural history is not quite so ominous, as many patients were found to spontaneously stop having these attacks; many patients had only one or more attacks and had no further trouble; some patients continued to have attacks for long periods and some rapidly developed cerebral infarction (1,24,32,33,35,40,41,57). In Figure 4, it can be seen that study of the natural history of untreated transient ischemic attacks, reveals that there is a wide variation in the data concerning the number of patients who will ultimately have a cerebral infarction within five years, the range being 25% to 40% of patients. It is likely that about one third of the patients who develop true transient ischemic attacks will go on to have a cerebral infarction. A third may stop having attacks and a third of the patients may continue to have attacks without developing cerebral infarction. It is now generally accepted that in a five year period, one third of the patients who have transient ischemic attacks will have a cerebral infarction giving an incidence of about 5% per year (55). The chance of having a cerebral infarction following the onset of transient ischemic attacks is not uniformly spread throughout this 5 year period. Cerebral infarction is most likely during the first year following the onset of the attacks, the period of the greatest danger. In the first year, one half of the patients will have a cerebral infarction within the first thirty days after the onset. Despite the fact that the chance of developing a cerebral infarction following the onset of transient ischemic attacks is greatest during the first few weeks after their onset, those patients who have these attacks still have an approximately 5% chance per year of having a stroke. This is about five times the expected rate of stroke for a similar age and sex matched population.

NATURAL HISTORY OF PATIENTS WITH TIA

25-40% of patients have a stroke in 5 years

20% of strokes occur in first 30 days after
    onset of TIA

5% per year will have stroke after the first
    6 months

FIGURE 4

The occurrence of transient ischemic attacks is an important warning symptom identifying those individuals who are at considerable risk of developing a cerebral infarction and serious permanent neurological disability. Unfortunately, as valuable as this set of warning symptoms is, it has not been particularly helpful in dealing with the overall problem of cerebral infarction. Frequently, the attacks are followed so quickly by cerebral infarction and neurologic disability that there is no chance for a therapy to be started which will effectively change the course of events. Often, the interpretation of the symptoms by the patient is that they are benign because they usually are rapidly self correcting and nothing is done about them. In the past there has been some lack of awareness of the importance of these attacks by physicians so that even after they have been reported by a patient, they have not been followed by careful evaluation and treatment. A rough estimate suggests if one half of the patients who develop nonembolic ischemic stroke have had something resembling a transient ischemic attack, that one half of that half will have a stroke so soon after the attacks begin that there would be no chance to intervene with an effective therapy. This leaves about 25% of the population who will develop cerebral infarction as potential candidates for preventive treatment which might stop the transient ischemic attacks and as a result reduce the chance of a subsequent cerebral infarction. In this remaining 25% of the total, a significant percentage of patients who have the attacks ignore the symptoms or they are not properly evaluated by physicians. This leaves about 10% to 15% of the total population of patients who are going to have cerebral infarction for whom suitable preventive therapy could be applied, a relatively small percentage of patients. Most importantly current data do not help to distinguish who in this group is likely to fall into one of the natural history courses and become most suitable for anticoagulants as a preventive treatment. This makes selection of patients for the study of treatment effect even more difficult and the numbers of patients needed for definitive studies becomes quite large.

The understanding of the mechanisms which produce transient ischemic attacks has undergone a number of changes since the concept was accepted by the neurological community in the early 1950's. The changes in concepts about the cause of attacks has made it difficult to evaluate therapies, as suggestions for the most suitable therapy have changed. When these changes in the concept of proper therapy have occurred during the conduct of a particular study, it has made it difficult to obtain adequate numbers of patients to conclude a previous study satisfactorily.

The earliest conception of transient ischemic attacks, using Gowers' statement, is that they were due to arterial disease which caused an interference of blood supply in one portion of the brain and thereby giving rise to symptoms. Later arterial spasm was considered as a possible cause but this was never well supported by clinical evidence and the attacks were not relieved by agents which at the time were believed to reduce cerebral arterial spasm. With the demonstration of significant arterial obstruction in the carotid and vertebral basilar arteries in the both large and small branches, following the development of safe arteriography, it was postulated if there were fluctuations in blood pressure that distal to such obstructions, there could be significant reductions in cerebral blood flow, to the level where focal cerebral ischemia could occur. This concept, that internal carotid artery obstruction or middle cerebral artery obstruction might be significant enough to make blood flow through an obstruction marginal, following alterations in blood pressure was accepted early, as the a likely cause of transient ischemic attacks. It gave support to the idea that surgical correction of obstructions was the most suitable treatment. It was demonstrated experimentally that the obstruction of the arterial lumen needed to be nearly total or at least more than 75% before flow was significantly impaired. It was also rare, to observe patients during a transient ischemic attack who had major reductions in blood pressure. Experiments to reduce blood pressure, in patients known to have transient

ischemic attacks, to levels which interfered with cerebral blood,
generally produced evidence of generalized cerebral blood flow deficiency
with syncope rather than focal neurologic deficits. This concept of
marked arterial obstruction causing distal reductions in cerebral blood
flow as a result of changes in blood pressure, was never well supported.
It was used as a reason for using anticoagulants, as it was postulated
that in those arterial beds distal or proximal to the obstruction where
changes in cerebral blood pressure might produce major changes in flow,
slow or stagnant flow would occur and that Coumadin anticoagulation would
be beneficial in reducing the chances of thrombosis in these vessels.

With the observation in some patients who were having transient
ischemic attacks, especially those with visual complaints, that one might
actually observe emboli moving through the retinal arterial system, the
notion that transient ischemic attacks might be embolic in origin was
formulated. It was reported by vascular surgeons who were opening carotid
arteries, that the corroded surface of the internal carotid artery removed
at operation often contained friable loosely attached collections of
platelets, cholesterol and thrombi which could easily be detached and
enter the circulation floating downstream to plug cerebral arteries (26).
It was concluded from the these observations that most attacks of
transient cerebral ischemia were embolic in origin. The effect of
anticoagulants in this instance was believed to be prevention of thrombus
formation on denuded areas. Although it was known that thrombotic clots
rarely formed in high flow and high pressure systems such as cerebral
arteries. Emboli from atherosclerotic ulcers on arterial walls were
usually made up of collections of platelets which had adhered to damaged
arterial surfaces. This concept led to the exploration of agents which
prevented platelet accumulation on these areas on blood vessel walls and
started the studies of aspirin, and other medications such as dipyridamole
and sulfinpyrazone as possible therapies for terminating transient
ischemic attacks and preventing stroke.

Despite this change in the concepts of causation of TIA, it was still
concluded that it was useful to use Heparin and Coumadin anticoagulants in
patients to prevent coagulation of blood in arterial systems with low
blood flow distal or proximal to an obstruction by an embolus as this
might be effective in either reducing the size of the infarction or
preventing it altogether. The possibility that cerebral emboli could
cause a transient ischemic attack has come under some criticism. The most
cogent argument against it is that the symptoms of transient ischemic
attacks frequently are exactly the same from attack to attack which is
hard to explain using the concept that emboli are the cause.

It is still not settled why particular patients have transient
ischemic attacks. Some must be due to flow changes due to atherosclerotic
obstruction of arteries, some are due to embolic debris from the heart or
from ulcerated atherosclerotic disease in vessels leading to the brain,
and for some, the cause may never be exactly determined. Patients with
transient ischemic attacks are most often those in the age group where
atherosclerotic cerebral vascular disease is most prevalent. Most
patients with TIA when studied, have evidence of cerebral and cardiac
atherosclerotic vascular disease.

Since the first suggestion that anticoagulants might be effective in
cerebrovascular disease it has been difficult to explain how this might
happen (23). The idea that thrombosis in vessels distal to an arterial
obstruction or in the "dammed back" area immediately proximal to an
obstruction could be reduced by Coumadin anticoagulants or heparin can
help explain how they might be effective in stopping a progressing stroke.
It does not help to explain how transient ischemic attacks might be

stopped and stroke prevented unless the effect on thrombosis development in the heart or ulcerated areas on arteries leading to the brain is reduced by such therapy.

Anticoagulants as treatment for transient ischemic attacks have been studied in a variety of ways. First there were reports on small numbers of (8,9,13,14,15,21,36,37,38,39,46,51) patients followed by anecdotal reports of larger series (8,14,15). When the natural history of these attacks was better appreciated, it was found that more careful evaluation would be needed using random selection of patients for treatment or no treatment, and a more vigorous definition of criteria for diagnosis. Later when surgery for obstructive arterial disease became widely used, the value of anticoagulant therapy and surgical treatment were compared. Still later, anticoagulant therapy was compared with the effects of aspirin. Also Coumadin anticoagulants have been evaluated in long term follow-up studies using life table analysis of treated patients compared to the general population using TIA and stroke as end points. The results of long-term follow-up of patients who were observed for periods on and off treatment have also been used.

ANTICOAGULANT TREATMENT FOR TIA
NONRANDOMIZED STUDIES

Date	Author	Patients	Total Infarcts	TIA Continued	Deaths Infarct
1958	Fisher				
	T	29	1	1	0
	C	23	8	4	0
1969	Siekert				
	T	175	7	44	3
	C	160	51	77	18
1969	Friedman				
	T	21	1	NS	NS
	C	23	7	NS	NS
1970	Toole				
	T	21	6	0	5
	C	56	7	15	2

NS=not stated

FIGURE 5

Anticoagulants were early suggested as a treatment for progressing stroke to prevent thrombosis in the collateral circulation and reduce infarct size and also to prevent transient ischemic attacks and future stroke. Anecdotal reports began in the early 1950's, Figure 5. Among early reports is that of Fisher in 1958 when he reported on a series of 52 patients, 29 patients were treated and 23 served as controls (16). He found that there was a reduction in the frequency of transient ischemic attacks and cerebral infarction among treated patients when compared to controls. The study was not randomized, and the numbers of patients who actually had stroke was small and the follow-up period was short. In 1963, Siekert and Millikan reported a large study of over 300 patients who had transient ischemic attacks some of whom were treated with anti-coagulants (48). The patients were not randomized for treatment. One hundred seventy-five were treated, 160 served as controls and the follow-up was a period of five years. In this group, the stroke frequency among treated patients was 4% while that among control patients it was 32%. The results were impressive but raised the possibility that they could have been the result of selection for treatment of those least likely to have recurrent attacks or future stroke. The large number of patients included in the series reduces but does not abolish that possibility.

Random selection of patients for treatment was considered necessary to prove that anticoagulants were effective especially as their use was not without considerable risk of serious side effects. A number of randomized control studies were reported beginning with the reports of Baker et al of the Veteran's Administration's study in 1961 and a number of others which followed over the next few years (52). See Figure 6. All of these studies are difficult to evaluate largely because of the small number of patients included, the variable differences in the length of follow-up (2,3,4,5,12,17,18,20,27,44) following the onset of anticoagulant treatment and the definition of effect. All studies used clinical evidence of reduction of TIA frequency and cerebral infarction as end points and some studies used overall death rates. In some, a detail of hemorrhagic complications in treated and nontreated is included and in others reports of such complications are general and nonspecific. References were usually made that bleeding was more common in patients who were treated. There was limited standardization of the methodology of anticoagulant treatment. In most of these reports, the prothrombin time elevation was higher (2-2½ times control) than what is now believed to be desirable. In analyzing these data, the duration of treatment is not considered here. This was done because the duration was different in each study but in all studies, both those with and without randomized controls, anticoagulants were given for the period when stroke is reported most likely to occur, and for a long enough period that an effect on recurrent TIA could become evident.

ANTICOAGULANT TREATMENT FOR TIA
RANDOMIZED CONTROLLED STUDIES

Date	Author	Patients	Total Infarcts	TIA Continued	Deaths Infarct
1961	V.A.				
	T	15	0	1	NS
	C	22	1	8	NS
1962	Baker				
	T	24	1	7	0
	C	20	4	25	1
1965	Pearce				
	T	17	1	10	0
	C	20	2	9	1
1966	Baker				
	T	30	2	10	0
	C	30	4	14	0

FIGURE 6

The interesting thing about these studies is that in all there is a decrease in the frequency of cerebral infarction among the treated compared with the control patients. The differences while not great are consistently in the direction of stroke prevention. Also in all, the number of TIA was reduced following adequate anticoagulation. None of the results of these studies on statistical evaluation provide significant evidence that anticoagulants do what they are believed to do, that is, stop TIA's and reduce the chance of future stroke. The number of patients with end points of TIA and stroke in all studies was relatively small and the differences between treated and control while not great in actual numbers in percentage differences, sometimes, they are striking. It is extremely unlikely that if anticoagulants had no effect on stopping TIA's and preventing stroke, that all studies would come out with some evidence of benefit. If there was no effect, one would expect more studies showing no evidence of effect and some studies showing that anticoagulants increased changes of ischemic attacks and stroke.

In these studies the diagnosis of a transient ischemic attack was based on clinical findings and only in a few were patients further studied by angiography to determine the amount of atherosclerotic disease in cerebral vessels. Cerebral hemorrhage was ruled out by the presence or absence of blood in the cerebral spinal fluid. It is probable based on what we know now of CT scan evidence of cerebral infarction, that some of the patients in these studies had small intracerebral hemorrhages rather than cerebral infarctions.

While it is not possible to group these studies to obtain significant numbers because of differences in inclusion and exclusion criteria, the differences in treatment programs and the difference in length of follow-up, it is striking that there is a consistent difference between the frequency of cerebral infarction which is nearly always lower in the treated than in control patients.

Among the studies that were carried in the middle 1960's were those which studied patients treated with anticoagulants for the suppression of TIA's and then taken off anticoagulants. An early study is that of Marshall et al (36) who found in patients with TIA who had been treated with anticoagulants and then anticoagulants were stopped, that there was a significant recurrence of transient ischemic attacks. In a study of 26 patients who were treated with anticoagulants because of TIA, treatment was continued in 13 and 4 had further attacks, the treatment was stopped in 13 and 8 patients had a recurrence of attacks over two to eight weeks after stopping anticoagulants. The study suggested that there was some beneficial effect from using anticoagulants and supported the earlier concept that this was a useful treatment for patients with transient ischemic attacks.

With the introduction of surgical treatment for obstructive arterial disease, as a cause of transient ischemic attacks, and the development of the concept that small cerebral emboli made up of platelets were the cause of transient ischemic attacks and could be prevented by aspirin, studies on the use of Coumadin anticoagulants comparing treated and control patients virtually stopped. Most studies reported since 1970 are comparisons of the effectiveness of anticoagulants with surgical treatment or agents which suppress platelet clumping.

In one study of 104 patients, by Garde (22), 50 received anticoagulants and 54 received aspirin and were followed for 20 months. There was no difference in the frequency of recurrent transient ischemic attacks or the development of subsequent stroke in the two groups. Hemorrhage was more common with anticoagulants with one intracerebral hemorrhage in the aspirin treated group. In an other study by Buren (7) of 125 patients, 60 with transient ischemic attacks treated with anticoagulants and 65 patients received aspirin, the recurrent rate of transient ischemic attacks and the development of subsequent stroke was higher among patients who received aspirin but the differences were not striking. This and other studies did conclude that the stroke incidence in both groups was lower than the expected incidence of stroke for the age and sex of the population studied (43). Other studies reporting the frequency of recurrent transient ischemic attacks and the expected frequency of stroke using life table analysis, found that patients who had transient ischemic attacks and were treated with anticoagulants had a nearly normal life expectancy (50). Recent studies have used the frequency of stroke and the recurrence of rate of transient ischemic attacks during anticoagulant therapy compared with similar observations made after anticoagulants had been stopped, and concluded that chances of stroke and stroke death were considerably higher after stopping anticoagulants (36,42).

A comparison of the effect of surgery versus anticoagulants was attempted in 1971, compiling the data from a number of studies (19). This analysis came to the conclusion that anticoagulant treatment prevents transient ischemic attacks and stroke more effectively than the reports of carotid surgery available at that time. The differences were small and not significant. There was a 5% stroke occurrence among 246 patients treated with anticoagulants and an 11% occurrence among 169 surgically treated patients. There have been no subsequent comparisons because randomized controlled trials of carotid endarterectomy have not been done and compared to anticoagulants.

Those studies which included death as an important end point were done at a time when it was not fully appreciated that the most common cause of death among patients with transient ischemic attacks is not stroke but cardiac disease. The high frequency of death from cardiac disease could mask an effect of anticoagulants on the prevention of stroke. Those studies which separate stroke, stroke death and death from other causes show no effect of anticoagulants on death rates while often demonstrating a difference in stroke frequency among treated and control patients (53).

The analysis has left out a concomitant analysis of the complication rate associated with use of anticoagulants in these studies. It is clear from all of them that cerebral hemorrhage was more common among patients who were being treated with anticoagulants. Less serious bleeding problems, as would be expected, were more frequent in patients treated with anticoagulants. It is interesting that among patients who were not treated with anticoagulants that cerebral hemorrhage also occurred with some frequency. This suggests the possibility that some of the patients in both groups may have had small cerebral hemorrhages which could account for their symptoms rather than infarction.

It is necessary to look at the complication rates to see whether the treatment is benign enough to warrant its use. In some studies, major bleeding occurred in as many as half of the patients while in others it was reported to be at an acceptable level. In the Veteran's Administration study of 1961, one half of the treated patients had major bleeding episodes and virtually all had some minor bleeding. In the large series of Millikan and Siekert, among treated patients there was a 7% incidence of cerebral hemorrhage with a 4% incidence among the controls. They do not state exactly what percentage of patients had minor bleeding episodes except to point out that such episodes were much more common in treated patients. In most reports bleeding, major and minor, occurred in 5 to 10% of patients.

Since the early studies, more has been learned about the use of anticoagulants. The prolongation of Prothrombin Times has been shortened as well as the duration of treatment. Unfortunately, no large randomized study has been done using less prolongation of Prothrombin Time and shorter periods of anticoagulation. Based on the reports of Whisnant et al, the most important time for treatment if it is to be offered, is during the first three to six months following onset of TIA. It is now generally accepted that most patients who are started on anticoagulants should continue on them for a period of approximately three to six months and the Prothrombin Time should rarely prolonged more than two times of control value, more preferably to one and one half times control. Whether careful study would support the efficacy of this program of treatment with limited complications, is not clear. Anticoagulant treatment of transient ischemic attacks is not an easy or trivial matter and must be carried with careful control by an experienced physician and a reliable laboratory. To be clearly effective, anticoagulant treatment would need a hemorrhagic complication rate of 5% or less. This would require a serious complication rate of less than 2% and nonserious of 3%. Whether this is possible with contemporary management of Coumadin anticoagulation remains to be studied.

It is of interest that in one reported study of the use of Heparin as the initial treatment for TIA, that the neurologic complications of Heparin given intravenously for as long as two to three weeks was .8% (45). There is no general agreement on whether or not hemorrhagic complications of anticoagulant therapy are more common among patients who have more marked prolongations of Prothrombin Times as compared to those who do not. In a recent review by Hirsch et al (29), no evidence was found that hemorrhagic complications were associated with the degree of Prothrombin Time prolongation while in other studies this has been believed to be the case (54).

Conclusions regarding the current usefulness of Coumadin anticoagulants must always be considered in the light of the effectiveness of other forms of therapy with potentially less risk. If surgery is considered the treatment of choice, the fact that the statistical evidence that carotid endarterectomy is effective in reducing the frequency of transient ischemic attacks and the prevention of future strokes is shaky at best, must be considered. The use of aspirin for the prevention of recurrent ischemic attacks and the prevention of future strokes, although done on a larger number of patients and under better designed programs of study, is clearly not free from flaws and there is controversy between a number of studies that have been carried out as to whether the results indicate that aspirin provides protective treatment.

It can probably be concluded with some degree of safety that a relatively small number of patients with TIA probably less than 10% of the total stroke population could be considered for anticoagulant treatment hoping for a reduction of the frequency of transient ischemic attacks and prevention of stroke. If other treatment strategies such as endarterectomy or antiaggregant agents are contra indicated or not effective, anticoagulants under careful control by experienced individuals should be used. They should be continued for no more than three to six months, with the expectation that transient ischemic attacks will be stopped and that during the period of most likely occurrence of stroke, the chance of stroke will be considerably reduced. Hemorrhagic risk is there and is certainly significant but is difficult to calculate using old data to guide current concepts of degree and duration of anticoagulation. With the current use of CAT Scan, the chances of anticoagulant being given to a patient who has a small intracerebral hemorrhage have been virtually eliminated. It is probable if there is no evidence of cerebral hemorrhage, that the chance of producing one with anticoagulants in a patient with TIA may be considerably reduced. Selection of patients for

Coumadin anticoagulation is important and risk factors which increase risk should be carefully sought.

Among all the suggested therapies for stopping recurrent transient ischemic attacks and most importantly reducing the chance of a future stroke, Coumadin anticoagulants may be as effective as any of the other suggested treatments. The fact that aspirin can be given with impunity with less concern about risk and that it has some beneficial effect has made Coumadin anticoagulation with its problems of frequent laboratory analysis and careful supervision by physicians less practical than it once was. Still the effectiveness of this form of treatment, I believe, has enough data to support it that it should always be seriously considered by physicians treating patients who have transient ischemic attacks.

REFERENCES

1. Acheson J, Hutchinson EC: Observations on the natural history of transient cerebral ischemia.
    Lancet 2:871-874, 1964.

2. Baker RN, Broward JA, Fang HC, et al: Anticoagulant therapy in cerebral infarction.
    Neurol 12:823-835, 1962.

3. Baker RN, Ramseyer JC, Schwartz WS: Prognosis in patients with cerebral ischemic attacks.
    Neurol 18:1157-1165, 1968.

4. Baker RN, Schwartz WS, Rose AS: Transient ischemic attacks.
    Neurol 16:841-847, 1966.

5. Bradshaw P, Brennan S: Trial of long-term anticoagulant therapy in the treatment of small stroke associated with a normal carotid angiogram.
    J Neurol Neurosurg & Psychiatry 38:642-647, 1975.

6. Browne TR, Poskanzer DC: Treatment of strokes.
    N Engl J Med 284:594-602, 1969.

7. Buren A, Ygge J: Treatment program and comparison between anticoagulants and platelet aggregation inhibitors after transient ischemic attack.
    Stroke 12:578-580, 1981.

8. Campbell MH: Basilar artery syndrome.
    Canad Med Ass J 69:314-315, 1953.

9. Deyken D: Warfarin therapy.
    N Engl J Med 283:691-694, 1970.

10. Duncan GW, Pessin MS, Mohr JP, Adams RD: Transient cerebral ischemic attacks.
    Advances in Internal Medicine 21:1-20, 1976.

11. Easton JD, Byer JA: Transient cerebral ischemic medical management. pp. 41-47. In current concepts in cerebrovascular disease. (eds.) McDowell FH, Sonnenblick EH, Lesch M. Grune & Stratton, New York, 1980.

12. Eriksson SE: Evaluation of anticoagulants in patients with cerebral infarction with slight to moderate neurological deficit.
    ACTA Neurol Scand 68:96-106, 1983.

13. Feiring EH: Spontaneous occlusion of the internal carotid artery.
    Neurol 4:405-421, 1954.

14. Fisher CM: Occlusion of the internal carotid artery.
    Arch Neurol & Psych 65:346-377, 1951.

15. Fisher CM, Cameron DG: Concerning cerebral vasospasm.
    Neurol 3:468-473, 1953.

16. Fisher CM: The use of anticoagulants in cerebral thrombosis.
    Neurol 8:311-332, 1958.

17. Fisher CM: Anticoagulant therapy in cerebral thrombosis and cerebral embolism - A national cooperative study, interim report. Neurol 11(4 part 2):119-131, 1961.

18. Fisher CM: Anticoagulant therapy. pp. 86-89. Third Conference on cerebral vascular diseases. (ed.) Millikan CH, Siekert RG, Whisnant JP. Grune & Stratton, New York, 1961.

19. Frank G: Comparison of antigoagulation and surgical treatments of T.I.A. A review and consolidation of recent natural history and treatment studies. Stroke 2:369-377, 1971.

20. Friedman GD, Wilson WS, Mosier JM, et al: Transient ischemic attacks in a community. JAMA 210:1428-1434, 1969.

21. Gallhofer B, Ladurner G, Lechner H: Prognosis of prophylactic anticoagulant treatment in ischaemic stroke. Eur Neurol 18:145-148, 1979.

22. Garde A, Samuelsson K, Fahlgren H, Hedberg E, Hjerne LG, Ostman J: Treatment after transient ischemic attacks, a comparison between anticoagulant drug and inhibition of platelet aggregation. Stroke 14:677-681, 1983.

23. Genton E, Barnett HJM, Fields WS, Gent M, Hoak JC: Cerebral Ischemia: The Role of Thrombosis and of Antithrombotic Therapy. Stroke 8:150-175, 1977.

24. Goldner LC, Whisnant JP, Taylor WF: Long Term Prognosis of Transient Cerebral Ischemic Attacks. Stroke 2:160-167, 1971.

25. Gowers WR: A Manual of Diseases of the Nervous System. p. 432. Blakiston, Philadelphia, 1893.

26. Gunning AJ, Pickering GW, Robb-Smith AHT, et al: Mural thrombosis of the internal carotid artery and subsequent embolism. Q J Med 33:155-193, 1964.

27. Hill AB, Marshall J. Shaw DA: A controlled clinical trial of long-term anticoagulant therapy in cerebrovascular disease. Q J Med 29:597-609, 1959.

28. Hunt JR: The role of the Carotid Arteries in the Causation of Vascular Lesions of the Brain with Remarks on Special Features of the Symptomology. Am J Med Sci 147:704-713, 1914.

29. Levine M, Hirsh J: Hemorrhagic Complications of Long Term Anticoagulants Therapy for Ischemic Vascular Disease. Stroke 17:111-116, 1986.

30. Link H, Lebram G, Johansson I, Radberg C: Prognosis in patients with infarction and TIA in carotid territory during and after anticoagulant therapy. Stroke 10:529-532, 1979.

31. McDowell FH: Transient cerebral ischemic diagnostic considerations. pp. 7-22. In current concepts in cerebrovascular disease. (eds.)

McDowell FH, Sonnenblick EH, Lesch M. Grune & Stratton, New York, 1980.

32. Marshall J, Meadows EC: The natural history of amaurosis fugax. Brain 91:419-434, 1968.

33. Marshall J, Wilkinson IMS: The prognosis of carotid transient ischaemic attacks in patients with normal angiograms. Brain 94:395-402, 1971.

34. Marshall J, Reynolds EH: Withdrawal of anticoagulants from patients with transient ischemic cerebrovascular attacks. Lancet 2:5-6, 1965.

35. Marshall J: The natural history of transient ischaemic cerebro-vascular attacks. Q J Med 33:309-324, 1964.

36. Millikan CH, Whisnant JP: Anticoagulant therapy in cerebro-vascular disease - current status. J Amer Med Ass 166:587-592, 1958.

37. Millikan CH, Siekert RG, Schick RM: Studies in cerebrovascular disease V. The use of anticoagulant drugs in the treatment of intermittent insufficiency of the internal carotid arterial system. Proc Mayo Clin 30:578-586, 1955.

38. Milliken CH, Siekert RG, Schick RM: Studies in cerebrovascular disease III. The use of anticoagulant drugs in the treatment of insufficiency or thrombosis within the basilar artery system. Proc Mayo Clin 30:116-126, 1955.

39. Millikan CH: Reassessment of Anticoagulant Therapy in Various Types of Occlusive Cerebrovascular Disease. Stroke 2:201-208, 1971.

40. Millikan CH: Transient cerebral ischemia definition and natural history. pp. 1-6. In current concepts in cerebrovascular disease. (eds.) McDowell FH, Sonnenblick EH, Lesch M. Grune & Stratton, New York, 1980.

41. Millikan CH, McDowell FH: Treatment of transient ischemic attacks. Stroke 9:299-308, 1978.

42. Olsson JE, Muller R, Bernali S: Long-term anticoagulant therapy for T.I.As. and minor strokes with minimum residuum. Stroke 7:444-451, 1976.

43. Olsson JE, Brechter C, Backlund H, Krook H, Muller R, Nitelius E, Olsson O, Tornberg A: Anticoagulant vs anti-platelet therapy as prophylactic against cerebral infarction in transient ischemic attacks. Stroke 11:4-9, 1980.

44. Pearce JMS, Gabbay SS, Walton J: Long-term anticoagulant therapy in transient cerebral ischemic attacks. Lancet 1:6-9, 1965.

45. Ramirez-Lassepass M, Quinones MR: Heparin Therapy for Stroke Hemorrhagic Complications and Risk Factors for Intracerebral Hemorrhage.

Neurol 34:114-117, 1984.

46. Rose WM: Anticoagulants in the management of cerebral infarction: A record of the poor result obtained.
    Med J Aust 1:503-504, 1950.

47. Siekert RG, Millikan CH, Whisnant JP: Anticoagulant therapy in intermittent cerebrovascular insufficiency.
    JAMA 176:19-22, 1961.

48. Siekert RG, Whisnant JP, Millikan CH: Surgical and Anticoagulant Therapy of Occlusive Cerebrovascular Disease.
    Ann Intern Med 58:637-641, 1963.

49. Schmidley JW, Caronna JJ: Transient cerebral ischemic pathophysiology. pp. 23-40. In current concepts in cerebrovascular disease. (eds.) McDowell FH, Sonnenblick EH, Lesch M. Grune & Stratton, New York, 1980.

50. Terent A: The outcome of patients with transient ischemic attacks and stroke treated with anticoagulants.
    ACTA Med Scand 208:359-365, 1980.

51. Toole JF, Janeway R, Choi R, et al: Transient ischemic attacks due to atherosclerosis, a prospective study of 160 patients.
    Arch Neurol 32:5-13, 1975.

52. Veterans Administration Cooperative Study of Atherosclerosis Neurology Section: An Evaluation of Anticoagulant Therapy in the Treatment of Cerebrovascular Disease.
    Neurol 11:132-138, 1961.

53. Warlow C: Transient ischaemic attacks, current treatment concepts.
    Drugs 29:474-482, 1985.

54. Weksler BB, Lewin M: Anticoagulation in cerebral ischemia.
    Stroke 14:658-663, 1983.

55. Whisnant JP, Matsumoto N, Elveback LR: The effect of anticoagulant therapy on the prognosis of patients with transient cerebral ischemic attacks in a community.
    Mayo Clin Proc 48:844-848, 1973.

56. Wilson SA, Bruce AN. (ed.)
    Neurology, p.1088. Edward Arnold, London, 1940.

57. Ziegler DK, Hassanein RS: Prognosis in patients with transient ischemic attacks.
    Stroke 4:666-673, 1973.

EPILOGUE

Stanford Wessler

Department of Medicine
New York University School of Medicine
New York, N.Y.

Carl G. Becker

Department of Pathology
Cornell University Medical College
New York, N.Y.

Yale Nemerson

Departments of Medicine and Biochemistry
Mount Sinai School of Medicine
of the City University of New York
New York, N.Y.

Introduction

An epilogue, according to the dictionary, is "the final part that serves typically to round out or complete the design of a ... work" or provides "an afterword." The editors thought an epilogue might be more appropriate than a summary of the papers of distinguished colleagues most of whom had, in any event, provided their own summaries or conclusions.

It is our goal, in short, to emphasize and extend some of the material presented: to suggest avenues of future research, identify technical issues in prothrombin time regulation, offer comment on drug dosage, and provide recommendations that may favorably affect .patient care now and in the future. Some of what follows includes speculation for which the editors share equally in responsibility. This afterword is intended primarily, however, to be helpful, occasionally provocative, never dogmatic.

Further observations on the mechanism of warfarin action

The mechanism of action of warfarin is now well understood, at least with respect to the carboxylation of coagulation proteins in the liver. However, the mechanism that directs the carboxylase towards a specific glutamic acid residue is unclear. In particular, unlike certain other post-translational modifications of proteins, such as glycosylation, the target residues are not contained within a "consensus sequence." Recently, however, sequence data on the cDNA for several gla-containing proteins has indicated the presence of a "propeptide" region between the amino terminus of the mature protein and the leader peptide sequence.[1,2] Thus, the regulation of carboxylation may be accomplished by a region on each gene which directs the enzymatic machinery, but which is not itself translated into the secreted protein.[3]

While it is a worthwhile goal to derive a unitary view of the regulation of carboxylation, and, perforce, the mechanism of action of vitamin K and warfarin, certain interesting anomalies must be dealt with and perhaps exploited. It is, for example, perfectly clear that warfarin-induced reduction in the activity of clotting factors can readily be reversed by vitamin K, whereas the induced changes in the gla-containing bone protein, osteocalcin, cannot (Chapter 5). The explanation for this seemingly incongruous finding likely resides in the observation that there are two enzymes in the liver capable of reducing vitamin K epoxide to its active form. Thus, in the presence of low (i.e. normal) levels of vitamin K, the poisoning of one pathway results in insufficient concentrations of the active vitamin. Upon the addition of large amounts of vitamin K, however, the second, warfarin-insensitive pathway can generate sufficient active vitamin K to enable carboxylation of the coagulation proteins to proceed normally.

In the case of the bone protein, however, only a single, warfarin-sensitive epoxidase is present. Thus, the addition of excess vitamin K does not result in increased levels of the active vitamin with its consequent carboxylation reactions. Accordingly, animals can be maintained with normal coagulation proteins while having greatly reduced concentrations of the gla-containing bone protein. This remarkable finding allows for the investigation of the long-term effects of warfarin apart from its action on coagulation factors. It is presently unknown whether the gla-containing proteins of sperm[4] and kidney are similarly responsive; however, if they prove to be, then the long term consequences of warfarin administration can readily be ascertained without concomitant bleeding simply by treating animals with warfarin plus vitamin K.

It is of considerable interest that half a century after the discovery of vitamin K and warfarin, and a decade after the recognition of gamma-carboxylation, the role of the gla residues in coagulation is still unclear. One view derives from the following observations: 1) in the absence of vitamin K, there is no carboxylation of the coagulation proteins; 2) in the absence of the gla residues, the proteins do not bind calcium ions; 3) in the absence of bound calcium ions there is impaired binding to phospholipid; 4) in this setting coagulation rates are markedly reduced. Ergo: gla is required for lipid-binding which, in turn, enhances coagulation rates. While this view may be correct, it should be kept in mind that the activation of factor X by the coagulant enzyme from Russell's viper venom requires the presence of carboxylated factor X. Inasmuch as this reaction does not require lipids (indeed, it is inhibited by phospholipid vesicles), it is certainly clear that the role of gla is not limited to lipid binding. Further, the actual role of membrane lipids in coagulation is still debatable. In chapter 3, it is emphasized that the lipids concentrate the substrate thus presenting increased substrate concentrations to the lipid-bound catalytic complex (factors Xa and Va). In contrast, in chapter 7 it is noted that acidic lipids actually change the affinity of the catalytic complex (tissue factor and factor VII) and that the true substrate pool is free in solution. Although it is certainly possible that the role of gla residues and acidic phospholipids differ for different reactions, it is likely that only one of these proposed mechanisms will prove to be correct.

Inherent in the concept of hypercoagulability is the issue of whether some patients who develop thrombosis have an increased tendency to clot and, if so, whether this is simply a clinical impression or a definable and predictable state before the thrombotic event. Hypercoagulability can be divided functionally into two categories: initiators and facilitators of thrombosis. In the former, tissue injury is the principle etiologic factor. Examples abound: trauma, surgery, prosthetic heart valves, acute myocardial infarction, vasculitis, cancer, infection, tobacco, snake venoms, homocystinuria. These conditions can be thought of as initiators of thrombosis in the sense that they have activated the coagulation sequence.

Whether initiation of coagulation results in overt thrombosis, however, depends not only on the intensity of the activating mechanism, but also on the status of the normal defense system against thrombogenesis. It is the impairment in these defense reactions that represents the second category of hypercoagulable states. These, while not themselves causing coagulation, facilitate its progress once initiated. Clinical conditions conforming to this latter definition include: deficiencies of antithrombin III, protein C, protein S and heparin co-factor II; the presence of high titers of substances that inhibit plasminogen activation, low fibrinolytic response; the presence of defective plasminogen, the administration of estrogens and, the example par excellence, retarded blood flow.

One can, however, overemphasize the distinction between initiators and facilitators of thrombosis for several reasons. First, because normally there may be a continual, low-level activation of the coagulation sequence; second, because it is possible that some of those states identified as facilitators may be associated with subliminal activation that rarely, if ever, progress alone to overt thrombosis; and, finally, in many if not most instances of thrombosis both initiators and facilitators are operative. The advantage of these categories is not that they appear to provide a simpler yet all-encompassing terminology, but rather that they offer operational definitions that in many instances are experimentally verifiable.

It is possible that the extrinsic system may be the major pathway leading to the initiation of arterial thrombosis. Evidence favoring this hypothesis is found in experiments demonstrating that a variety of substances (lipopolysaccharide, interleukin-1, tissue necrosis factor) can stimulate expression of tissue factor by vascular endothelial cells and that in hypercholesterolemia there is increased traffic of blood monocytes into the arterial wall providing for a local source of considerable quantities of tissue factor.[5,6] This, of course, does not exclude the participation of the Hageman factor-dependent pathway in arterial thrombosis.

In 1980 an epidemiological study in Great Britain revealed that plasma levels of factor VII were highly predictive of myocardial infarction, particularly in the near future.[7] This observation has been confirmed[8], but not yet explained. In particular, and in common with other data of this type, it is not clear whether this increase is causative or epiphenominal. It is obviously of enormous importance to make this determination, because, if causal, it would follow that warfarin therapy would be indicated as a preventive measure in the population at risk of myocardial infarction. Indeed, because it would be relatively easy to reduce factor VII with low-dose and therefore low-risk oral anticoagulation, it would be critical to make this determination. Epidemiological evidence, in fact, implicates factor VII to be causally connected because "If high clotting-factor levels were secondary to atheroma, men with ischemic or hypertensive ECGs might be expected to have higher values than those without, but our ECG data do not bear this out."[7] This reasoning notwithstanding, owing to the magnitude of the increase (factor VII levels of 116% in those who died vs. 102% in survivors), it is difficult to hypothesize a mechanism relating death to quantitative factor VII levels alone.

However, inasmuch as factor VII, unlike other clotting factors, can circulate in an active state[9,10], it is at least possible that the increase is due not to an increased mass of factor VII, but rather to a small amount of activated factor VII. The latter might, in fact, be disproportionately active in hemostasis (and perhaps in thrombosis) as preliminary data have shown activated factor VII to be effective in arresting hemorrhage in hemophiliacs.[11] Indeed, evidence exists that among populations with atherosclerosis some activated factor VII does circulate;[12] alternatively, the suggestion has been made that factor VII in the presence of ischemic heart disease is lipid-bound and "hyperactive".[13] Thus, the suggestion that factor VII is causally related to cardiovascular death ought to be given prompt and careful consideration.

Enigmas among risk factors for thrombosis

Epidemiologic studies of myocardial infarction have identified a number of risk factors associated with the external or internal environment including cigarette smoking, hypercholesterolemia, diabetes, hypertension, and maleness. However, in autopsy-based epidemiologic studies of atherosclerosis, when cases were stratified according to race, sex, age, and disease there remained striking individual variation in the extent of raised atherosclerotic lesions in the aorta, coronary and cerebral arteries.[14] Further, some individuals sustain heart attacks that cannot be identified with any major risk factors.[15,16] The number of such patients is not precisely known, but may be as high as 50%.[17] Studies aimed at determining this number might provide the basis for the recognition of additional, and perhaps modifiable, risk factors that are at present unknown. Such studies might also help to define and possibly explain the variation in lesion severity among individuals already in recognized risk groups. For example, it has been established that young and middle-aged smokers are at greater risk of a heart attack than older smokers.[18] Identification of the mechanisms underlying the susceptibility of certain individuals to cardiovascular disease might permit more specific approaches to its prevention or amelioration. Such studies should be designed to determine those aspects of individual risk that contribute to the pathogenesis of atherosclerosis as well as those that contribute to acute events such as thrombus formation in a coronary artery or arrhythmia and sudden death in the absence of a thrombus.

Determination of the prothrombin time

Several papers at this symposium have referred to the performance of the prothrombin time and it may therefore be useful to state our own views on this subject. A present weakness in the overall prothrombin time procedure is not only the quality of the thromboplastin reagent, but also the nature of the blood collecting system itself. We would strongly support the view that organizations responsible for the approval of clinical laboratories require that bloods for prothrombin times be collected in "clinical grade" polymer-lined tubes, such as polypropylene and not in glass or imperfectly siliconized glass vessels. The availability of a "clean" polymer vacuum tube containing sodium citrate would facilitate the practicality of this recommendation. The artifactual shortening of the prothrombin time when blood is collected in most siliconized tubes begins within one hour and is marked within 2 - 4 hours after venipuncture: this phenomenon can lead to drug overdosage (Chapter 9). In many hospitals blood collected from patients may easily remain in their glass tubes for several hours before the test is performed and this certainly is true of outpatient blood samples sent to reputable clinical laboratories. Blood for partial thromboplastin times can also be collected in polymer-lined tubes. Resistance to efforts to implement this suggestion must reckon with the fact that, for the forseeable future, the prothrombin time will remain the effective means of regulating the dose of warfarin - the drug of choice for many thousands of patients at risk of venous and arterial thromboembolism.

Although the rabbit thromboplastins currently available in the U.S. provide acceptable endpoints both as to antithrombotic efficacy and safety from hemorrhage, it should, in time, become the reporting responsibility of the clinical laboratory to provide clinicians with a single INR number for warfarin dose regulation.[19,20] The INR system has the advantage that it is independent of the thromboplastin reagent as well as the recording instrument employed. Until this system is implemented in the U.S., however, clinical laboratories, in our opinion, are remiss if they do not at least report out their control values in seconds with each patient's prothrombin time. In addition, the ratio of the patient's prothrombin time to the control value should also be reported, because that is the actual piece of information (like the INR number) upon which dosage should be based.

Attention has been drawn to the recent unavailability of tissue thromboplastin derived from the human brain due to fear of transmission of HIV to laboratory personnel and the problems this has presented for standardization. In our view, the availability of sensitive and accurate means for detecting the presence of antibodies to HIV removes this threat. It has been clearly demonstrated that anti-HIV testing, coupled with adequate history taking, has provided a safe blood supply. It follows that the same criteria of careful history taking and HIV antibody testing of antemortem or postmortem blood, which, when also tested for antibodies to hepatitis B, would provide human brain thromboplastin that posed no threat to laboratory personnel.

The potential production of tissue factor from recombinant DNA might not only provide a uniformly standard product; but, if produced and distributed at affordable cost, would permit absolute standardization of the thromboplastin reagent. Availability of both recombinant tissue factor and "clean" polymer-lined vacuum tubes for blood collection would provide for more accurate, reproducible and reliable determination of prothrombin times than are presently obtainable. While awaiting the former, however, there is no justification in delaying the development and implementation of "clinical grade" polymer-lined vacuum tubes for blood collection.

Prudent warfarin regimens

As reported in Chapter 11, it is reasonable, using U.S. rabbit brain thromboplastins, to divide warfarin regimens into three degrees of intensity: low dose (PT ratio of 1.5, range 1.3 - 1.7), medium dose (PT ratio of 1.7, range 1.5 - 1.9) and high dose (PT ratio of 2, range 1.8 - 2.1). The corresponding INR ranges for low, medium and high intensities are 2.0 - 3.5, 3.0 - 4.2, and 3.9 - 5.0 respectively. The higher the ratio, the greater not only the antithrombotic power but also the risk of hemorrhage. After reviewing the variables inherent in the prothrombin time assay itself, in the many parameters that may promote bleeding, in the knowledge that administration may involve a life-time of use, and that many of the patients most needing long-term prophylaxis are in their seventies and eighties; we would urge that the high dose regimen, as defined above, no longer be considered for patient administration. Most patients can probably be managed at the low-dose, whereas some may require the medium-dose range: if the latter fails (as will inevitably occur with any antithrombotic agent, when on rare occasions, the thrombogenic stimulus is too great), one should then try a modality other than a high-dose warfarin regimen.

It is clear from clinical trials that a low-dose protocol is adequate to prevent a recurrence of venous thromboembolism (Chapter 16). What is not yet established is whether low dose warfarin can prevent embolic strokes from mural thrombi especially atrial thrombi. For atrial fibrillation, in which much of the thrombus resembles in composition a stasis or venous thrombus, low-dose warfarin may be adequate. We believe such a recommendation is justified at the present time, but wish to emphasize that more conclusive evidence must await future clinical trials.

The choice of the terms "low-risk" and "high-risk" depends both on the accumulated risk factors that the patient brings to the present illness and on the degree of thrombogenicity caused by the present illness be it a medical or a surgical insult. For patients in whom the combined risk factors add up to a low or medium risk, a low-dose regimen may be adequate. For high-risk patients, the medium-dose range may be necessary. The latter can be justified so long as it is appreciated that a greater risk of bleeding is entailed.

In view of the fact that many of the patients needing warfarin will be receiving a low-dose regimen, it would be advantageous for patients to have available a one mg. warfarin tablet.

Is there any advantage to an ultra-low-dose protocol, that is ratios of 1.2 and below?[21,22] Present evidence does not justify such levels either for its antithrombotic efficacy or because there is excessive bleeding in the low-dose range. The role of regimens with prothrombin ratios at or below 1.2 is of importance, however, and answers should be sought in the near future.

Tissue necrosis

Tissue necrosis is an exceedingly rare phenomenon associated with warfarin therapy. Recent observations indicate that many cases are associated with deficiencies in levels of protein C (Chapter 4, 20). It is our present opinion that this complication might be minimized by determining whether the patient or blood relatives have had previous thrombotic episodes or occurrences of skin necrosis associated with either warfarin or heparin therapy.

In patients without such a history, combining heparin with lower initial doses of warfarin might reduce the likelihood of skin necrosis.[23] In patients with such a history, however, a trial of concurrent administration of fresh frozen plasma with warfarin may ameliorate lesion development, since it has been reported that administration of fresh frozen plasma with warfarin was associated with non-recurrence of skin necrosis.[24]

In either event, during the induction period of warfarin therapy, it is incumbent upon the physician to examine each patient adequately during the first several days of therapy for evidence of local erythema, particularly in adipose and dependent regions. If such erythema is found, consideration should be given to the administration of fresh frozen plasma and to the options of discontinuing warfarin or substituting heparin for the oral anticoagulant.

The pathogenesis of tissue necrosis is still poorly understood. The mechanism deserves further research not only because it may be a preventable complication of warfarin therapy, but because its elucidation may provide additional insight into the process of intravascular coagulation and thrombosis.

Warfarin and cancer

An increasing body of data has established that fibrin is a regular stromal component of both authochthonous and transplantable tumors and that this fibrin is covalently cross linked.[25] The establishment of stromal matrices may hinder lymphocytes and other inflammatory cells from reaching tumor cells and attacking them. These observations raise the possibility that prolonged treatment with warfarin might be associated with a lower apparent incidence of certain cancers or of overt metastatic disease in individuals who developed tumors while taking warfarin. Data from studies in which large numbers of patients were treated with warfarin should be carefully examined for this result and prospective studies should address this question.

REFERENCES

1) G. L. Long, R. M. Belagaje and R. T. A. MacGilivray, Cloning and sequencing of liver cDNA coding for bovine protein C. Proc Natl Acad Sci U.S.A. 81:5653 (1984).

2) L. C. Pan and P. A. Price, The propeptide of rat bone gamma-carboxyglutamic acid protein shares homology with other vitamin K-dependent protein precursors. Proc Nat Acad Sci U.S.A. 82:6109 (1985).

3) J. W. Suttie, J. A. Hoskins, J. Engelke, A. Hopfgartner, H. Ehrlich, N. U. Bang, R. M. Belagaje, B. Schoner, and G. L. Long, Vitamin K-dependent carboxylase: possible role of the "propeptide" as an intracellular recognition site (gamma-carboxyglutamic acid/ protein C), Proc Natl Acad Sci U.S.A. (1987) in press.

4) B. A. M. Soute, W. Muller-Esterl, M. A. G. de Boer-van den Berg, M. Ulrich and C. Vermeer, Discovery of a gamma-carboxyglutamic acid-containing protein in human spermatozoa. FEBS 190:137 (1985).

5) A. Faggiotto, R. Ross, L. Harker, Studies of hyperchloresterolemia in the non-human primate. I. Changes that lead to fatty streak formation. Arteriosclerosis 4:323 (1984).

6) A. Faggiotto, R. Ross, L. Harker, Studies of hyperchloresterolemia in the non-human primate. II. Changes that lead to fatty streak conversion to fibrous plaque. Arteriosclerosis 4:341 (1984).

7) T. W. Meade, W. R. S. North, R. Chakrabarti, Y. Stirling, A. P. Haines, S. G. Thompson and M. Brozovic, Haemostatic function and cardiovascular death: early results of a prospective study. Lancet I: 1050 (1980).

8) T. W. Meade, Y. Stirling, S. G. Thompson, M. V. Vickers, L. Woolf, A. B. Ajdukiewicz, G. Stewart, J. F. Davidson, I. D. Walker, A. S. Douglas, et al., An International and Interregional comparison of Haemostatic Variables in the study of Ischaemic Heart Disease. Report of a Working Group. Int J Epidemiology 15:331 (1986).

9) M. Zur, R. D. Radcliffe, J. Oberdick and Y. Nemerson, The dual role of factor VII in coagulation: initiation of coagulation by a zymogen. J Biol Chem 257:5623 (1982).

10) U. Seligsohn, C. K. Kasper, B. Osterud, S. I. Rapaport, Activated Factor VII: Presence in Factor IX concentrates and persistance in the circulation after infusion. Blood 53:828 (1979).

11) V. Hedner and W. Kisiel, Use of human factor VIIa in treatment of two haemophiliac A patients with high titer inhibitors. J Clin

Invest 71:1836 (1983).

12) G. J. Miller, S. J. Walter, Y. Stirling, S. G. Thompson, M. P. Esnouf, T. W. Meade, Assay of Factor VII activity by two techniques: evidence for increased conversion of VII to alpha VIIa in hyperlipidaemia, with possible implications for ischaemic heart disease. Brit J Haematology 59:249 (1985).

13) K. Dalaker, I. Hjermann, H. Prydz, A novel form of Factor VII in plasma for men at risk for cardiovascular disease. Brit J Haematology 61:315 (1985).

14) L. A. Salberg and J. P. Strong, Risk factors and atherosclerotic lesions: a review of autopsy studies. Arteriosclerosis 3:187 (1983).

15) T. Gordon, M. R. Garcia-Palmieri, A. Kagan, W. E. Kannel, and J. Schiffman, Differences in coronary heart disease in Framingham, Honolulu and Puerto Rico. J Chronic Dis 27:329 (1974).

16) J. Stamler and F. H. Epstein, Coronary heart disease: risk factors as guides to preventive action. Prev Med 1:27 (1972).

17) H. C. McGill, Jr., Risk factors in atherosclerosis. Adv Exp Med Biol 104:273 (1978).

18) The Framingham Study: an epidemiologic investigation of cardiovascular disease. Monograph sections 26-27. DHEW Publication. National Heart Institute (1970,71).

19) J. Hermans, T. van den Besselaar, E. A. Loeliger, E. A. van der Veide, A collaborative calibration study of reference materials for thromboplastin. Thromb Haemost 50:712 (1983).

20) J. A. Koepke and D. A. Triplett, Standardization of the prothrombin time - finally. Arch Path Lab Med 109:800 (1985).

21) R. G. Berger and N. N. Hadler, Treatment of calcinosis universalis secondary to dermatomyositis or scleroderma with low dose warfarin. Presented at the annual meeting of the American Rheumatism Association, San Antonio, Texas. June 1-4, 1983.

22) M. M. Bern, A. Bothe, Jr., B. Bistrian, C. D. Champagne, M. S. Keane, G. L. Blackburn, Prophylaxis against central vein thrombosis with low-dose warfarin. Surgery 99:216 (1986).

23) M. Samama, M. H. Horellou, J. Soria, J. Conrad, G. Nicholas, Successful progressive anticoagulation in a severe protein C deficiency and previous skin necrosis at the initiation of oral anticoagulant treatment. Thromb Haemost 51:132 (1984).

24) P. Zauber and M. W. Stark, Successful warfarin anticoagulation despite protein C deficiency and a history of warfarin necrosis. Ann Int Med 104:659 (1986).

25) H. F. Dvorak, Tumors: Wounds that do not heal. Similarities between tumor stroma generation and wound healing. New Eng J Med 315:1650 (1986).

CONTRIBUTORS

Becker, Carl G.
Department of Pathology
Cornell Medical School
New York, New York 10021

Broekmans, A.W.
Department of Hematology
University Hospital Leiden and
Leiden Thrombosis Centre
The Netherlands

Dalen, James E.
Department of Medicine
University of Massachusetts
Worcester, MA 01605

Deykin, Daniel
Cooperative Studies Program (151-I)
V.A. Medical Center
Boston, MA 02130

Esmon, Charles T.
Thrombosis/Hematology
Oklahoma Medical Research Foundation
and Department of Medicine
University of Oklahoma Health Sciences
Center
Oklahoma City, OK 73104

Genton, Edward
Department of Cardiology
Ochsner Clinic
New Orlean, LA 70121

Gralnick, Harvey R.
Hematology Service
Clinical Pathology Department
National Institutes of Health
Bethesda, MD 20892

Hirsh, Jack
Department of Medicine
McMaster University
Hamilton, Ontario L8N 3Z5

Kuller, Lewis H.
University of Pittsburgh
Department of Epidemiolog
Pittsburgh, PA 15261

Kurachi, Kotoku
Department of Human Genetics
University of Michigan Medical
School
Ann Arbor, MI 48109

Mann, Kenneth G.
University of Vermont
Department of Biochemistry
Burlington, VT 05405

Marciniak, Ewa
Department of Medicine
University of Kentucky College
of Medicine
Lexington, KY 40536

Marder, Victor J.
Department of Medicine
University of Rochester
School of Medicine
Rochester, NY 14642

Moser, Kenneth, M.
Department of Medicine
University of California
San Diego, CA 92103

McDowell, Fletcher H.
The Burke Rehabilitation Center
785 Mamaroneck Avenue
White Plains, NY 10605

Nemerson, Yale
Department of Medicine
Mt. Sinai School of Medicine
New York, NY 10029

O'Reilly, Robert A.
Department of Medicine
Santa Clara Valley Medical Center
San Jose, CA 95128

Poller, Leon
UK Reference Laboratory for
Anticoagulant Reagents & Control
Withington Hospital
Manchester M20 8LR
United Kingdom

Price, Paul
Department of Biology
University of California at San Diego
La Jolla, CA 92093

Salzman, Edwin W.
Department of Surgery
Harvard Medical School
Beth Israel Hospital
Boston, MA 02215

Sherman, David G.
Department of Medicine (Neurology)
University of Texas Health Science
Center
San Antonio, TX 78284

Sherry, Sol
Department of Medicine
Thrombosis Research Center
Temple University School of Medicine
Philadelphia, PA 19140

Suttie, John W.
Department of Biochemistry
University of Wisconsin-Madison
Madison, WI 53706

Wessler, Stanford
Department of Medicine
NYU School of Medicine
New York, NY 10016